SpringerWienNewYork

Beat Hintermann

Total Ankle Arthroplasty

Historical Overview, Current Concepts
and Future Perspectives

SpringerWienNewYork

Prof. Dr. Beat Hintermann
Orthopädische Universitätsklinik, Universitätsspital, Basel, Switzerland

This work is subject to copyright.
All rights are reserved, whether the whole or part of the material is concerned, specifically those of translation, reprinting, re-use of illustrations, broadcasting, reproduction by photocopying machines or similar means, and storage in data banks.

Product Liability: The publisher can give no guarantee for all the information contained in this book. This does also refer to information about drug dosage and application thereof. In every individual case the respective user must check its accuracy by consulting other pharmaceutical literature. The use of registered names, trademarks, etc. in this publication does not imply, even in the absence of a specific statement, that such names are exempt from the relevant protective laws and regulations and therefore free for general use.

© 2005 Springer-Verlag/Wien
Printed in Austria

SpringerWienNewYork is part of Springer Science + Business Media
springeronline.com

Typesetting and Printing: Theiss GmbH, 9431 St. Stefan, Austria

Printed on acid-free and chlorine-free bleached paper
SPIN: 10993453

With numerous Figures

Library of Congress Control Number: 2004111515

ISBN 3-211-21252-3 SpringerWienNewYork

*To my wife Daniela,
and my children Sabrina, and Mathias,
for their support, love, and care
that have made this all possible.*

FOREWORD

"Obviously, there are many secondary problems associated with ankle arthrodesis, and this procedure cannot be recommended for the treatment of end-stage arthritis without concerns. Respecting anatomy and biomechanics, the search for a viable alternative, such as total ankle replacement, must continue."

This was the main conclusion at the end of my 18-month research fellowship at the University of Calgary in December 1992. Upon returning home, I carefully evaluated my end-stage osteoarthritis patients with a view to offering them a treatment other than arthrodesis. It was a long time until I was convinced that I had a patient with ideal indications for total ankle replacement. In the interim, I also visited some experts, including *Hakon Kofoed,* to whom I am extremely grateful for giving and sharing his experience, and broadening my knowledge of how to replace the ankle joint. Finally, in February 1995, I did my first total ankle replacement, and the surgery went extremely well. Ten years later, that first patient is still very satisfied with the obtained result. In retrospect, it was really a "winning ankle," with perfect alignment, stability, and bone stock.

As time passed, more difficult cases presented in my outpatient clinic, and it became obvious that replacing the destroyed surface was not always sufficient to solve the problem. The more total ankle replacement became a part of the reconstructive surgery of the hindfoot, the more important was the achieved alignment and stability at the end of surgery.

Lifelong documentation of cases is a tremendous amount of work, but it may be mandatory in order to recognize and gain insight into the many underlying processes that can affect the final result. In fact, when studying the cases in my database, the "bad" cases, not surprisingly, evidenced many more technical mistakes in positioning of implants and/or ankle realignment than did the "good" cases. By learning from this, my results have become much better, and thus more predictable for my patients. In addition, ongoing improvements in instruments and implant design have helped to make total ankle arthroplasty better and safer.

Now that total ankle arthroplasty is a more routine treatment option, the adverse clinical and biomechanical consequences of ankle arthrodesis are far more apparent. What is also interesting is how the spectrum of ankle and extensive hindfoot arthrodesis procedures has become more evident. This, in turn, makes the surgeon's decision regarding his treatment approach for the management of ankle osteoarthritis more difficult, and requires him to have a more thorough understanding of all treatment options. This is particularly true for total ankle arthroplasty. This book is an attempt to give an overview not only of the available knowledge about ankle replacement, but also of the available scientific data. In this way, it addresses the apprentice as much as the more experienced foot and ankle surgeon.

Teaching and sharing our experience with others may be one of the highest privileges we have as surgeons. The effort invested in the preparation of this book has been immense, but the learning process has been a most rewarding experience. If *Total Ankle Arthroplasty* offers useful information to my colleagues and provides a new platform of knowledge from which others can advance the further evolvement of total ankle arthroplasty, I will have reached my goal.

October 2004   *Beat Hintermann*

ACKNOWLEDGEMENTS

First, I would like to thank my wife, *Daniela,* and my children, *Sabrina* and *Mathias,* for providing me with the atmosphere, the support, and above all, the acceptance that allowed me to write this book in my home environment.

I am deeply indebted to my dear friend and colleague, *Victor Valderrabano,* for his continual contribution to total ankle replacement research, and for his assistance with searching of literature and editing this book. His support was invaluable. My gratitude is further extended to *Claire Huene* for correcting and improving the quality of language of the manuscript. My special thanks are extended to my head secretary, *Brigitte Thaler,* and to my head surgical nurse, *Mierta Huonder,* for organizing the illustration material from X-rays and surgeries. In addition, I would like to thank my friend and professor of biomechanics, *Benno M. Nigg,* who deeply encouraged my dedication to the ankle joint, and my chief and colleague, *Walter Dick,* who allowed me to follow my dedication to reconstructive surgery of the hindfoot, and especially to proceed with total ankle replacement in our clinic. Finally, I would like to thank my friend and colleague, *James Nunley,* for all I have learned from him, and particularly for writing the preface.

The production of a book is truly a team effort, and therefore I am also very grateful to the editor at Springer-Verlag Wien/Austria, *Renate Eichhorn,* for her kind and encouraging support.

October 2004

Beat Hintermann

PREFACE

Arthritis of the ankle continues to be a significant problem for patients and its prevalence, at least post-traumatic arthritis, appears to be increasing. Currently there is a great deal of interest within the orthopaedic foot and ankle community concerned with treating patients with arthritis of the ankle. Traditional teaching has indicated that ankle arthrodesis is a satisfactory procedure to solve the pain of ankle arthritis and yields reliable results. Yet, as our orthopaedic knowledge has expanded and the length of our follow-up of ankle arthrodesis patients has lengthened, we see that there are many secondary problems associated with ankle arthrodesis. Thus, this timely text addresses a significant problem for patients and their physicians.

In the 1970s as surgeons began routine replacement of the hip and knee joints, many believed that replacement of the ankle would be easy and would yield results similar to the excellent results seen with total hips and total knees. Unfortunately, as we have learned, these early promising ankle results deteriorated quite rapidly and the first generation total ankle replacements were largely unsuccessful. Over the last decade there has been significant progress made in the understanding of biomaterials, biomechanics, and much progress has been made in extending the excellent results of total joint replacement throughout the body. Moreover, recently there has been a resurgence of interest among foot and ankle surgeons in finding a way to replace the ankle joint. Thus, this book by Hintermann on Total Ankle Replacement is a timely addition to the foot and ankle surgeon's armamentarium and to the orthopaedic surgeon who must treat these difficult problems, for it is only through study of our past history of ankle replacement surgery that one can avoid the mistakes of the past into the future. Hintermann has clearly indicated through his historical review of previous ankle replacements the mistakes of the past. With this as a knowledge base, he then proceeds to outline for us the current state of affairs into the future.

Chapter 2 is particularly useful as it illustrates the characteristics of post-traumatic ankle arthritis. Many orthopaedic surgeons having performed anatomic open reduction internal fixation of ankle fractures truly believe that the patient will be sparred the development of post-traumatic arthritis in the future. Nevertheless, as Hintermann illustrates, even well done open reduction internal fixation will frequently lead to a post-traumatic arthritis and a significant problem for the patient. Thus, we should anticipate that in the future we will continue to see an increase prevalence of this problem as more and more trauma victims are surviving with these devastating ankle fractures.

Chapter 4, which deals with the anatomy and biomechanics of the ankle joint, is a "must read" for any serious student of foot and ankle surgery. It is only through an understanding of the complex anatomy and biomechanics that we can address many disorders of the ankle. Hintermann is recognized as a world authority on biomechanics and ligamentous stability of the ankle. This beautifully illustrated chapter takes us through the importance of the bony restraints, ligamentous anatomy, fixation of the prosthesis, contact area, and biomechanics of this complex joint. Once one has an understanding of these basics, designing a total ankle replacement becomes an easier task.

To give us an overview of what is currently available, Chapter 6 is an excellent addition as it shows all of the current total ankle designs that are used worldwide and allows the reader to become familiar both with the design and characteristics of the individual prostheses. This chapter also addresses the surgical technique and the published results for each of the ankle replacements. This is an outstanding accumulation of all of the current literature and the bibliography is a wonderful resource.

With his thoughtful approach to ankle and ankle arthritis, Hintermann takes us through the current indications and contraindications for ankle replacement. He particularly draws attention to malalignment of the extremity as this has caused a problem for surgeons both at the hip and at the knee and certainly has plagued ankle surgeons in the past. With this understanding of alignment, adjacent joint arthritis, and the previous chapter on anatomy and biomechanics, one can easily understand the indications and contraindications for total ankle arthroplasty.

One of the true strengths of this text is the beauty of its illustrations. This is a massive collection of cases and case material which Hintermann accumulated through his lifelong study of ankle instability and ankle arthritis. The chapter on techniques is beautifully designed to allow the surgeon to understand the intricacies of this procedure.

Certainly the most thought provoking and impressive chapter is the one on the possibilities. Through creative thought and sound reasoning, Hintermann has illustrated how to perform osteotomies of the tibia above the ankle while simultaneously performing total ankle arthroplasty or conversely performing osteotomies and fusions below the ankle joint and simultaneously correcting foot and limb malalignments. The depth of this chapter is breathtaking and some of the surgical results could probably not be reproduced many places in the world.

To add overall balance, the chapter on complications brings us back to the many nuances that must be considered when one undertakes such a difficult procedure.

I find this book to be extremely timely. I believe it is an accumulation of a lifelong effort in collecting cases and thinking about and improving on techniques related to the treatment of ankle arthritis. This will become a "must textbook" for all serious foot and ankle surgeons and will certainly help our understanding of this complex joint.

October 2004

James A. Nunley,
Duke University Medical Center,
Durham, USA

CONTENTS

Chapter 1
Introduction 11

1.1 Why Total Ankle Arthroplasty? 11
1.2 Poor Success Rate with Early Attempts 12
1.3 Where Are We Today? 12

Chapter 2
Characteristics of the Diseased Ankle 15

2.1 Epidemiology 15
2.2 Characteristics of Ankle Arthritis 15
    2.2.1 Primary Osteoarthrosis 18
    2.2.2 Post-Traumatic Osteoarthrosis 18
    2.2.3 Systemic Arthritis 19
2.3 Conclusions 19

Chapter 3
Ankle Arthrodesis 21

3.1 Historical Background 21
3.2 Biomechanical Considerations 22
    3.2.1 Isolated Ankle Arthrodesis 23
    3.2.2 Extensive Hindfoot Fusions 23
3.3 Techniques and Results 23
    3.3.1 Ankle Arthrodesis without Internal Fixation 24
    3.3.2 Ankle Arthrodesis with Internal Fixation 24
    3.3.3 Functional Outcome after Ankle Arthrodesis 27
    3.3.4 Degenerative Changes after Ankle Arthrodesis 27
    3.3.5 Ankle Arthrodesis versus Total Ankle Arthroplasty 29
3.4 Conclusions 31

Chapter 4
**Anatomic and Biomechanical Characteristics of the Ankle Joint
and Total Ankle Arthroplasty 35**

4.1 Anatomic Considerations 35
    4.1.1 Bony Configuration 35
    4.1.2 Ligamentous Configuration 37
4.2 Ankle Joint Motion 39
    4.2.1 Axis of Rotation 39
    4.2.2 Range of Ankle Motion 40
    4.2.3 Restraints of Ankle Motion 40
4.3 Bone Support at the Ankle 41
4.4 Contact Area and Forces at the Ankle 44
    4.4.1 Contact Area 44
    4.4.2 Axial Load and Stress Forces of the Ankle 44
4.5 Fixation of Total Ankle Prostheses 45
4.6 Limitations of Polyethylene 47
4.7 Component Design 47
4.8 Conclusions 49

Chapter 5
History of Total Ankle Arthroplasty 53

5.1 Classification of Total Ankle Arthroplasties 53
5.2 First-Generation Total Ankle Arthroplasty – Cemented Type 55
    5.2.1 Pioneers in Total Ankle Arthroplasty 55
    5.2.2 Short-Term Results 57
    5.2.3 Mid- to Long-Term Results 57
    5.2.4 Specific Problems with Early Use of Total Ankle Implants 58
5.3 Second-Generation Total Ankle Arthroplasty – Uncemented Type 59
    5.3.1 Basic Biomechanical Considerations in New Prosthetic Designs 59
    5.3.2 Two-Component Designs 60
    5.3.3 Three-Component Designs 61
    5.3.4 First Results 61
    5.3.5 Critical Issues in Second-Generation Total Ankle Replacement 62
5.4 Conclusions 63

Chapter 6
Current Designs of Total Ankle Prostheses 69

6.1 AES® Ankle 69
    6.1.1 Background and Design 69
    6.1.2 Results 70
    6.1.3 Concerns 70
6.2 AGILITY™ Ankle 71
    6.2.1 Background and Design 71

Contents   XV

        6.2.2 Results   72
        6.2.3 Concerns   73
6.3 Buechel-Pappas™ Ankle   74
        6.3.1 Background and Design   74
        6.3.2 Results   75
        6.3.3 Concerns   76
6.4 ESKA Ankle   78
        6.4.1 Background and Design   78
        6.4.2 Results   78
        6.4.3 Concerns   80
6.5 HINTEGRA® Ankle   80
        6.5.1 Background and Design   80
        6.5.2 Results   81
        6.5.3 Concerns   81
6.6 Ramses Ankle   85
        6.6.1 Background and Design   85
        6.6.2 Results   87
        6.6.3 Concerns   87
6.7 SALTO® Ankle   88
        6.7.1 Background and Design   88
        6.7.2 Results   88
        6.7.3 Concerns   88
6.8 S.T.A.R. Ankle   90
        6.8.1 Background and Design   90
        6.8.2 Results   91
        6.8.3 Concerns   92
6.9 TNK Ankle   94
        6.9.1 Background and Design   94
        6.9.2 Results   94
        6.9.3 Concerns   97
6.10 Conclusions   97

Chapter 7
Preoperative Considerations for Total Ankle Arthroplasty   101

7.1 Indications   101
7.2 Contraindications   102
7.3 Considerations Specific to Total Ankle Replacement Surgery   103
        7.3.1 Rheumatoid Arthritis and Inflammatory Arthropathy   103
        7.3.2 Infection   103
        7.3.3 Osteopenia and Osteoporosis   105
        7.3.4 Weight Restrictions   105
        7.3.5 Adjacent Joint Arthritis   107
        7.3.6 Lower Limb, Ankle, or Hindfoot Malalignment   108
        7.3.7 Hindfoot-Ankle Instability   108
        7.3.8 Heel Cord Contracture   111
        7.3.9 Soft-Tissue Considerations   111

7.3.10 Age Considerations 111
7.3.11 Activity Limitations 112
7.3.12 Smoking 113
7.4 Conclusions 113

Chapter 8
Surgical Techniques 115

8.1 Preoperative Planning 115
8.2 Surgical Approach to the Ankle 115
8.2.1 Anterior Approach to the Ankle 115
8.2.2 Lateral Approach to the Ankle 118
8.2.3 Complications 118
8.3 Surgical Preparation of the Ankle 118
8.4 Insertion of the Implants 123
8.5 Wound Closure 126
8.6 Additional Surgeries 127
8.6.1 Lateral Ligament Reconstruction 127
8.6.2 Peroneal Tendon Transfer 129
8.6.3 Dorsiflexion Osteotomy of the First Metatarsal 129
8.6.4 Valgisation Osteotomy of the Calcaneus 130
8.6.5 Medial Ligament Reconstruction 130
8.6.6 Medial Sliding Osteotomy of the Calcaneus 130
8.6.7 Hindfoot Fusion 130
8.6.8 Heel Cord Lengthening 131
8.7 Conclusions 131

Chapter 9
Postoperative Care and Follow-up 137

9.1 Postoperative Care 137
9.2 Rehabilitation Program 138
9.3 Follow-up Examination 138
9.3.1 Clinical Assessment 138
9.3.2 Radiographic Measurements 139
9.4 Conclusions 143

Chapter 10
What is Feasible in Total Ankle Arthroplasty? 145

10.1 Reconstruction of the Malaligned Ankle 145
10.1.1 Varus Malalignment 145
10.1.2 Valgus Malalignment 146
10.1.3 Sagittal Plane Malalignment 151
10.2 Reconstruction of the Post-Traumatic Hindfoot and Ankle 151

Contents

        10.2.1 Fibular Malunion   152
        10.2.2 Tibiofibular Instability (Syndesmotic Incompetence)   153
        10.2.3 Calcaneal Malunion   154
10.3 Specific Articular Pathologies and Disorders   160
        10.3.1 Systemic Inflammatory Arthritis   160
        10.3.2 Clubfoot Deformity   162
        10.3.3 Post-Polio Foot Deformity   162
        10.3.4 Avascular Necrosis   162
        10.3.5 Septic Arthritis   165
10.4 Disarthrodesis   168
10.5 Revision Arthroplasty (for Failed Primary Arthroplasty)   169
10.6 Conclusions   172

Chapter 11
Complications of Total Ankle Arthroplasty   173

11.1 Characteristics of Ankle Osteoarthritis   173
        11.1.1 Primary Osteoarthrosis of the Ankle   173
        11.1.2 Post-Traumatic Osteoarthrosis of the Ankle   173
        11.1.3 Rheumatoid Arthritis of the Ankle   173
11.2 Patient Selection   175
        11.2.1 Age of the Patient   175
        11.2.2 Weight of the Patient   175
11.3 Preoperative Conditions and Planning   175
        11.3.1 Soft-Tissue Conditions   175
        11.3.2 Malalignment and Malunion   175
        11.3.3 Preoperative Foot Deformity   177
11.4 Implant- and Implantation-Related Complications   178
        11.4.1 Problems with First-Generation Total Ankle Prostheses   178
        11.4.2 Problems with Second-Generation Total Ankle Prostheses   178
11.5 Early Postoperative Complications   185
        11.5.1 Wound Healing Problems   185
        11.5.2 Swelling   186
        11.5.3 Infection   186
        11.5.4 Deep Venous Thrombosis   186
        11.5.5 Syndesmotic Nonunion / Instability   186
        11.5.6 Fractures of Malleoli   186
11.6 Late Postoperative Complications   186
        11.6.1 Loss of Motion   186
        11.6.2 Aseptic Loosening   188
        11.6.3 Subsidence   190
        11.6.4 Polyethylene Wear   191
11.7 Salvage of Failed Total Ankle Arthroplasty   191
11.8 Conclusions   191
        11.8.1 Requirements for Successful Total Ankle Arthroplasty   193
        11.8.2 Surgeon Experience, Skill, and Training   193

Chapter 12
Future Directions   195

12.1. Current Concerns to be Addressed   195
        12.1.1. Prospective Studies   195
        12.1.2. Prosthetic Design   195
        12.1.3. Preoperative Planning and Implantation Technique   195
        12.1.4. Polyethylene Wear   196
        12.1.5. Stability of Bone-Implant Interface   196
12.2. Further Success will Increase Patient Demand   196
12.3. Further Research   196
12.4. Conclusions   197

Subject Index   199

Chapter 1

INTRODUCTION

Treatment of the end-stage osteoarthritic ankle is often complicated by associated problems such as scarring of the thin soft-tissue envelope, stiffness, malalignment, and degenerative changes in the subtalar and talonavicular joints that may result in instability, deformity, and changes in the biomechanics of the joint(s). An isolated arthrodesis of the ankle may address the immense pain at the ankle, but may not sufficiently address the associated problems and ongoing changes in the neighboring joints. This may become particularly problematic in young patients who have a long life expectancy (Fig. 1.1).

1.1 Why Total Ankle Arthroplasty?

In an era of joint replacement surgery, ankle procedures have failed to achieve what has been accomplished with other joints. An example that to some extent typifies the "ankle replacement experience" to date is that of British orthopedic surgeon John Charnley, who, frustrated by the failure of his compression arthrodesis, turned to hip arthroplasty and successfully pioneered procedures in that specialty. Decades after Charnley's failed efforts, ankle arthrodesis is still the most commonly used procedure for the painful arthritic ankle. Although unilateral ankle arthro-

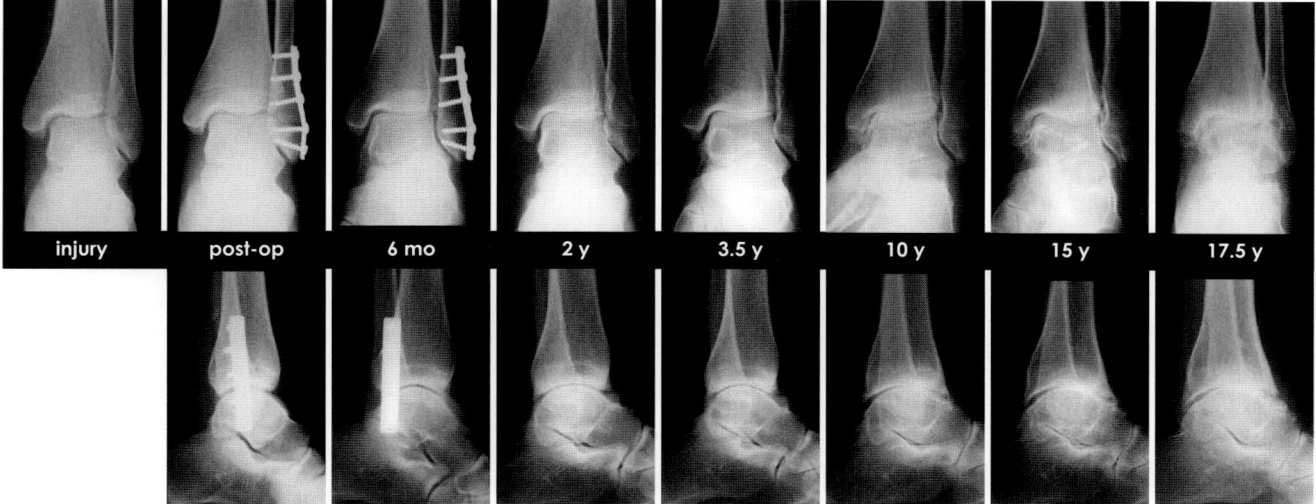

Fig. 1.1. Development of post-traumatic osteoarthrosis.
This 36-year-old female patient with post-traumatic osteoarthrosis sustained a complex ankle sprain while playing volleyball at the age of 19 years. The X-ray evidenced a nondisplaced fracture of the fibula (lateral view lost), and open reduction and internal fixation (ORIF) was made four days after injury. The implants were removed after eight months because of local discomfort. Painful limitation of dorsiflexion persisted despite arthroscopic decompression of the anterior ankle after 3.8 years. In the last five years, progressive pain under loading has limited sports activities to zero; in fact, the patient experiences pain even at rest. The lateral X-rays show a progressive widening of the tibiotalar contact area after 3.5 years with osteophyte formation, decrease in the joint space, incongruency, and subchondral sclerosis. Degenerative disease of the subtalar and talonavicular joints occurred in the same period, which may explain a 50% decrease in pronation/supination with respect to the contralateral side

desis may result in acceptable function (provided that the subtalar and midtarsal joints are normal and provide a compensatory mechanism), the disadvantages are, at least in the long term, significant.

In the longest follow-up after ankle arthrodesis (23 years, range 20 to 33 years), Fuchs et al [10] reported that half of the 18 patients followed considered themselves slightly or not limited in activities of daily living, although 61% had suffered a post-surgical complication. Fifteen feet had an equinus deformity: seven (39%) had a deformity of 5° to 10°, and eight (44%) had a deformity of 11° to 20°. There were seven varus deformities and one valgus hindfoot. One-third considered their professional handicap as "moderate" and one-third as "significant." The SF-36 for physical function, emotional disturbance, and bodily pain revealed significant deficits. The radiological assessment showed signs of hindfoot arthritis (subtalar and talonavicular joint) in 95% of the cases. Coester et al [7], in a 12- to 44-year follow-up (mean 22 years) of 23 patients, found moderate to severe osteoarthritic changes in the subtalar joint of 21 patients (91.3%), and in the talonavicular joint of 13 patients (56.6%). These findings were supported by the reports of others [1, 4, 21]. When a young patient undergoes ankle arthrodesis, there is a significant likelihood that he or she will develop hindfoot arthritis during the next 20 years, and will have to be treated for this secondary degenerative change (see Chap. 3: Ankle Arthrodesis). Increased stiffness of the foot and additional arthrodesis of the arthritic joint(s) is the likely outcome.

Evidence for the superiority of arthroplasty over arthrodesis has been provided by Koefoed and Stürup [20]. In a series of 26 patients treated for osteoarthritis of the ankle, 13 patients with 14 arthrodeses were compared with 13 patients with 14 total ankle replacements. The median follow-up was 84 months. Total ankle arthroplasty gave better pain relief, better function, and a lower infection rate without the development of subtalar arthritis.

1.2 Poor Success Rate with Early Attempts

Multiple problems were encountered during the early use of total ankle implants in the 1970s.

Appropriate surgical instruments were often lacking or poorly designed, and this resulted in poor or inaccurate positioning of the implants. Soft-tissue balancing was initially not addressed, because most implants were used in ankles that had worn out in neutral position. No attempts were made to replace joints that had any significant varus or valgus deformity, thus excluding a great number of patients. Methyl methacrylate was used for fixation in most implants, and multiple difficulties were encountered both in cementing techniques and in retrieving cement from behind the implant. Fractures of both malleoli occurred because of inaccurate sizing and poor instrumentation. Excessive traction in the skin during surgery resulted in a high incidence of skin complications [3]. Excessive bone removal (for example, up to 17 mm on the tibial side and up to 7 mm on talar side) resulted in the implant being seated on soft cancellous bone that could not support the bone-cement interface. This caused subsidence with weight-bearing [8]. Non-anatomically shaped, undersized implants of the tibia also tended to subside into the soft cancellous bone [12].

The design of total ankle arthroplasty implants has varied substantially from the early constrained designs that supplemented ankle ligament support completely [23]. Newer semiconstrained and nonconstrained designs require ligament stability but permit increased axial rotation [5, 17, 22]. The most recent, least constrained three-component designs require less bone resection and have improved (cementless, porous coat) fixation techniques. Promising intermediate results [14, 15, 18, 19, 24], however, remain tempered by the poor track record of earlier (constrained and mainly cemented) prostheses, the difficulty of perfecting the surgical technique, troublesome complications, and the difficulty of salvage and revision [9].

1.3 Where Are We Today?

Increasing success with arthroplasty of joints such as the knee and hip, along with concerns about the long-term outcomes of ankle arthrodesis [7, 10], has created renewed interest in total ankle arthroplasty over the last decade. New implants have been designed with attention to reproducing normal ankle anatomy, joint kinematics, ligament stability, and mechanical alignment. Two- and three-component designs are used to allow for sliding and rotational motions at the ankle joint. Newer prostheses also include metal backing with porous surfaces that allow for biological fixation, thereby decreasing the amount of bone resection necessary for implantation.

There is reason to believe that total ankle arthroplasty has evolved from an experimental and occasionally successful procedure into a worthwhile and durable solution. No arthroplasty, however, can be assessed without a minimum five-year follow-up. Time is needed for the true picture to emerge, but there is an expectation that ankle arthroplasty will soon take its place alongside other well-tried and accepted procedures in the knee and hip. It is hoped that the superiority of total ankle arthroplasty, in contrast to arthrodesis, will become firmly established, and that the procedure will become a standard part of the orthopedic surgeon's repertoire.

Encouraging intermediate clinical results for second-generation arthroplasties hold promise for patients with end-stage ankle arthritis [2, 6, 16, 18, 19, 22, 25, 26]. The unique physiological and mechanical characteristics of the ankle joint, however, remain a challenge. Failures of ankle implants are, to date, still higher than implants in other joints. To a certain extent, this may be related to the inability of a surgeon to adequately restore the critical stabilizing role of the ligaments, as well as to poor reproduction of the normal mechanics of the ankle joint, and to the lack of involvement of the underlying subtalar joint in the coupled motion pattern of the entire ankle joint complex [11, 13]. However, adequate patient selection, careful preoperative planning, appropriate treatment of associated disorders (for example, instability, malalignment, and arthritis of adjacent joints), and minimizing perioperative complications will help to maximize the chance for a successful outcome.

This book attempts to provide an update of current knowledge on the arthritic ankle and the treatment of end-stage arthritis of the ankle. Biomechanical considerations are specifically addressed with regard to the need for successful total ankle arthroplasty. It also includes an extensive review of the literature, with an emphasis on objective analysis of the clinical results in order to help define and delineate the role of total ankle arthroplasty.

References

[1] Ahlberg A, Henricson AS (1981) Late results of ankle fusion. Acta Orthop Scand 52: 103–105

[2] Anderson T, Montgomery F, Carlsson A (2003) Uncemented STAR total ankle prosthesis. Three to eight-year follow-up of fifty-one consecutive ankles. J Bone Joint Surg Am 85: 1321–1329

[3] Bolton-Maggs BG, Sudlow RA, Freeman MA (1985) Total ankle arthroplasty. A long-term review of the London Hospital experience. J Bone Joint Surg Br 67: 785–790

[4] Boobbyer GN (1981) The long-term results of ankle arthrodesis. Acta Orthop Scand 52: 107–110

[5] Buechel FF, Pappas MJ, Iorio LJ (1988) New Jersey low contact stress total ankle replacement: biomechanical rationale and review of 23 cementless cases. Foot Ankle 8: 279–290

[6] Buechel FFS, Buechel FF, Pappas MJ (2003) Ten-year evaluation of cementless Buechel-Pappas meniscal bearing total ankle replacement. Foot Ankle Int 24: 462–472

[7] Coester LM, Saltzman CL, Leupold J, Pontarelli W (2001) Long-term results following ankle arthrodesis for post-traumatic arthritis. J Bone Joint Surg Am 83: 219–228

[8] Demottaz JD, Mazur JM, Thomas WH, Sledge CB, Simon SR (1979) Clinical study of total ankle replacement with gait analysis. A preliminary report. J Bone Joint Surg Am 61: 976–988

[9] Easley ME, Vertullo CJ, Urban WC, Nunley JA (2002) Total ankle arthroplasty. J Am Acad Orthop Surg 10: 157–167

[10] Fuchs S, Sandmann C, Skwara A, Chylarecki C (2003) Quality of life 20 years after arthrodesis of the ankle. A study of adjacent joints. J Bone Joint Surg Br 85: 994–998

[11] Giannini S, Leardini A, O'Connor JJ (2000) Total ankle replacement: review of the designs and of the current status. Foot Ankle Surg 6: 77–88

[12] Gill LH (2002) Principles of joint arthroplasty as applied to the ankle. AAOS Instructional Course Lectures 13: 117–128

[13] Hamblen DL (1985) Editorial. Can the ankle joint be replaced? J Bone Joint Surg Br 67: 689–690

[14] Hintermann B (1999) Die STAR-Sprunggelenkprothese. Kurze und mittelfristige Erfahrungen. Orthopäde 28: 792–803

[15] Hintermann B, Valderrabano V (2001) Endoprothetik am oberen Sprunggelenk. Z Arztl Fortbild Qualitätssich 95: 187–194

[16] Hintermann B, Valderrabano V, Dereymaeker G, Dick W (2004) The HINTEGRA ankle: rationale and short-term results of 122 consecutive ankles. Clin Orthop 424: 57–68

[17] Kofoed H (1995) Cylindrical cemented ankle arthroplasty: a prospective series with long-term follow-up. Foot Ankle Int 16: 474–479

[18] Kofoed H, Lundberg-Jensen A (1999) Ankle arthroplasty in patients younger and older than 50 years: a prospective series with long-term follow-up. Foot Ankle Int 20: 501–506

[19] Kofoed H, Sorensen TS (1998) Ankle arthroplasty for rheumatoid arthritis and osteoarthritis: prospective long-term study of cemented replacements. J Bone Joint Surg Br 80: 328–332

[20] Kofoed H, Stürup J (1994) Comparison of ankle arthroplasty and arthrodesis. A prospective series with long-term follow-up. Foot 4: 6–9

[21] Morgan CD, Henke JA, Bailey RW, Kaufer H (1985) Long-term results of tibiotalar arthrodesis. J Bone Joint Surg Am 67: 546–550

[22] Pyevich MT, Saltzman CL, Callaghan JJ, Alvine FG (1998) Total ankle arthroplasty: a unique design. Two to twelve-year follow-up. J Bone Joint Surg 80-A: 1410–1420

[23] Saltzman CL (2000) Perspective on total ankle replacement. Foot Ankle Clin 5: 761–775

[24] Schernberg F (1998) Current results of ankle arthroplasty: European multi-center study of cementless ankle arthroplasty. In: Current status of ankle arthroplasty (Kofoed H, ed) Springer, Berlin, pp 41–46

[25] Valderrabano V, Hintermann B, Dick W (2004) Scandinavian total ankle replacement: a 3.7-year average follow-up of 65 patients. Clin Orthop 424: 47–56

[26] Wood PL, Deakin S (2003) Total ankle replacement. The results in 200 ankles. J Bone Joint Surg 85-B: 334–341

Chapter 2

CHARACTERISTICS OF THE DISEASED ANKLE

There is essentially one bone above the ankle and 26 bones and as many joints below it that can affect alignment and functioning of the ankle joint. The normal soft-tissue envelope around the ankle is thin, and because of possible antecedent trauma and initial surgical repairs, this envelope often is scarred and inelastic. These same issues, combined with the post-traumatic period of immobilization, lack of physical therapy, chronic pain, and progressive periarticular bone formation, often lead to significant loss of ankle joint motion. In addition, progressive joint incongruency, destruction of the articular surfaces, and talar dislocation out of the ankle mortise may cause alteration of ankle joint mechanics, malalignment of the hindfoot, and destabilization of the ankle joint complex. Careful investigation is, therefore, mandatory in order to identify the potential problems that may be encountered during and after total ankle replacement.

2.1 Epidemiology

Many sports-related ankle injuries have been associated with biomechanical deficits such as static or dynamic malalignment of the skeleton [2, 6]. Hindfoot disorders, and especially ankle and hindfoot arthritis, have gained great epidemiological and social-preventive importance in recent years. It has been stated that ankle and hindfoot arthritis will increase in the future decades, due to increasing incidence of trauma, involvement in sports activities, and longer life expectancy [1, 6, 9].

2.2 Characteristics of Ankle Arthritis

To understand the particular problems with total ankle replacement, it is first necessary to under-

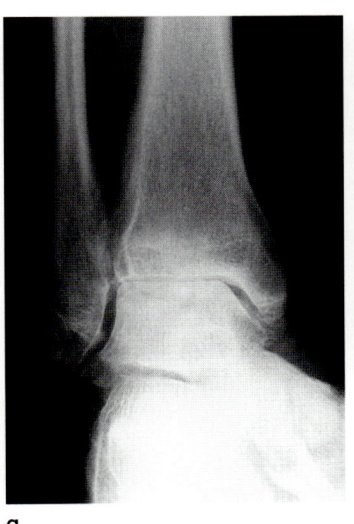
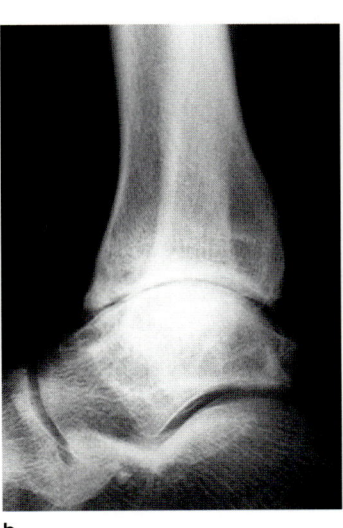
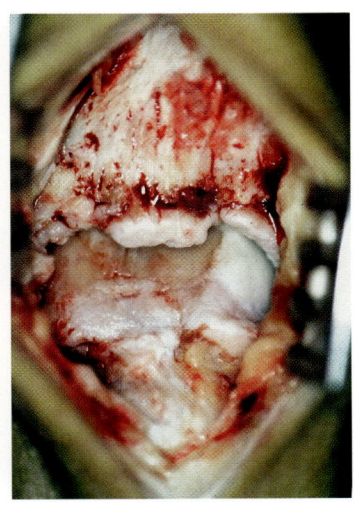

a b c

Fig. 2.1. Primary osteoarthrosis.
Forty-nine-year-old male patient with primary osteoarthrosis: correct alignment and stability, dorsi-/plantar flexion 10° – 0° – 30°, typical radiological changes (see text) and cartilage wear. Weight-bearing X-rays (**a, b**). Intra-operative *situs* (**c**)

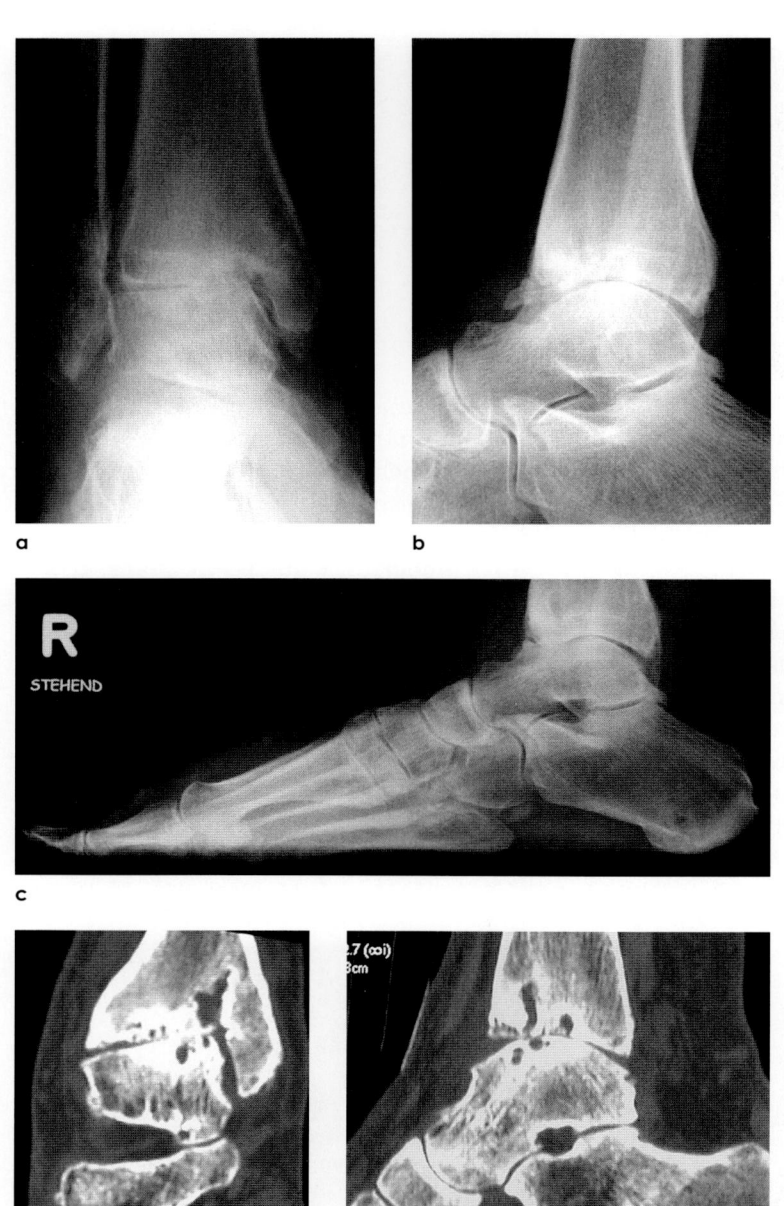

Fig. 2.2. Severe post-traumatic osteoarthrosis.
Forty-three-year-old female patient with post-traumatic osteoarthrosis (**a, b**) 3.5 years after surgically treated ankle fracture: joint incongruency, varus malalignment, subchondral sclerosis and cyst formation, dorsi-/plantar flexion 10° – 0° – 20°. Notice the effect of loading in the lateral view (**c**). The CT scan evidences more articular changes and destruction than radiologically expected, particularly in the anteromedial part of the ankle (**d, e**)

2.2 Characteristics of Ankle Arthritis

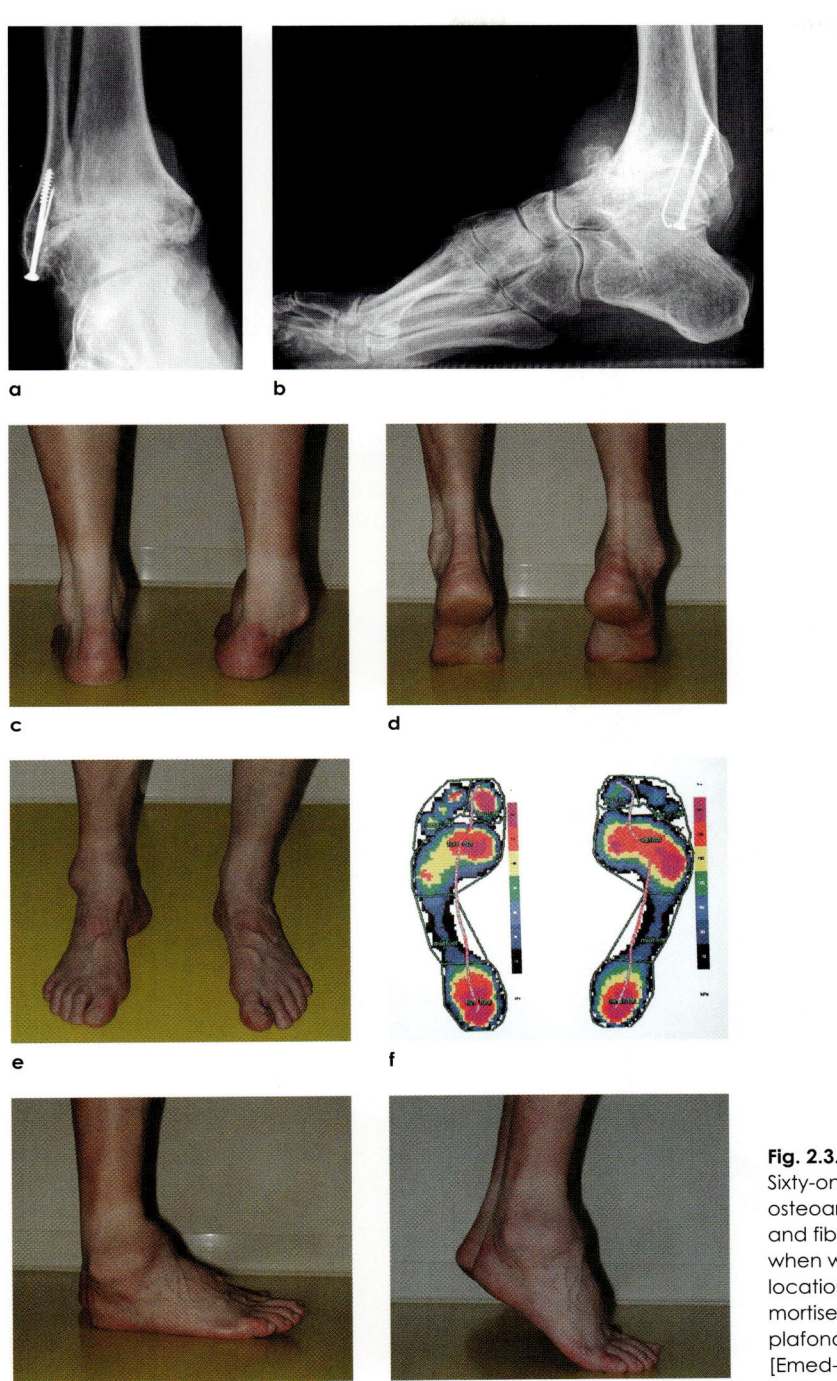

Fig. 2.3. Severe post-traumatic varus osteoarthrosis. Sixty-one-year-old male patient with post-traumatic osteoarthrosis (**a, b**) after multiple ankle sprains, tenodesis, and fibula fracture, complaining of instability and pain when weight-bearing on the foot: anterolateral dislocation and varus malalignment of the talus in the ankle mortise (**c–e**), breakdown of the anteromedial tibial plafond, cavus deformity (**f**, dynamic pedobarography [Emed-System, Novel, Munich, Germany]), dorsi-/plantar flexion 5° – 0° – 30° (**g, h**)

stand the basic problem: namely, the pathology and varieties of ankle arthritis. Ankle arthritis includes primary and secondary arthritis (post-traumatic osteoarthritis and systemic arthritis [neuropathic arthropathy, inflammatory arthritis, and, rarely, infectious arthritis]). Osteoarthrosis is probably a better descriptive term for primary and post-traumatic arthritis conditions, as it minimizes the inflammatory component of this disorder.

2.2.1 Primary Osteoarthrosis

Primary osteoarthrosis is characterized by loss of joint cartilage and hypertrophy of bone. The exact mechanisms have not been defined, but subchondral bone injury and mechanical stress contribute to the damage [9]. The radiographic hallmarks are joint-space narrowing (which correlates with loss of joint cartilage), osteophyte formation, subchondral bone cysts, and subchondral sclerosis. [5] There is usually an absence of juxta-articular osteoporosis in primary osteoarthrosis (Fig. 2.1).

2.2.2 Post-Traumatic Osteoarthrosis

While hip and knee osteoarthrosis is predominantly of degenerative etiology and seen in older patients, 80% of ankle arthritis is post-traumatic in origin [3], and occurs, therefore, mostly in younger patients. Post-traumatic osteoarthrosis usually occurs secondary to an intra-articular fracture of the weight-bearing ankle joint (Fig. 2.2) [4, 8, 10].

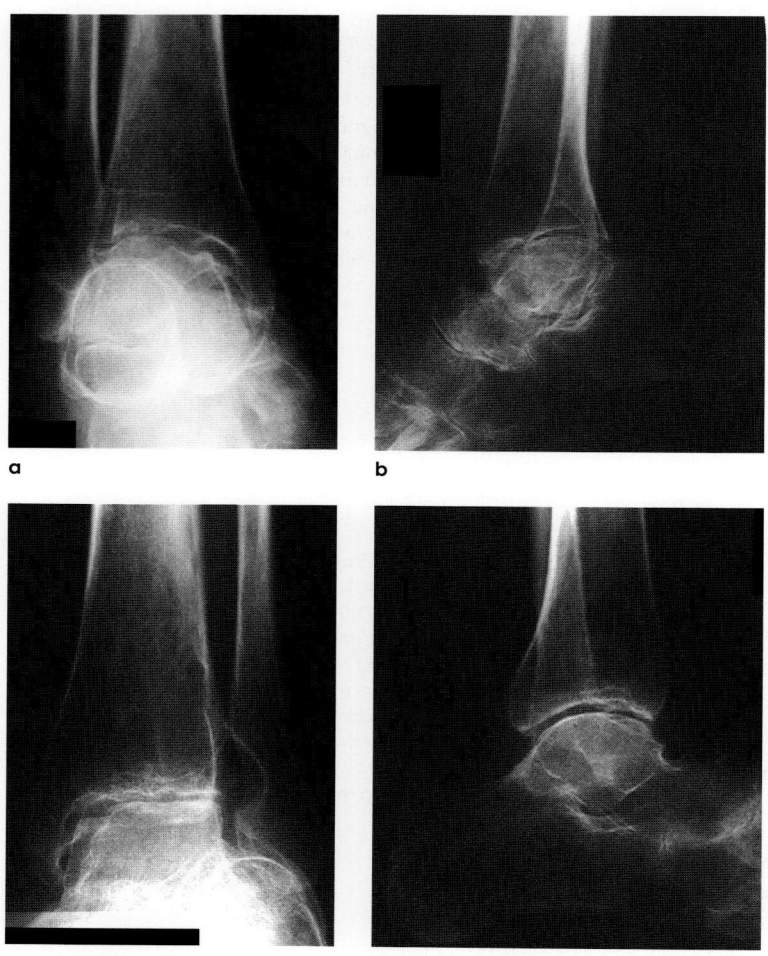

Fig. 2.4. Bilateral rheumatoid arthritis of the ankle. Forty-one-year-old female patient with bilateral rheumatoid arthritis of the ankle, right leg (**a, b**), left leg (**c, d**): valgus malalignment, bone cyst formation, concomitant talonavicular and subtalar arthritis

In addition to fractures, severe ligament lesions (chronic ankle instability) and dislocation injuries can also cause this entity (Fig. 2.3). In such cases, the soft-tissue envelope around the ankle is typically involved, often becoming scarred and inelastic. Chronic pain and progressive periarticular formation of new bone often lead to significant loss of ankle joint motion. In addition to the changes seen in primary osteoarthrosis (that is, joint-space narrowing, osteophyte formation, subchondral bone cysts, and subchondral sclerosis), radiographically, post-traumatic osteoarthrosis also potentially includes joint incongruency, malalignment, and dislocation.

2.2.3 Systemic Arthritis

The category of systemic or inflammatory arthritis includes the various presentations of rheumatoid arthritis, mixed connective-tissue disorders, and synovial inflammatory conditions of unknown etiology [10]. Septic arthritis, psoriatic arthritis, arthritis associated with spondyloarthropathy, and Reiter's syndrome are also in this category. Rheumatoid arthritis is characterized by the formation of hyperplastic synovium that may destroy the underlying articular cartilage, subchondral bone, and supportive musculotendinous and ligamentous tissues [7, 9]. Radiographically, inflammatory arthritis is characterized by symmetric joint-space narrowing, joint subluxation secondary to the imbalance of opposing muscle groups about a joint, juxta-articular erosions, and osteopenia (Fig. 2.4) [9, 11].

2.3 Conclusions

In recent years, ankle arthritis has increased in frequency due to increased incidence of trauma during sports activities and increased life expectancy. The pathology of ankle arthritis involves cartilage degeneration, joint deformity, pain, and a decreased of range of motion that often leads to malalignment, limp, and gait abnormality. Ankle arthritis can be sub-classified into three groups: primary osteoarthrosis, post-traumatic osteoarthrosis, and systemic arthritis. In relative terms, the post-traumatic group is the largest.

References

[1] Baumhauer JF, Alosa DM, Renstroem PA, Trevino S, Beynnon B (1995) A prospective study of ankle injury risk factors. Am J Sports Med 23: 564–570
[2] Clement DB, Taunton JE, Smart GE, McNicol KL (1981) A survey of overuse running injuries. Phys Sports Med 9: 47–58
[3] Conti SF, Wong YS (2001) Complications of total ankle replacement. Clin Orthop 391: 105–114
[4] Hefti F, Baumann J, Morscher EW (1980) Ankle joint fusion: determination of optional position by gait analysis. Arch Orthop Trauma Surg 96: 187–192
[5] Hintermann B, Valerrabano V (2003) Total ankle replacement. Foot Ankle Clin 8: 375–405
[6] James B, Bates B, Osterning L (1978) Injuries in running. Am J Sports Med 6: 40–50
[7] Kean WF, Forestier F, Kassam Y, Buchanan WW, Rooney PJ (1985) The history of gold therapy in rheumatoid disease. Semin Arthritis Rheum 14: 180–186
[8] Morrey BF, Wiedermann GP (1980) Complications and long-term results of ankle arthrodesis following trauma. J Bone Joint Surg Am 62: 777–784
[9] Praemer A, Furner S, Rice DP (1992) Arthritis. In: Musculoskeletal conditions in the United States (Park Ridge I, ed), 1st ed. American Academy of Orthopaedic Surgeons
[10] Quill GE (2000) An approach to the management of ankle arthritis. In: Foot and ankle disorders (Myerson MS, ed). Saunders, Philadelphia, pp 1059–1084
[11] Vahvanen V (1969) Arthrodesis of the talocalcaneal or pantalar joints in rheumatoid arthritis. Acta Orthop Scand 40: 642–652

Chapter 3

ANKLE ARTHRODESIS

Arthrodesis of the hindfoot has been used to treat a variety of neuromuscular and degenerative foot disorders for more than 100 years [4]. Techniques have evolved over time, and well-designed biomechanical studies have provided guidance regarding the desirable ranges of hindfoot alignment during arthrodesis [10, 29, 57]. As contemporary implants have made osseous union more reliable, indications and techniques for the fusion of selected joints have evolved and offer the promise of improved function [71, 83]. Nonetheless, the underlying principles of careful tissue handling, meticulous joint alignment, and attentive aftercare remain important in these complex procedures.

3.1 Historical Background

For many years, the most frequent indication for surgical arthrodesis of the foot and ankle was the treatment of flaccid paralysis resulting from a variety of neuromuscular conditions, particularly poliomyelitis [35, 37, 47, 48]. Because orthoses used to restore stability to flail lower extremities were heavy, cumbersome, and uncomfortable [98], many procedures were developed to make paralytic limbs into useful, plantigrade appendages suitable for weight-bearing. Early attempts at soft-tissue procedures failed because of attenuation and insufficient motor strength after tendon transfer in the paralytic extremity [15]. Extra-articular bone-block procedures [56, 12, 37] were ineffective because of the subsequent increase in deformity, destruction of the adjacent joints, and resorption of the bone block.

Hindfoot and ankle arthrodeses, by contrast, were effective at providing stability for paralytic extremities because they allowed the foot to be controlled by more proximal, less affected musculature. Internal fixation was initially performed using boiled cadaver allograft struts, ivory, fibular autograft, or sutures to hold the bone in position long enough to apply a cast [12]. Such techniques required prolonged periods of immobilization and restricted weight-bearing in order to minimize the nearly inevitable consequence of fibrous union [96]. A wide variety of ankle and foot fusion techniques has been described in the literature [15, 35, 47, 52, 78, 85], however, most reports consist of anecdotal series of case reports, without controls or consistent methods of patient assessment.

As techniques evolved and the success rates for arthrodeses increased, surgical indications expanded accordingly to post-traumatic osteoarthrosis [21], Charcot-Marie-Tooth disease [54, 82], osteonecrosis [92], clubfoot deformity [64], sequelae of posterior tibial tendon dysfunction [8, 26, 36], diabetic neuropathy [69], and cerebral palsy [89]. The use of arthrodesis to treat conditions other than neuromuscular disease has, however, required a reassessment of joint alignment [29, 57]. The 10° to 20° of equinus, which was useful with polio patients to force the knee into extension, yielded poor results in nonparalytic limbs [54].

More modern surgical techniques increased the rate of fusion. Charnley [13] introduced an external compression fixator. Not satisfied with this method, Pfahler et al [73] achieved better functionality and a significant reduction in time to fusion using compression screw fixation. In an experimental setup, screw fixation was found to be superior to an external fixator with regard to dorsiflexion/plantar flexion; whereas, the external fixator was superior to screw fixation with regard to tibial rotation [90]. Since then, use of the principles of AO interfragmentary compression (AO: Arbeitsgemeinschaft für Osteosynthesefragen / Association for the Study of Internal Fixation) has resulted in considerable improvement in the rate of osseous union [2, 61, 66,

76, 87, 91] More recently, modified blade plate [84] and tibiocalcaneal intramedullary nails [41, 75] were added to the list of internal fixation techniques. In addition, arthroscopically assisted ankle fusion has been employed to further reduce morbidity and to reduce the time to healing (Table 3.1) [16, 19, 20, 25, 65, 66, 67, 91, 102].

3.2 Biomechanical Considerations

Several studies about ankle arthrodesis and other hindfoot fusions have shown results that include limited range of motion, pathological gait, as well as limitation of other biomechanical variables.

Table 3.1. Results: open versus arthroscopic techniques

Author(s)	Year	No. of Ankles		Type of Fusion	Fusion Time [weeks]	Fusion Rate	Results Good-Excellent	Complications
Open techniques								
Morgan et al [62]	1985	101		Screws	12	95%	90%	5 nonunions 3 infections 6 hardware removals
Lynch et al [53]	1988	62	33 15 14	Charnley Anterior graft Gallie / dowel	†	86%	†	9 nonunions 6 infections
Helm [30]	1990	47		Pins & clamps	†	85%	†	3 amputations 9 infections 7 nonunions 4 malpositions
Maurer et al [56]	1991	47	35 12	Screws Charnley	12 †	100% 83%	† †	1 infection 2 nonunions 5 infections
Myerson and Quill [65]	1991	16		Screws	15.5	100%	†	1 infection 1 delayed union
Moeckel et al [60]	1991	40	27 13	Screws & anterior graft Screws	†	90%	93%	2 nonunions 2 delayed unions 5 stress fractures
		28	19 7 2	Charnley Hoffmann Calandruccio	†	79%	93%	6 nonunions 4 delayed unions 1 stress fracture
Stranks et al [87]	1994	20		Screws and dowel	12.5	95%	85%	1 nonunion 6 hardware removals
Anderson et al [5]	2002	30	16 14	Screws Charnley	†	90%	†	3 nonunions
Mini-open techniques								
Paremain et al [70]	1996	15		Screws	6	100%	†	2 hardware removals
Arthroscopic techniques								
Myerson and Quill [65]	1991	17		Screws	8.7	94%	†	1 nonunion 1 malposition
Ogilvie-Harris et al [67]	1993	19		Screws	10.8	89%	84%	2 nonunions
Corso and Zimmer [16]	1995	16		Screws	9.5	100%	87%	None
Turan et al [91]	1995	10		Screws	10	100%	†	None
Glick et al [25]	1996	34		Screws	9	97%	86%	1 nonunion 1 malunion
Zvijac et al [102]	2002	21		Screws	8.9	95%	95%	1 nonunion

† Data not reported

3.2.1 Isolated Ankle Arthrodesis

Arthritis that is localized solely in the ankle is treated effectively by tibiotalar fusion. The appropriate position of an ankle arthrodesis (shown by gait analysis) is neutral flexion, slight valgus, and slight external rotation [10, 29, 57]. Neutral alignment of the foot in the coronal and sagittal planes altered subtalar and talonavicular joint characteristics the least, compared with normal controls [97].

After tibiotalar fusion, Takakura et al [88] reported a loss of dorsiflexion from a mean of 10.5° preoperatively to 4.2° at follow-up of seven years, and a mean loss of plantar flexion from 24.7° to 14°. *In vitro*, ankle arthrodesis reduced dorsiflexion by 50% and plantar flexion by 70%, whereas motion in the coronal plane was decreased by 30% [24], which confirmed the results of others [33, 34, 100]. In a recent *in vitro* study using 3-D motion analysis, ankle-joint fusion reduced the range of motion in dorsiflexion/plantar flexion by 30.4° to 12.5°, and in tibial rotation by 6.7° to 14.7°, whereas it only decreased slightly by 4.4° to 14.4° in eversion/inversion of the foot [93]. In the same experimental setup, during dorsiflexion/plantar flexion of the foot, ankle-joint fusion increased the movement transfer to tibial rotation by a factor of 2.4, and to eversion/inversion by a factor of 18.5, as compared with the normal ankle [94]. As the range of motion at the tibiotalar joint is decreased, damage may occur because neighboring structures have to provide movement for which they are not suited [24, 32]. If movement transfer is increased, then increased articular stress forces may occur at the neighboring joints, causing joint degeneration and secondary arthritis [33, 34]. Additionally, changes in range of motion and/or movement transfer may affect the actual movement pattern [24], producing changes in the gait pattern.

Gait analysis of patients with a fused ankle shows:
– decreased knee flexion before heel strike,
– less time in single-limb stance,
– reduced sagittal ground-reaction force (which is important only with barefoot walking), and
– increased external rotation when the ankle is fused in equinus.

There is also a decreased time between heel-off and toe-off and an elevation of the center of gravity during stance phase, with an abrupt depression at terminal stance [10, 29, 42, 99].

In patients with ankle arthrodesis walking barefoot, researchers found a 16% decrease in gait velocity, a 3% increase in oxygen consumption, and an overall decrease of 10% in gait efficiency [95], whereas hip and knee joint movement were not found to be significantly changed [10, 29, 57, 86].

3.2.2 Extensive Hindfoot Fusions

Triple arthrodesis (that is, fusion of the subtalar, talonavicular, and calcaneocuboid joints) results in a 12° to 15° decrease in sagittal plane motion, even though the tibiotalar joint is not fused. Coronal plane motion is decreased by 60%, which is a result of the subtalar portion of the arthrodesis [24]. The loss of motion in the coronal plane is well tolerated in level gait on a flat outdoor surface while wearing appropriate footgear, but it makes ambulation on uneven surfaces much more difficult [77]. Since there are no biomechanical studies that specifically address the effects of subtalar, tibiotalocalcaneal, or pantalar arthrodeses on gait, energy expenditure, or alterations in adjacent joint motions, resultant changes in these parameters can be extrapolated only from existing studies. As an example, after subtalar fusion, two-thirds of patients may be affected while walking on uneven ground [21].

3.3 Techniques and Results

In the last century, countless ankle arthrodesis techniques have been developed, including external fixation, internal fixation, screw fixation, plate fixation, nail fixation, open technique, semi-open technique, and arthroscopic technique. The results vary from positive mid-term results (ability to participate in demanding activities, sports activities) to negative long-term results (including non- and malunion, degeneration of neighboring joints, and disability).

3.3.1 Ankle Arthrodesis without Internal Fixation

Isolated ankle fusions were rarely performed before the routine use of internal fixation. In 1953, Barr and Record [7] reviewed and reported on 55 procedures performed between 1947 and 1951. The procedures used a technique with medial and lateral incisions, malleolar osteotomy, and placement of a cortico-cancellous peg across the tibiotalar joint through the anterior tibial harvest site. Neither duration of follow-up nor the criteria outcome assessment were described. The authors were very satisfied with the results, and they concluded that it "is not particularly difficult to obtain solid bony union of the ankle joint [7]."

Lance et al [48] reviewed a total of 168 patients after seven months to 11 years. Anterior arthrodesis (similar to the technique used in the cases reviewed by Barr and Record) [7] was used in 36 patients. Transfibular arthrodesis, in which the distal fibula was osteomized for joint preparation and reattached as a strut graft, was used in 44 patients. In another study, compression with a Charnley clamp [13] was used in 21 patients, and distraction/compression was used in 50 patients. Excellent results, defined as "no significant distinction made by the patient between the operated and contralateral healthy ankle," were found in 30 patients (18%), and good results, defined as "occasional mild symptoms," in 89 patients (53%). The remaining 49 patients (29%) were rated as unsatisfactory because of permanent pain and disability or because of a major revision operation. There was a 94% rate of osseous union in the group operated on using the compression technique, which was markedly higher than in all other groups. Overall, nonunion occurred in 20% of the patients, but of the patients operated on for neuromuscular disease, two-thirds failed to unite. Another source of failure was technical mistakes. Complications included infection, skin necrosis, neuroma formation, loss of position, and fractures. A major limitation of this study was that in 58% of all patients, the surgery was performed as a part of a staged pantalar arthrodesis.

Morrey and Wiedermann [63] studied ankle arthrodesis for post-traumatic osteoarthrosis in a series of 60 patients. Nineteen (32%) of the patients were, however, lost to follow-up. The remaining patients were contacted by questionnaire after a mean of 7.5 years (range, one to 34 years), and 30 of the 41 patients were also interviewed in the office. The Charnley external compression fixator [13] was used in most patients. Both a solitary lateral incision and a transverse incision resulted in unacceptably high rates of complications, including nonunions and infections. The use of two incisions decreased the complication rate by a factor of three. Although 75% of patients reported some level of persistent pain, an overall satisfaction rate of 83% was achieved. Radiographic progression of osteoarthrosis to adjacent joints was observed in half of the patients studied, and appeared to increase with duration of follow-up. The high number of patients lost to follow-up, however, limits the strength of that conclusion. Hagen [28], after using the ICLH (Imperial College of London Hospital) device in eight patients and the Charnley external compression fixator in nine patients, reported union in 11 patients (65%), with an average immobilization period of five months. The nonunion group of six patients (35%), with an average of 10 months of immobilization, included two patients who were treated by below-knee amputation.

3.3.2 Ankle Arthrodesis with Internal Fixation

A variety of techniques using internal fixation for ankle fusion have been investigated in an attempt to increase the rate of fusion in primary procedures (Fig. 3.1) [2].

Symmetric chevron cuts of the tibial and talar articular surfaces, in conjunction with distal displacement of the medial malleolus, were used to obtain three flat surfaces in two planes to maximize bone contact. Marcus et al [55] reported on 13 adult patients (followed for 2.5 to 9.5 years) and found a 77% success rate. There was one nonunion, one fatigue fracture, one superficial infection, and one patient with continued pain.

Monroe et al [61] reported on 29 adult patients, followed for four to 48 months, who underwent open joint preparation using a transfibular approach and percutaneously placed screws. Primary fusion resulted in 93% of cases, achieving osseous union at nine weeks.

3.3 Techniques and Results

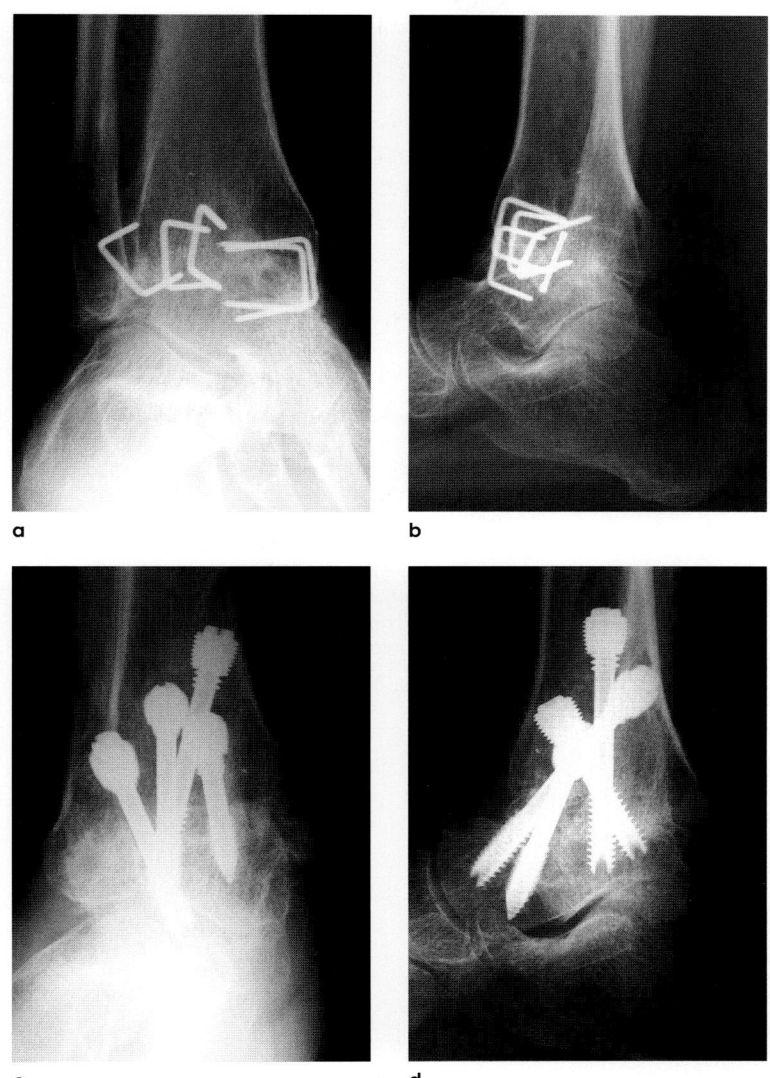

Fig. 3.1. Correctional osteotomy and re-arthrodesis after malpositioned ankle arthrodesis.
Ankle fusion was achieved in this 32-year-old male patient by using staples and cast immobilization for 16 weeks. Obtained equinus and supinatus position was, however, not satisfactory (**a, b**); therefore, correctional osteotomy and re-arthrodesis were performed after nine years. Fusion was achieved after eight months by using an improved compression technique with I.CO.S. screws (Ideal Compression Screw, Newdeal®, Lyon, France) (**c, d**)

In the absence of significant deformity, arthroscopic or arthroscopically assisted techniques may be advantageous (Table 3.1). Glick et al [25] reported on 34 adult patients followed for a mean of eight years (range, five to 11 years) and found rapid bone union and a low incidence of complications. Successful union occurred in 33 patients (97%), with good or excellent results in 29 patients (86%). Complications included one nonunion and one malunion. Zvijac et al [102] analyzed the results after arthroscopically assisted ankle arthrodesis in 21 patients after a mean of 34 months (range, 18 to 60 months). Successful union occurred in 20 patients (95%), and the average time to clinical and radiographic union was 8.9 weeks (range, seven to 14 weeks). The single failure had a preoperative diagnosis of extensive avascular necrosis involving approximately 50% of the talus. The authors of both reports concluded that arthroscopic ankle fusion is favorable to open techniques when selection criteria are met, and that it may shorten the time for fusion.

Although compression screw fixation is generally reliable in producing union, failures have been reported (Figs. 3.2 and 3.3) [50]. Revision essentially consists of repeating the ankle fusion with additional bone graft and meticulous technique.

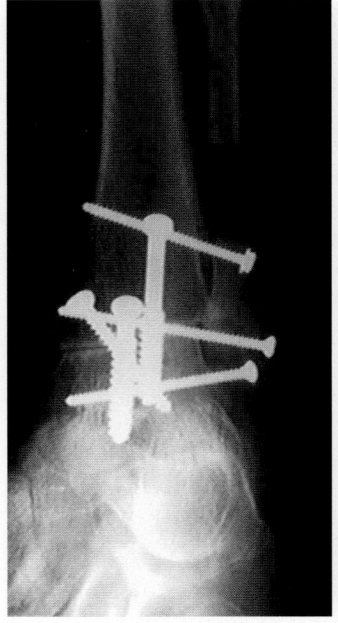
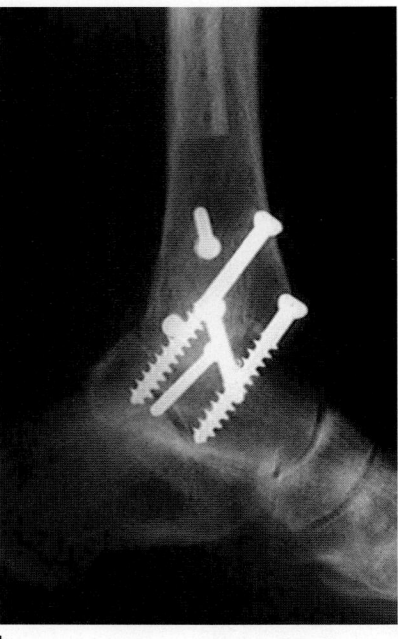

Fig. 3.2. Nonunion and malpositioning after ankle arthrodesis.
Painful nonunion and equinus malpositioning of the ankle arthrodesis after 12 months in a patient with symptomatic post-traumatic osteoarthrosis following ankle fracture (**a, b**). As a consequence of pain and instability, this 69-year-old female needs crutches for ambulation. Flat resection, inappropriate compression, and equinus malposition may have caused nonunion

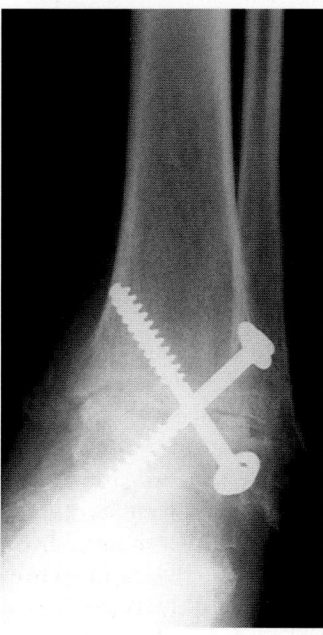
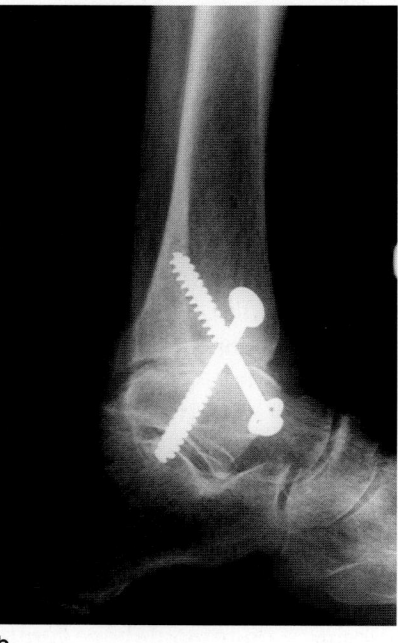

Fig. 3.3. Nonunion and malpositioning after ankle arthrodesis.
Painful nonunion and varus malalignment of the ankle arthrodesis after 16 months in a patient with symptomatic post-traumatic osteoarthrosis following ankle fracture (**a, b**). As a consequence of pain and instability, this 71-year-old male needs crutches for ambulation. Inappropriate compression and achieving stability with two screws may have caused nonunion and varus malalignment

Union in greater than 95% of nonunions treated can be expected [27, 50]. Compression by external fixator may be used when available bone stock does not permit repeated internal fixation.

In a retrospective analysis of 78 adult patients followed for two to 15 years, Frey et al [22] noted that concomitant medical conditions (including smoking two or more packs of cigarettes per day), open injuries, infection, avascular necrosis, and certain fractures all result in an increased risk of nonunion. Tibial plafond fractures, talus fractures, and combined talus and plafond fractures resulted in nonunions 59% to 75% of the time, and more than one-third of Weber C ankle fractures developed nonunions. A history of open fracture as a cause for post-traumatic osteoarthrosis had a significant effect upon nonunion rates, and the presence of other risk factors caused a trend toward nonunion in patients who smoke tobacco, have diabetes, use alcohol or illegal drugs, or have a psychiatric history [72].

3.3.3 Functional Outcome after Ankle Arthrodesis

Most ankle arthrodeses do relieve pain, and most patients are able to walk and perform daily activities more easily, at least in the short term [14]. Many reports, however, describe short-term and long-term problems for patients with ankle arthrodeses [48, 53, 57, 62], such as climbing stairs, getting out of a chair, walking on uneven surfaces, and running. Additionally, the patients' level of satisfaction is often reported as being unsatisfactory, because decreased functional ability often causes the need for ambulatory aids and/or permanent shoe modifications [9, 29, 57].

In other studies, ankle arthrodesis did not appreciably alter hip and knee motion [29, 57], and gait was thought to be 90% efficient in terms of oxygen consumption [95]. While wearing shoes, patients who had had an ankle arthrodesis exhibited excellent gait characteristics, with lost ankle motion compensated for by ipsilateral small-joint motion and altered motion within the foot on the contralateral side [57].

At a mean of 12.3 years, Ahlberg and Henricson [3] found pain in the subtalar joint in two-thirds of the 31 patients followed. Seventy-five percent of the patients needed special footwear, and 84% had difficulty walking on uneven ground.

In a retrospective clinical and radiological study, Coester et al [14] reviewed 23 patients who had had an isolated ankle arthrodesis for the treatment of painful post-traumatic osteoarthrosis. At a mean of 22 years (range, 12 to 42 years), the majority of patients had substantial and accelerated arthritic changes in the ipsilateral foot, but not the knee. Twenty-two patients (96%) had a slight-to-moderate limp, nine patients (39%) had varus malalignment, and eight patients (35%) had valgus malalignment. The ranges of motion of ipsilateral and contralateral knees were comparable. Twenty patients (87%) had full and painless motion of the uninvolved ankle. The ipsilateral subtalar range of motion was decreased in every case, with 0% range of motion in nine patients (39%), 10% to 50% range of motion on the contralateral side in 13 patients (57%), and more than 50% range of motion on the contralateral side in one patient. Most patients were limited functionally by foot pain. The authors concluded that, although ankle arthrodesis may provide good early relief of pain, it is associated with premature deterioration of other joints of the foot, and eventual osteoarthrosis, pain, and dysfunction.

In the longest follow-up after ankle arthrodesis (23 years; range, 20 to 33 years), Fuchs et al reported that half of the 18 patients followed considered themselves slightly or not limited in activities of daily living, although 61% had suffered a post-surgical complication [22]. Fifteen feet had an equinus deformity: seven (39%) had a deformity of 5° to 10°, and eight (44%) had a deformity of 11° to 20°. There were seven varus deformities and one valgus hindfoot. All patients, except one with spinal cord injury, were still employed; 44% returned to their pre-injury occupation, while others changed to lighter employment, although still undertaking manual labor. One-third considered their professional handicap as "moderate" and one-third as "significant." The SF-36 for physical function, emotional disturbance, and bodily pain revealed significant deficits, however, there was a significant correlation between the functional outcome as determined by the clinical score (Olerud Molander Ankle [68]) and the SF-36 score, and between the clinical score and the radiological degree of osteoarthrosis in the subtalar and transverse tarsal joints. There was, by contrast, no significant correlation between the radiological parameters and the quality of life score. On the whole, the correlation analysis revealed a high significance between the clinical outcome and the quality of life, whereas degenerative changes in the adjacent joints (especially the subtalar) had a significant impact on the clinical result (and thereby also on quality of life), but did not directly correlate with the quality of life. A similar result was reported by Morgan et al [62], who reviewed 101 patients at a mean of 10 years after ankle arthrodesis. While most of the unsatisfactory results were related to a nonunion or symptomatic arthritis of the ipsilateral foot, they found no association between the radiographic evidence of the arthritis and the severity of the symptoms.

3.3.4 Degenerative Changes after Ankle Arthrodesis

Ankle arthrodesis is not without risk, including prolonged periods of immobilization with resultant loss of subtalar motion, ultimate breakdown of midfoot joints, pseudarthrosis in 10% to 35% of cases, and persistent pain in a high percentage of cases, even after successful arthrodesis [14, 63]. In a 7.5-year follow-up analysis of 18 patients, Said et al [79] noted that 16 patients (89%) had a stiff subtalar joint. Wu et al [99] showed a reduced range of motion and a generalized stiffness of the hindfoot, whereas an overall increased range of motion was noted in the forefoot. Mazur et al [57], in an eight-year follow-up analysis of 12 patients, found radiographic changes of osteoarthrosis in the subtalar and midtarsal joints in all of the patients. Jackson and Glasgow [38], in a one- to 25-year follow-up analysis of 37 patients, found radiographic degenerative changes in the tarsal joints of 22 patients (59%), and a stiff subtalar joint in all 37 patients. Takakura et al [88], in a 7.3-year follow-up (range, two to 15 years), found progressive osteoarthrosis in the transverse tarsal joints of 16% of their 43 patients, and in the subtalar joint of 33% of the patients. Nonunion occurred in three patients (7%), and tibial stress fractures in two patients (5%). Coester et al [14], in a 12- to 44-year follow-up (mean 22 years) of 23 patients, found moderate to severe osteoarthritic changes in the subtalar joint of

Table 3.2. Complications and problems after ankle arthrodesis

Author(s)	Year	No. of Ankles	Average Follow-up [yr]	Major Complications* [%]	Hindfoot Continued Pain [%]	Joint Degeneration [%]
Said et al [79]	1978	36	8	24	†	>50
Mazur et al [57]	1979	12	8	†	25	100
Jackson and Glasgow [38]	1979	37	10	†	†	100
Morrey and Wiedermann [63]	1980	41	8	48	76	50
Ahlberg and Henricson [3]	1981	41	12	32	68	44
Boobbyer [9]	1981	58	9	21	†	†
Morgan et al [62]	1985	101	10	10	†	†
Marcus et al [55]	1983	13	6	23	8	†
Lynch et al [53]	1988	62	7	34	†	†
Leicht and Kofoed [49]	1992	27	6	43	46	39
Frey et al [22]	1994	78	4	56	†	†
Glick et al [25]	1996	34	8	6	†	†
Takakura et al [88]	1999	43	7	12	†	48
Coester et al [14]	2001	23	22	†	83	>91
Anderson et al [5]	2002	25	4	15	†	†
Fuchs et al [23]	2003	18	23	61	†	94
Average		41	10	30	51	66
Standard deviation		24	5	18	30	28

* Deep infection, nonunion, or amputation
† Data not reported

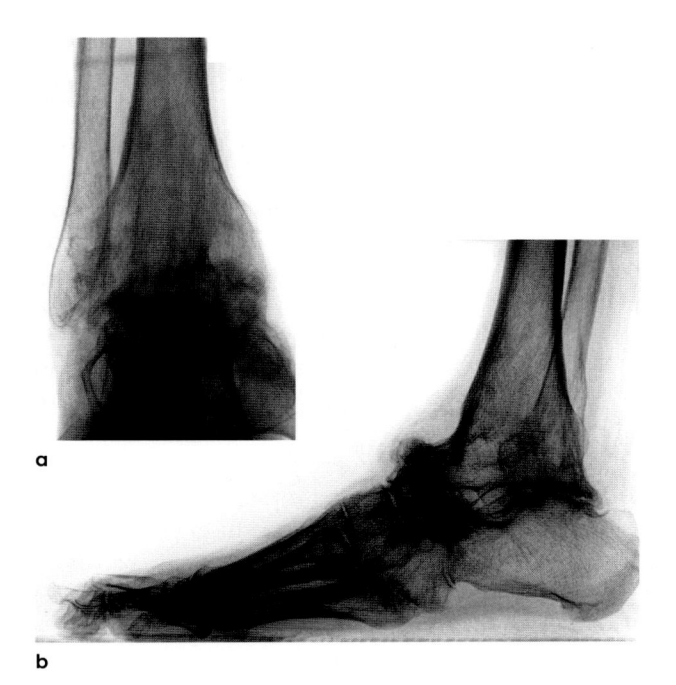

Fig. 3.4. Degeneration of adjacent hindfoot joints after ankle arthrodesis. Eight years after ankle fusion for symptomatic post-traumatic osteoarthrosis after fracture, this 59-year-old female patient complains of pain and disability while walking, despite shoe modifications. Clinical evaluation reveals an equinus position of 12°, and the X-rays evidence severe degenerative changes at the subtalar and talonavicular joints (a, b)

21 patients (91.3%), and in the talonavicular joint of 13 patients (56.6%). Lidor et al [51], in a study of 13 patients, found a tibial stress fracture in 12 patients, and a fibular stress fracture in one patient after arthrodesis of the ankle or foot. Seven patients had an isolated tibiotalar arthrodesis, and six had an arthrodesis of both the tibiotalar and subtalar joint (pantalar arthrodesis). Only six of the 13 patients had a malunion at the arthrodesis site; the other seven fractures were in patients who were thought to have optimum positioning after the arthrodeses.

Based on literature reports [3, 9, 62] (Table 3.2), there is a long-term probability of 68% ± 28% for hindfoot joint degeneration after ankle arthrodesis. In practical terms, when a young patient undergoes ankle arthrodesis, there is a significant likelihood that he or she will develop hindfoot arthritis during the next 20 years (Fig. 3.4), and will have to be treated for this secondary degenerative change. Increased stiffness of the foot and additional arthrodesis of the arthritic joint(s) is the likely outcome. Recent studies employing gait analysis and validated functional outcome measures to study patients with isolated ankle arthrodesis have demonstrated that even the most satisfied patients have major physical limitations compared with healthy controls [17].

Despite the high level of satisfaction with the results of ankle arthrodesis, it is a salvage procedure with limitations (Fig. 3.5) [3, 9, 14, 22, 53, 81]. If the expected outcome of treatment for end-stage arthritis or osteoarthrosis of the ankle is the restoration of normal physical function, then preservation of ankle motion is essential. The widespread advocacy of ankle arthrodesis as the final treatment for ankle arthritis or osteoarthrosis thus seems imprudent.

3.3.5 Ankle Arthrodesis versus Total Ankle Arthroplasty

Since the first reports of its successful use in the 19th century, ankle arthrodesis has become the standard surgical treatment for painful end-stage arthritis of the ankle. As techniques evolved and the success rates for arthrodeses increased, surgical indications expanded accordingly to post-traumatic osteoarthrosis. Although positive results have been reported in the literature [1, 9, 40], a few problems seem to endanger the future of this treatment, for example:

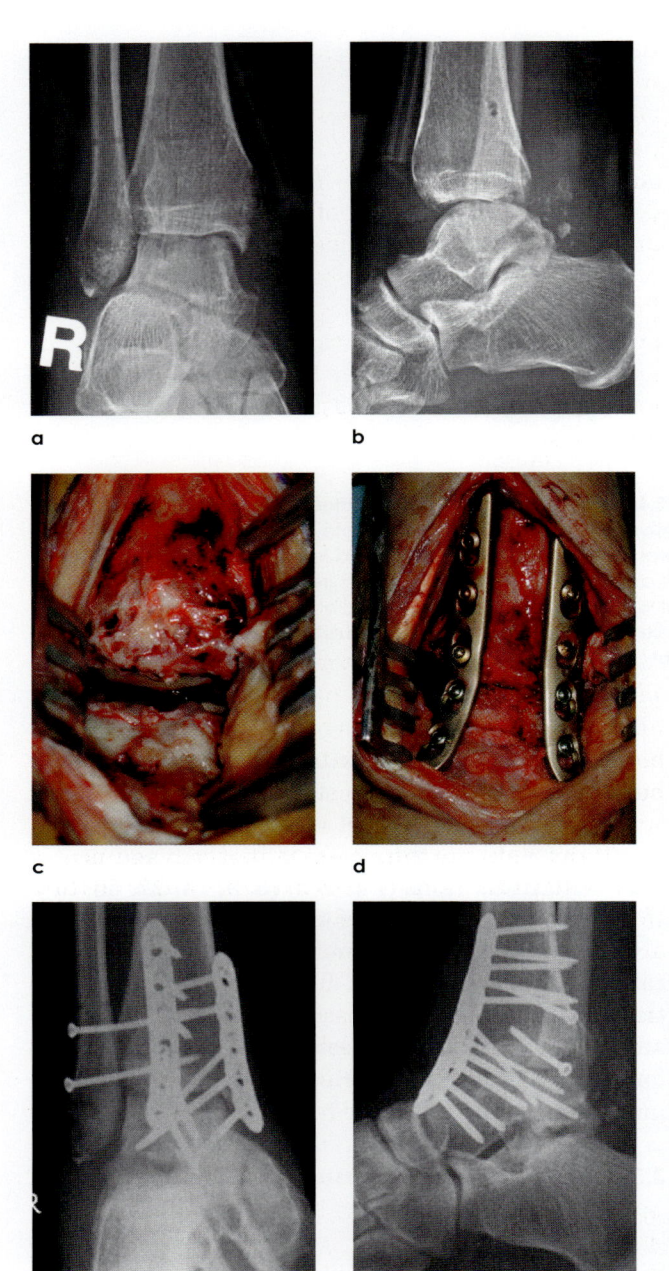

Fig. 3.5. Post-primary ankle fusion after post-traumatic articular infection.
This 42-year-old male mountain climber fell into a crevasse and sustained an open fracture of his right ankle, which resulted in severe infection and destruction of the ankle joint (**a, b**). An anterior approach was made to expose the joint (**c**), and after joint debridement, ankle fusion was achieved by using two plates (**d**). The postoperative X-rays show a plantigrade position of the foot with preservation of the subtalar joint (**e, f**). This technique has preserved the anatomy of the ankle joint as much as possible, which will potentially allow the fusion to be for taken apart for ankle arthroplasty when painful degeneration at the subtalar and/or transverse tarsal joints makes further fusion necessary

- compensatory overload (and therefore degeneration of neighboring hindfoot joints) [14, 23],
- gait changes [10, 17, 29, 42, 57, 99],
- decreased functional ability of patients due to pain and limp,
- high rates of pseudarthrosis, and
- long rehabilitation period [3, 9, 14, 22, 46, 48, 62, 95].

Further, biomechanical studies have shown that ankle arthrodesis results in a marked increase of tibial rotation [34, 94], thus leading (in extreme situations) to tibial stress fractures [51, 59, 88].

Although still controversial [11, 39, 43, 80, 81, 92, 101], total ankle arthroplasty may be a potentially viable treatment alternative [31, 44, 45, 74] to ankle arthrodesis. Further, in the opinion of the author, total ankle arthroplasty is a particularly exciting possibility for patients with ankle degeneration after an extensive hindfoot arthrodesis (that is, conversion of painful ankle arthrodesis to total ankle arthroplasty), because pantalar fusion has yielded unsatisfying results in nonparalytic extremities [69].

There are only a very few reports in the literature that compare total ankle arthroplasty with ankle arthrodesis [18, 46, 58]. Demottaz et al [18] noted that, at an average of only 14.7 months postoperatively, 88% of 21 total ankle arthroplasties of various designs had progressive radiolucent lines. Only four of the 21 patients (19%) were pain free. In the ankle arthrodesis group, nine of 12 patients (75%) remained pain free for up to 15 years. In the arthroplasty group, Demottaz et al [18] found abnormal gait patterns in speed, stride dimension, and temporal aspects of gait, as well as considerable muscle weakness about the ankle. The gait performance of the arthrodesis group was found to be superior, though this could be a result of longer adaptation over the years.

Kofoed and Stürup [46] reported on two groups of 13 patients (14 ankles) that were matched according to age, sex, diagnosis, and occupation. The Charnley external compression fixator was used in the arthrodesis group, and a cemented experimental ankle device was used in the prosthesis group. After a mean follow-up of 84 months (58 to 116 months), ankle arthroplasty gave significantly better pain relief, better function, and lower infection rate, without development of subtalar osteoarthrosis. One prosthesis was removed because of persistent pain, and union occurred within five months for the subsequent arthrodesis. The only other series dealing with comparison of ankle arthrodesis and arthroplasty was a retrospective series (25 arthroplasties and 18 arthrodeses), in which indications for one or the other procedure were not clearly stated [58]. The complication rate was 32% in the arthroplasty group (mean follow-up of 3.8 years), and 62% in the arthrodesis group (mean follow-up of 3.3 years).

3.4 Conclusions

The widespread advocacy of ankle arthrodesis as the final treatment for ankle arthritis seems imprudent.

For decades, ankle arthrodesis has been the principal option for treating debilitating end-stage osteoarthrosis or arthritis of the ankle, and it may continue to be a standard operative treatment for selected cases of severe post-traumatic ankle osteoarthrosis.

Many patients who were initially presumed to have been successfully treated with ankle arthrodesis have, during ensuing decades, developed arthritis of the subtalar and transverse tarsal joints. The prevalence of this adjacent joint arthritis increases with time. Further, following the conversion of an ankle arthrodesis to either a tibiocalcaneal or pantalar arthrodesis, the load shifts anteriorly to the midfoot and forefoot. Therefore, when counseling patients with regard to the potential long-term effects of ankle arthrodesis, one should explain that if the patient lives long enough, he or she can expect to develop symptomatic osteoarthrosis in the other joints of the foot.

References

[1] Abdo RV, Wasilewski SA (1992) Ankle arthrodesis: a long-term study. Foot Ankle 13: 307–312

[2] Abidi NA, Gruen GS, Conti SF (2000) Ankle arthrodesis: indications and techniques. J Am Acad Orthop Surg 8: 200–208

[3] Ahlberg A, Henricson AS (1981) Late results of ankle fusion. Acta Orthop Scand 52: 103–105
[4] Albert E (1879) Zur Resektion des Kniegelenkes. Wien Med Press 20: 705–708
[5] Anderson T, Montgomery F, Besjakov J, Verdier H, Carlsson A (2002) Arthrodesis of the ankle for non-inflammatory conditions – healing and reliability of outcome measurements. Foot Ankle Int 23: 390–393
[6] Ansart MB (1951) Pan-arthrodesis for paralytic flail foot J Bone Joint Surg Br 33: 503–507
[7] Barr JS, Record EE (1953) Arthrodesis of the ankle joint: indications, operative technique and clinical experience. N Engl J Med 248: 53–60
[8] Beals TC, Pomeroy GP, Manoli A (1999) Posterior tendon insufficiency. J Am Acad Orthop Surg 7: 112–118
[9] Boobbyer GN (1981) The long-term results of ankle arthrodesis. Acta Orthop Scand 52: 107–110
[10] Buck P, Morrey BF, Chao EY (1987) The optimum position of arthrodesis of the ankle. A gait study of the knee and ankle. J Bone Joint Surg Am 69: 1052–1062
[11] Buechel FF, Pappas MJ, Iorio LJ (1988) New Jersey low contact stress total ankle replacement: biomechanical rationale and review of 23 cementless cases. Foot Ankle 8: 279–290
[12] Campbell WC (1929) Bone-block operation for drop-foot. J Bone Joint Surg 27: 317–324
[13] Charnley J (1951) Compression arthrodesis of the ankle and shoulder. J Bone Joint Surg Br 33: 180–191
[14] Coester LM, Saltzman CL, Leupold J, Pontarelli W (2001) Long-term results following ankle arthrodesis for post-traumatic arthritis. J Bone Joint Surg Am 83: 219–228
[15] Cook AG, Stern WG, Ryerson EW (1923) Report of the commission appointed by the American Orthopedic Association for the study of stabilizing operations on the foot. J Bone Joint Surg 21: 135–140
[16] Corso SJ, Zimmer TJ (1995) Technique and clinical evaluation of arthroscopic ankle arthrodesis. Arthroscopy 11: 585–590
[17] Daniels TR, Thomas RH, Parker K (2002) Gait analysis and functional outcomes of isolated ankle arthrodesis. Read at the 2nd IFFAS Triennial Scientific Meeting in San Francisco
[18] Demottaz JD, Mazur JM, Thomas WH, Sledge CB, Simon SR (1979) Clinical study of total ankle replacement with gait analysis. A preliminary report. J Bone Joint Surg Am 61: 976–988
[19] Dent CM, Patil M, Fairclough JA (1993) Arthroscopic ankle arthrodesis. J Bone Joint Surg Br 75: 830–832
[20] Fitzgibbons TC (1999) Arthroscopic ankle debridement and fusion: indications, techniques, and results. Instr Course Lect 48: 243–248
[21] Fjermeros H, Hagen R (1967) Post-traumatic arthrosis in the ankle and foot treated with arthrodesis. Acta Orthop Scand 133: 527–534
[22] Frey C, Halikus NM, Vu-Rose T, Ebramzadeh E (1994) A review of ankle arthrodesis: predisposing factors to nonunion. Foot Ankle Int 15: 581–584
[23] Fuchs S, Sandmann C, Skwara A, Chylarecki C (2003) Quality of life 20 years after arthrodesis of the ankle. A study of adjacent joints. J Bone Joint Surg Br 85: 994–998
[24] Gellman H, Lenihan M, Halikis N, Botte JM, Giordani M, Perry J (1987) Selective tarsal arthrodesis: An *in vitro* analysis of the effect on foot motion. Foot Ankle 8: 127–133
[25] Glick JM, Morgan CD, Myerson MS, Sampson TG, Mann JA (1996) Ankle arthrodesis using an arthroscopic method: long-term follow-up of 34 cases. Arthroscopy 12: 428–434
[26] Graves SC, Stephenson K (1997) The use of subtalar and triple arthrodesis in the treatment of posterior tibial tendon dysfunction. In: Adult flatfoot: Posterior tibial tendon dysfunction (Shereff JM, ed). Saunders, Philadelphia, pp 319–328
[27] Haddad SL, Myerson MS, Pell RF, Schon LC (1997) Clinical and radiographic outcome of revision surgery for failed triple arthrodesis. Foot Ankle Int 18: 489–499
[28] Hagen RJ (1984) Ankle arthrodesis. Problems and pitfalls. Clin Orthop 202: 152–162
[29] Hefti F, Baumann J, Morscher EW (1980) Ankle joint fusion: determination of optional position by gait analysis. Arch Orthop Trauma Surg 96: 187–192
[30] Helm R (1990) The results of ankle arthrodesis. J Bone Joint Surg Br 72: 141–143
[31] Hintermann B (1999) Die STAR-Sprunggelenkprothese. Kurz- und mittelfristige Erfahrungen. Orthopäde 28: 792–803
[32] Hintermann B, Nigg BM (1995) *In vitro* kinematics of the axially loaded ankle complex in response to dorsiflexion and plantar flexion. Foot Ankle Int 16: 514–518
[33] Hintermann B, Nigg BM (1995) Influence of arthrodeses on kinematics of the axially loaded ankle complex during dorsiflexion/plantar flexion. Foot Ankle Int 16: 633–636
[34] Hintermann B, Nigg BM, Cole GK (1994) Influence of selective arthrodesis on the movement transfer between calcaneus and tibia *in vitro*. Clin Biomech 9: 356–361
[35] Hoke (1921) An operation for stabilizing paralytic feet. Am J Orthop Surg 3: 494–507
[36] Horton GA, Olney BW (1995) Triple arthrodesis with lateral column lengthening for treatment of severe planovalgus deformity. Foot Ankle Int 16: 395–400
[37] Hunt JC, Brooks AL (1965) Subtalar extra-articular arthrodesis for correction of paralytic valgus deformity of the foot. J Bone Joint Surg Am 47: 1310–1314
[38] Jackson A, Glasgow M (1979) Tarsal hypermobility after ankle fusion – fact or fiction? J Bone Joint Surg Br 61: 470–473
[39] Jensen NC, Kroner K (1992) Total joint replacement: A clinical follow-up. Orthopaedics 15: 236–239
[40] Katcherian DA (1998) Treatment of ankle arthrosis. Clin Orthop 349: 48–57
[41] Kile TA, Donnelly RE, Gehrke JC (1994) Tibiocalcaneal arthrodesis with an intramedullary device. Foot Ankle Int 15: 669–673
[42] King HA, Watkins TB, Samuelson KM (1980) Analysis of foot position in ankle arthrodesis and its influence on gait. Foot Ankle 1: 44–49

References

[43] Kitaoka HB, Patzer GL (1996) Clinical results of the Mayo total ankle arthroplasty. J Bone Joint Surg Am 78: 1658–1664

[44] Kofoed H, Lundberg-Jensen (1999) Ankle arthroplasty in patients younger and older than 50 years: a prospective series with long-term follow-up. Foot Ankle Int 20: 501–506

[45] Kofoed H, Sorensen TS (1998) Ankle arthroplasty for rheumatoid arthritis and osteoarthritis: prospective long-term study of cemented replacements. J Bone Joint Surg Br 80: 328–332

[46] Kofoed H, Stürup J (1994) Comparison of ankle arthroplasty and arthrodesis. A prospective series with long-term follow-up. Foot 4: 6–9

[47] Lambrinudi C (1927) New operation of drop foot. Br J Surg 15: 193–200

[48] Lance EM, Paval A, Fries I, Larsen I, Patterson RL (1979) Arthrodesis of the ankle joint. A follow-up study. Clin Orthop 142: 146–158

[49] Leicht P, Kofoed H (1992) Subtalar arthrosis following ankle arthrodesis. Foot 2: 89–92

[50] Levine SE, Myerson MS, Lucas P, Schon LC (1997) Salvage of pseudarthrosis after tibiotalar arthrodesis. Foot Ankle Int 18: 580–585

[51] Lidor C, Ferris LR, Hall R, Alexander IJ, Nunley JA (1997) Stress fracture of the tibia after arthrodesis of the ankle or the hindfoot. J Bone Joint Surg Am 79: 558–564

[52] Liebolt FL (1939) Pantalar arthrodesis in poliomyelitis. Surgery 6: 31–34

[53] Lynch AF, Bourne RB, Rorabeck CH (1988) The long-term results of ankle arthrodesis. J Bone Joint Surg Br 70: 113–116

[54] Mann DC, Hsu JD (1992) Triple arthrodesis in the treatment of fixed cavovarus deformity in adolescent patients with Charcot-Marie-Tooth disease. Foot Ankle 13: 1–6

[55] Marcus RE, Balourdas GM, Heiple KG (1983) Ankle arthrodesis by chevron fusion with internal fixation and bone grafting. J Bone Joint Surg Am 65: 833–838

[56] Maurer RC, Cimino WR, Cox CV, Satow GK (1991) Transarticular cross-screw fixation: a technique of ankle arthrodesis. Clin Orthop 268: 56–64

[57] Mazur J, Schartz E, Simon S (1979) Ankle arthrodesis. Long-term follow-up with gait analysis. J Bone Joint Surg Am 61: 964–975

[58] McGuire MR, Kyle RF, Gustilo RB, Premer RF (1988) Comparative analysis of ankle arthroplasty versus ankle arthrodesis. Clin Orthop 226: 174–181

[59] Mitchell R, Johnson JE, Collier BD, Gould JS (1995) Stress fracture of the tibia following extensive hindfoot and ankle arthrodesis: a report of three cases. Foot Ankle Int 16: 445–448

[60] Moeckel BH, Patterson BM, Inglis AE, Sculco TP (1991) Ankle arthrodesis. A comparison of internal and external fixation. Clin Orthop 268: 78–83

[61] Monroe MT, Beals TC, Manoli A (1999) Clinical outcome of arthrodesis of the ankle using rigid internal fixation with cancellous screws. Foot Ankle Int 20: 227–231

[62] Morgan CD, Henke JA, Bailey RW, Kaufer H (1985) Long-term results of tibiotalar arthrodesis. J Bone Joint Surg Am 67: 546–550

[63] Morrey BF, Wiedermann GP (1980) Complications and long-term results of ankle arthrodesis following trauma. J Bone Joint Surg Am 62: 777–784

[64] Mulier E, deRijcke J, Fabray C (1990) Triple arthrodesis in neuromuscular disorders. Acta Orthop Belg 56: 557–561

[65] Myerson MS, Quill G (1991) Ankle arthrodesis. A comparison of an arthroscopic and an open method of treatment. Clin Orthop 268: 84–95

[66] O'Brien TS, Hart TS, Shereff MJ, Stone J, Johnson J (1999) Open versus arthroscopic ankle arthrodesis: a comparative study. Foot Ankle Int 20: 368–374

[67] Ogilvie-Harris DJ, Lieberman I, Fitsialos D (1993) Arthroscopically assisted arthrodesis for osteoarthritic ankles. J Bone Joint Surg Am 75: 1167–1174

[68] Olerud C, Molander H (1984) A scoring scale for symptom evaluation after ankle fracture. Arch Orthop Traum Surg 103: 190–194

[69] Papa J, Myerson MS, Girard P (1993) Salvage, with arthrodesis, in intractable diabetic neuropathic arthropathy of the foot and ankle. J Bone Joint Surg Am 75: 1056–1066

[70] Paremain GD, Miller SD, Myerson MS (1996) Ankle arthrodesis: results after miniarthrotomy technique. Foot Ankle Int 17: 247–252

[71] Patterson RL, Parrish FF, Hathaway EN (1950) Stabilizing operations on the foot: a study of the indications, techniques used, and end results. J Bone Joint Surg Am 32: 1–26

[72] Perlman MH, Thordarson DB (1999) Ankle fusion in a high risk population: an assessment of nonunion risk factors. Foot Ankle Int 20: 491–496

[73] Pfahler M, Krodel A, Tritschler A, Zenta S (1996) Role of internal and external fixation in ankle fusion. Arch Orthop Trauma Surg 115: 146–148

[74] Pyevich MT, Saltzman CL, Callaghan JJ, Alvine FG (1998) Total ankle arthroplasty: a unique design. Two to twelve-year follow-up. J Bone Joint Surg Am 80: 1410–1420

[75] Quill GE (1996) Tibiotalocalcaneal and pantalar arthrodesis. Foot Ankle Clin 1: 199–210

[76] Quill GE (2000) An approach to the management of ankle arthritis. In: Foot and ankle disorders (Myerson MS, ed). Saunders, Philadelphia, pp 1059–1084

[77] Russotti GM, Johnson KE, Cass JR (1988) Tibiocalcaneal arthrodesis for arthritis and deformity of the hind part of the foot. J Bone Joint Surg Am 70: 1304–1307

[78] Ryerson E (1923) Arthrodesing operations on the feet. J Bone Joint Surg 5: 453–471

[79] Said E, Hunka L, Siller TN (1978) Where ankle fusion stands today. J Bone Joint Surg Br 60: 211–214

[80] Saltzman CL (2000) Perspective on total ankle replacement. Foot Ankle Clin 5: 761–775

[81] Saltzman CL, McIff TE, Buckwalter JA, Brown TD (2000) Total ankle replacement revisited. J Orthop Sports Phys Ther 30: 56–67

[82] Santavira S, Turunen V, Ylinen P (1993) Foot and ankle fusions in Charcot-Marie-Tooth disease. Arch Orthop Traum Surg 112: 175–179

[83] Soren A, Waugh TR (1980) The historical evolution of arthrodesis of the foot. Int Orthop 4: 3–11

[84] Sowa DT, Krackow KA (1989) Ankle fusion: A new technique of internal fixation using a compression blade plate. Foot Ankle 9: 232–240

[85] Staples OS (1956) Posterior arthrodesis of the ankle and subtalar joints. J Bone Joint Surg Am 38: 50–58

[86] Stauffer RN, Chao EY, Brewster RC (1977) Force and motion analysis of the normal, diseased, and prosthetic ankle joint. Clin Orthop 127: 189–196

[87] Stranks GJ, Cecil T, Jeffrey ITA (1994) Anterior ankle arthrodesis with cross-screw fixation. A dowel graft method used in 20 cases. J Bone Joint Surg Br 76: 943–946

[88] Takakura Y, Tanaka Y, Sugimoto K, Akiyama K, Tamai S (1999) Long-term results of arthrodesis for osteoarthritis of the ankle. Clin Orthop 361: 178–185

[89] Tenuta J, Shelton YA, Miller F (1993) Long-term follow-up of the triple arthrodesis in patients with cerebral palsy. J Pediatr Orthop 13: 713–716

[90] Thordarson DB, Markolf KL, Cracchiolo A (1992) Stability of an ankle arthrodesis fixed by cancellous-bone screws compared with that by an external fixator. J Bone Joint Surg Am 74: 1050–1055

[91] Turan I, Wredmark T, Felländer-Tsai L (1995) Arthroscopic ankle arthrodesis in rheumatoid arthritis. Clin Orthop 320: 110–114

[92] Unger AS, Inglis AE, Mow CS, Figgie HEI (1988) Total ankle arthroplasty in rheumatoid arthritis: a long-term follow-up study. Foot Ankle 8: 173–179

[93] Valderrabano V, Hintermann B, Nigg BM, Stefanyshyn D, Stergiou P (2003) Kinematic changes after fusion and total replacement of the ankle, part 1: range of motion. Foot Ankle Int 24: 881–887

[94] Valderrabano V, Hintermann B, Nigg BM, Stefanyshyn D, Stergiou P (2003) Kinematic changes after fusion and total replacement of the ankle, part 2: movement transfer. Foot Ankle Int 24: 888–896

[95] Waters RL, Barnes G, Husserl T, Silver L, Liss R (1988) Comparable energy expenditure after arthrodesis of the hip and ankle. J Bone Joint Surg Am 70: 1032–1037

[96] Waugh TR, Wagner J, Stinchfield FE (1965) An evaluation of plantar arthrodesis – A follow-up study of one hundred and sixteen operations. J Bone Joint Surg Am 47: 1315–1322

[97] Wayne JS, Lawhorn KW, Davis KE, Prakash K, Adelaar RS (1997) The effect of tibiotalar fixation on foot biomechanics. Foot Ankle Int 18: 792–797

[98] Whitman R (1901) The operative treatment of paralytic talipes of the calcaneous type. Am J Med Sci 122: 593–601

[99] Wu WL, Su FC, Cheng YM, Huang PJ, Chou YL, Chou CK (2000) Gait analysis after ankle arthrodesis. Gait Posture 11: 54–61

[100] Wülker N, Stukenborg C, Savory KM, Alfke D (2000) Hindfoot motion after isolated and combined arthrodeses: measurements in anatomic specimens. Foot Ankle Int 21: 921–927

[101] Wynn AH, Wilde AH (1992) Long-term follow-up of the Conaxial (Beck-Steffee) total ankle arthroplasty. Foot Ankle 13: 303–306

[102] Zvijac JE, Lemak L, Schurhoff MR, Hechtman KS, Uribe JW (2002) Analysis of arthroscopically assisted ankle arthrodesis. Arthroscopy 18: 70–75

Chapter 4

ANATOMIC AND BIOMECHANICAL CHARACTERISTICS OF THE ANKLE JOINT AND TOTAL ANKLE ARTHROPLASTY

The ankle joint forms a functional unit with the subtalar joint that is fundamental for plantigrade, bipedal ambulation. The intact ankle efficiently dissipates the compressive, shear, and rotatory forces that are encountered while adapting to weight-bearing and ground reaction forces during different phases of the gait cycle. A large articular contact area provides inherent stability under static load, and dynamic stability is afforded by ligamentous support and balanced muscular forces. The mechanical efficiency of the ankle can be inferred from its relative resistance to primary degenerative joint disease. Cartilage and ligament injury or changes in alignment caused by trauma or inflammatory disease may, however, result in articular degeneration.

In recent decades, total ankle arthroplasty has become a viable alternative to fusion in the treatment of end-stage degenerative disease. To achieve successful results, however, proponents of total ankle replacement must consider the biomechanical properties of this unique and complex joint. This chapter will elucidate the anatomic and biomechanical characteristics of the ankle joint with a perspective on total ankle replacement.

4.1 Anatomic Considerations

The ankle joint is a highly congruent and dynamic joint consisting of three bones, collateral and syndesmotic ligaments, and surrounding tendons and muscles (Fig. 4.1). The talar body is held within a mortise formed by the distal tibia and fibula, and is bound by strong ligaments. It articulates superiorly with the tibial plafond, and on the medial side with the medial malleolus. On the lateral side, it articulates with the lateral malleolus. The facets of both the medial and lateral malleoli are parallel to corresponding facets of the talus [29]. Congruency of the corresponding malleolar and talar facets is provided throughout the entire range of motion [29]. Both the medial tibiotalar and fibulotalar contact areas are, however, found to increase significantly with weight-bearing and to be maximized at 50% of stance [11].

4.1.1 Bony Configuration

The talus is a truncated, cone-shaped bone that has a smaller medial and larger lateral radius (Fig. 4.2). The superior articular portion of the talus is wedge-shaped. The mediolateral width is

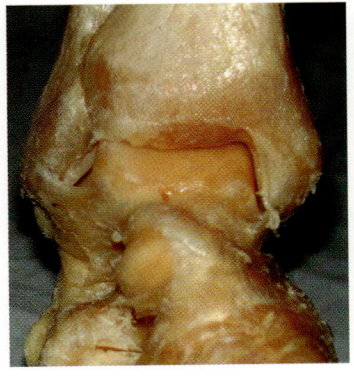

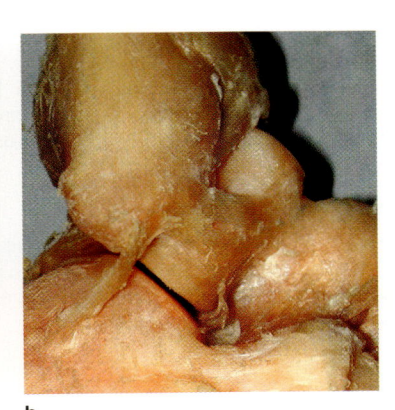

Fig. 4.1. Anatomy of the talocrural joint.
The ankle joint is highly congruent with close joint contacts. Each ligament has a well-defined isometric position to the joint, and some ligaments cross neighboring joints as well. (**a**) anterior view, (**b**) lateral view

widest anteriorly and converges asymmetrically to a narrow posterior process [1, 29]. In a cadaver study of 100 specimens [29], Inman determined that the medial angle of orientation of the talus (medial facet) measured 83.9°, with a range of 70° to 90°. The lateral angle of orientation (lateral facet) formed a lateral angle averaging 89.2°, with a range of 80° to 95°. From this data, Inman determined that the talus is not a cylinder, but rather a section of a frustum of a cone, the apex of which is directed medially.

Inman [29] also evaluated the fit of the talus in the mortise (Fig. 4.3). On the lateral side, the radius of the mortise curvature was within 1 mm of the talus, whereas on the medial side, the average difference was 2.1 mm ± 1.1 mm (range, 0 mm to 5 mm). In all specimens examined, the radius of the mortise curvature was larger than that of the talus, suggesting that this difference allows for some degree of horizontal rotation.

The tibial plafond serves as the most superior aspect of the ankle joint and articulates with the

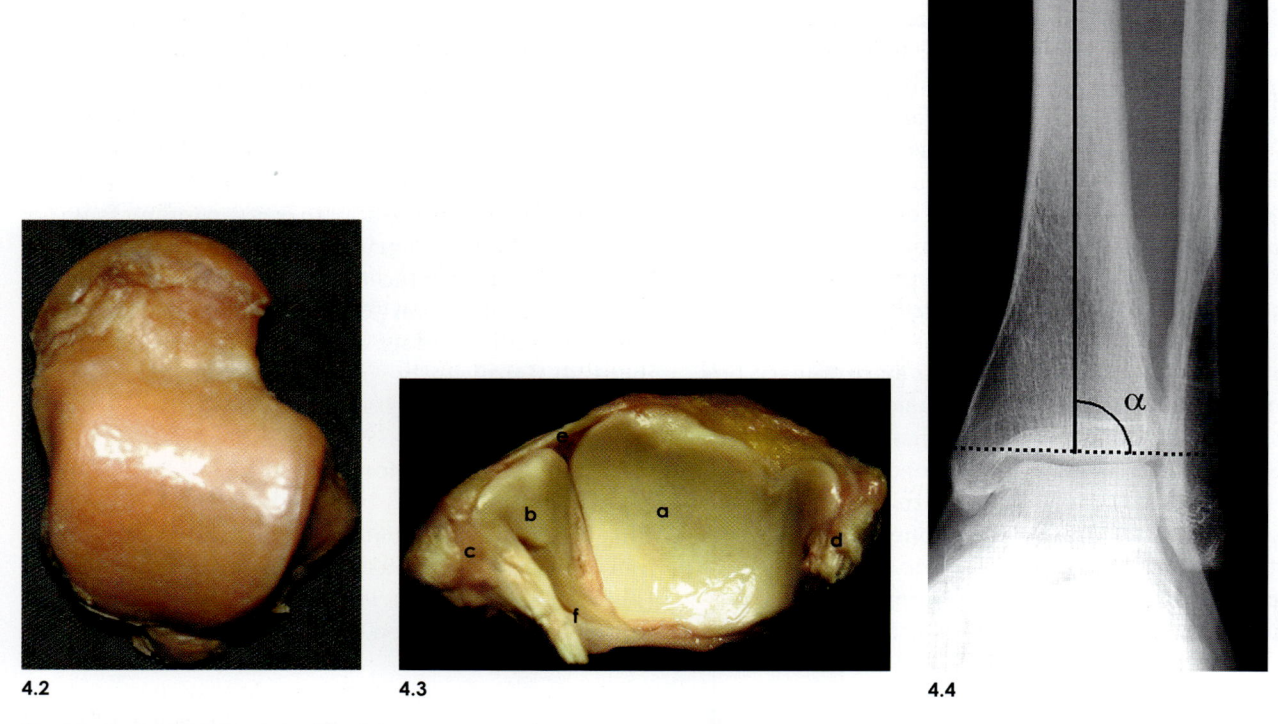

4.2 4.3 4.4

Fig. 4.2. Anatomical aspects of the talus.
Up to 60% of the talus is covered by cartilage, which is of utmost importance for its vascularization. The most important blood supply comes from posteromedially through the deltoid ligament and the talar neck. The talus is larger anteriorly than posteriorly, and the medial radius is smaller than the lateral radius (see text). This anatomical configuration implicates rotational movement of the talus during dorsiflexion/plantar flexion of the foot

Fig. 4.3. The ankle mortise.
The ankle mortise consists of two bones: the tibia (**a**) and fibula (**b**). In dorsiflexion, the ankle mortise is the main stabilizer for talus rotation. In plantar flexion, however, the mediolateral ligament complex (lateral, **c**; medial, **d**) is the main stabilizer (see Fig. 4.6). The syndesmotic ligament structures (anterior, **e**; posterior, **f**) at the inferior tibiofibular joint also stabilize and allow some dynamic play of the mortise

Fig. 4.4. Orientation of the distal tibial plafond.
Alpha (α) shows the tibiotalar angle with an angulation from distal lateral to proximal medial (see text)

4.1 Anatomic Considerations

dome of the talus. It is concave in the anteroposterior plane and elevated slightly on the medial side. This shape dictates an orientation of the distal tibial plafond that is slightly oblique from distal lateral to proximal medial. This forms, with respect to the longitudinal axis of the tibia, an angle averaging 93°, with a relatively small amount of variation (Fig. 4.4) [29]. Similar values were found in a recent radiographic study of 97 healthy volunteers, with the mean tibiotalar angle being 92.4° (SD 3.1°), and a range from 84° to 100° (Fig. 4.5) [32]. Females had a smaller tibiotalar angle (92.2°) than males (94.4°), and for both females and males, there was a slight increase in

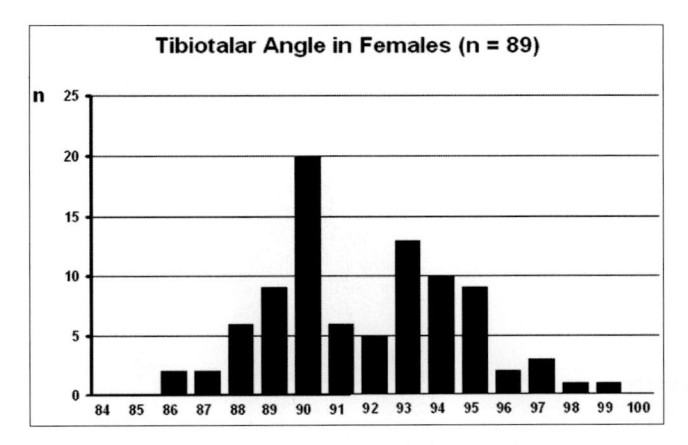

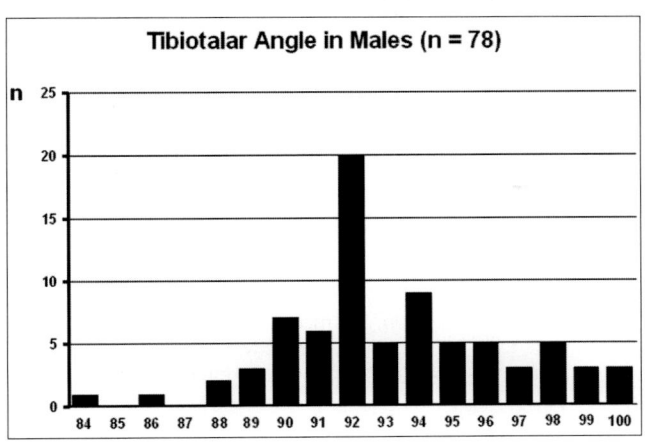

Fig. 4.5. Tibiotalar angle distribution in females and males.
These graphs depict the tibiotalar angle distribution in females and males (see also Fig. 4.4). In this study (see text), the mean tibiotalar angle was 92.4° with a range from 84° to 100°. Females had a smaller tibiotalar angle (92.2°) than males (94.4°), and for both females and males, there was a slight increase in this angle with age

this angle with age. In the group of 75 volunteers who agreed to have bilateral radiological investigation, an intraindividual difference of 1.08° (SD 1.09°) was found (range, 0° to 6°) between both legs.

The complex anatomic configuration, high congruency of the ankle joint, and complex dynamic nature of the ankle axis of rotation has important implications in the design of total ankle prostheses [17, 20].

4.1.2 Ligamentous Configuration

The anterior talofibular, calcaneofibular, and posterior talofibular ligaments constitute the lateral collateral ligaments of the ankle and stabilize the ankle laterally. Each of the lateral ligaments has a role in stabilizing the ankle and/or subtalar joint, depending on the position of the foot (Fig. 4.6). In dorsiflexion, the posterior talofibular ligament is maximally stressed and the calcaneofibular ligament is taut, while the anterior talofibular ligament is loose. In plantar flexion, however, the anterior talofibular ligament is taut, and the calcaneofibular and posterior talofibular ligaments become loose [16, 56, 62]. Some variation of this is allowed by the different patterns of divergence between the anterior talofibular and calcaneofibular ligaments.

Sequential sectioning of the lateral ligaments has demonstrated the function of these ligaments in different positions and under various loading conditions. Johnson and Markolf [30] studied laxity after sectioning the anterior talofibular ligament and found that most changes occur in plantar flexion. They found a smaller change in laxity in dorsiflexion, suggesting that the anterior talofibular ligament limits talar tilt throughout the full range of motion, but has greatest advantage in plantar flexion. Rasmussen and Tovberg-Jensen [55] further confirmed these findings, stating that talar tilt is limited in plantar flexion and neutral position by the anterior talofibular ligament, and in dorsiflexion by the calcaneofibular ligament plus the posterior talofibular ligament. Hollis et al [27], in a similar *in vitro* study, found that inversion motion of the ankle increased when the both the calcaneofibular ligament and the anterior talofibular ligament were sectioned.

Wide variations have been noted in the anatomic description of the medial ankle ligament complex (Fig. 4.7). Composed of superficial and deep portions

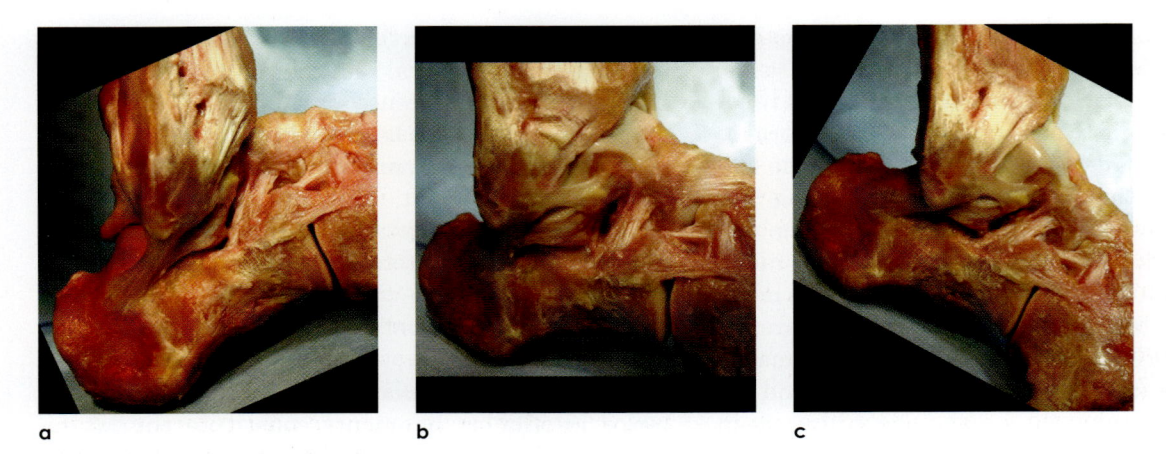

Chapter 4: Anatomic and Biomechanical Characteristics

Fig. 4.6. The lateral ankle ligament complex.
This series of pictures shows the position and tension of the lateral ankle ligament complex at (**a**) dorsiflexion, (**b**) neutral position, (**c**) plantar flexion of the foot

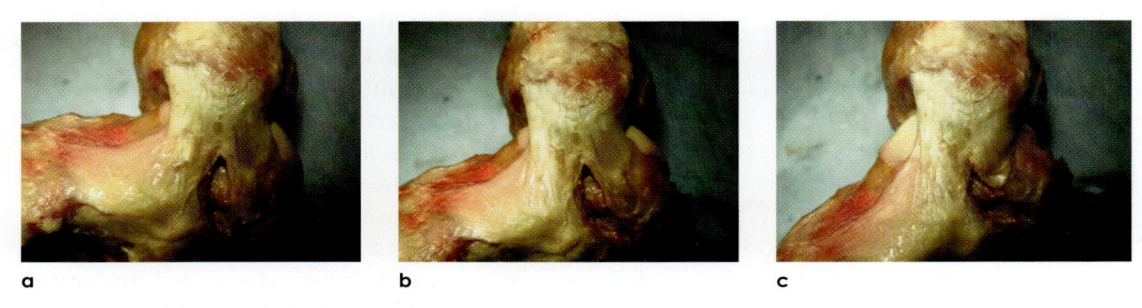

Fig. 4.7. The medial ankle ligament complex.
This series of pictures shows the position and tension of the medial ankle ligament complex at (**a**) dorsiflexion, (**b**) neutral position, (**c**) plantar flexion of the foot

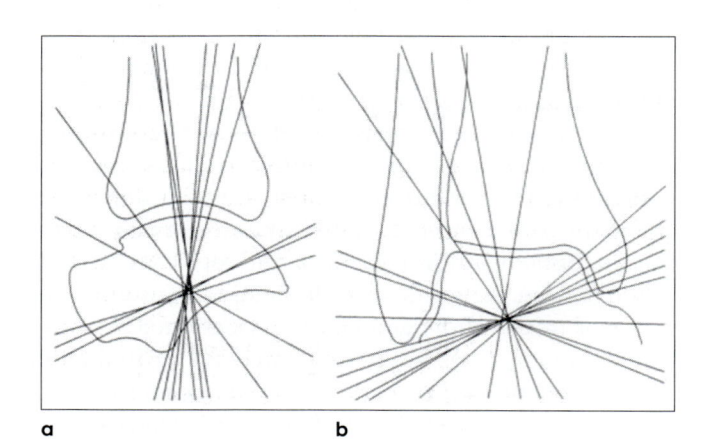

Fig. 4.8. The ankle joint: a uniaxial, modified hinge joint.
These pictures show the dynamic position of the ankle joint axis in eight healthy ankles for each 10°-interval from 30° of plantar flexion to 30° of dorsiflexion, projected (**a**) onto the sagittal plane, and (**b**) onto the frontal plane (From Lundberg A, Svensson OK, Nemeth G, 1989: The axis of rotation of the ankle joint. J Bone Joint Surg Br 71: 94–99; with permission)

of the deltoid ligament, it prevents valgus tilting and external rotation of the talus. The tibiocalcaneal (TCL), tibiospring (TSL), and tibionavicular (TNL) ligaments comprise the superficial portion and span the medial malleolus to insert broadly onto the sustentaculum tali (calcaneus), navicular, talar neck, and spring ligament [7, 22, 52]. The deep anterior tibiotalar (ATTL), superficial posterior tibiotalar (STTL), and deep posterior tibiotalar (PTTL) ligaments constitute the deep deltoid complex.

Close [15] found the deltoid ligament to be a strong restraint limiting talar abduction. With all lateral structures removed, he found that the intact deltoid ligament allowed only 2 mm of separation between the talus and medial malleolus. When the deep deltoid ligament was released, the talus could be separated from the medial malleolus by a distance of 3.7 mm. The tibiocalcaneal ligament (the strongest superficial ligament) specifically limits talar abduction, whereas the deep portions resist more external rotation as well [21, 55, 54].

4.2 Ankle Joint Motion

Anatomic and biomechanical studies have indicated that the ankle does not move as a pure hinge mechanism [1, 23, 43, 25]. Instead, ankle motion occurs in the sagittal, coronal, and transverse planes [43, 44].

4.2.1 Axis of Rotation

An early anatomic study pointed out that the wedge of the talus and differing medial and lateral talar dome radii of curvature implied that tibiotalar congruency could not be maintained through sagittal motion unless the talus exhibited coupled axial rotation [1]. The joint axis tends to incline downward laterally when projected onto a frontal plane and posterolaterally when projected onto a horizontal plane [2, 29, 43]. Because of this oblique orientation, dorsiflexion of the ankle results in eversion of the foot, whereas plantar flexion results in inversion. Dorsiflexion causes internal rotation of the leg, and plantar flexion causes external rotation of the leg, when the foot is fixed on the ground [1, 11, 42, 24, 59, 63, 70, 75]. This has been substantiated in kinematic tests of loaded cadaver ankle specimens [50, 70].

Sammarco [59] studied sagittal plane motion relative to the tibiotalar joint surface, and explained that the motion between the tibia and talus takes place about multiple instant centers of rotation. Ankles taken from plantar flexion to dorsiflexion showed a tendency toward distraction early in motion, followed by a sliding movement through the midportion, and ending in compression at the end of dorsiflexion. This process was reversed when the joint was moved in the opposite direction. Locations and patterns of instant centers varied among different individuals, direction of motion, weight-bearing states, and pathologic states. An unstable ankle demonstrated normal gliding during weight-bearing, but non-weight-bearing motion was grossly abnormal.

Using stereophotogrammetry, Lundberg et al [43] performed a three-dimensional evaluation of the ankle joint axis in eight healthy ankles. They explained that talar rotation occurs about a dynamic axis during sagittal plane movement of the ankle (Fig. 4.8), which in each subject lay close to the midpoint of a line between the tips of the malleoli. Plantar flexion axes were more horizontal, and inclined downward and medially compared with those of dorsiflexion. Most interestingly, no frontal plane movement occurred between the talus and the tibia during inversion/eversion of the loaded foot within a physiological range of motion.

Leardini et al [34] developed a mathematical model to explain the multiaxial motion of the ankle in the sagittal plane. These authors described a four-bar linkage model showing the talus/calcaneus and tibia/fibula rotating about one another on inextensible line segments that represent the calcaneofibular and tibiocalcaneal ligaments without resistance. Motion between the polycentric, polyradial trochlea consisted of a combination of "rolling" and "sliding" motions. In this model, rotation is dictated by the most anterior fibers of the anterior talofibular and calcaneofibular ligaments. Leardini [33] later observed that these specific fiber bundles were isometric through the range of sagittal motion of the ankle. The instant center of rotation translates from a posteroinferior to a superoanterior position, which is consistent with several studies that suggest that the ankle is incongruent and rotates about a transient center [60, 61, 63].

The complex and dynamic nature of the ankle's axis of rotation may be one reason for poor results in total ankle replacement surgery, and has important implications for the design of total ankle prostheses.

4.2.2 Range of Ankle Motion

Overall values found in the literature for normal range of motion in the ankle range from 23° to 56° of plantar flexion, and from 13° to 33° of dorsiflexion [23, 37, 38, 42, 53, 57, 58, 65, 69, 74, 75]. Ten degrees to 15° of plantar flexion and 10° of dorsiflexion are used during walking [58]. About 14° range of motion are used in the stance phase of gait, whereas 37° of motion are needed for ascending stairs, and 56° for descending stairs [65]. In the diseased ankle, dorsiflexion is typically decreased and limits daily activities, especially in the presence of pain. Ten degrees to 15° of dorsiflexion are all that is needed for daily activities in patients who do not rely on their ability to ascend and descend stairs [43]. The goal in total ankle replacement should be, therefore, to provide a minimum of 10° of dorsiflexion, as well as 20° of plantar flexion for an appropriate push-off.

Several factors influence sagittal plane motion of the ankle. Healthy older individuals demonstrate decreased plantar flexion [39, 53, 58]. Sagittal motion (primarily dorsiflexion) was found to significantly increase by assessing the subjects while weight-bearing, as compared with passive measuring [38, 57].

Rotation of the ankle in the transverse plane is usually reported relative to instability [46, 66], however, transverse plane motion is coupled with sagittal plane motion [41, 43, 49, 58, 15]. Transverse plane motion is also noted during normal gait [15, 41, 42, 63]. Lundberg et al [43] observed 8.9° of external rotation of the talus as the ankle moved from neutral position to 30° of dorsiflexion, whereas a small amount of internal rotation occurred with plantar flexion from neutral to 10°, followed by external rotation at terminal plantar flexion [42]. Michelson and Helgemo [49] reported that dorsiflexion resulted in an average of 7.2° ± 3.8° of external rotation of the foot relative to the leg with ankle dorsiflexion, and 1.9° ± 4.12° of internal rotation with plantar flexion. In unloaded specimens, some coupling between the ankle and subtalar joints was also observed with sagittal plane motion [63]. With dorsiflexion, there was internal rotation at the subtalar joint and external rotation at the ankle joint. The idea that this coupling is caused by tensioning of the deltoid ligament is supported by the findings of McCullough and Burge [46], who describe greater external rotation of the talus after deltoid ligament sectioning.

Coronal motion is described as varus or valgus rotation, but may also be described as inversion or eversion. Michelson et al [48] observed that plantar flexion of the ankle was associated with internal rotation and inversion of the ankle. They attributed coronal plane motion to the position of the deltoid ligament, showing that following progressive medial ankle destabilization, talar external rotation and inversion increased.

4.2.3 Restraints of Ankle Motion

The stability and integrity of the ankle joint depends on articular geometry and ligamentous attachments. Ankle ligaments have a passive tracking and stability effect on the ankle joint. On the medial side, the strong deep deltoid ligament is shown to be a secondary restraint against lateral and anterior talar excursion [7, 22, 56], whereas on the lateral side, the relatively weak anterior talofibular ligament is the only restraint against anterior talar excursion [35, 51, 56]. The anterior talofibular ligament is the ligament that is most susceptible to injury and subsequent insufficiency [5], often leading to anterolateral dislocation of the talus out of the mortise, and posterior dislocation of the fibula, respectively. In such a case, reconstruction of the anterior talofibular ligament (or "ligament balancing") may be advised when unconstrained prostheses are used for total ankle replacement.

Several studies [26, 64], have reported the effects of the lateral ligaments on axial rotation of the loaded ankle. Hintermann et al [26] observed that the rotation of the tibia that occurred after sectioning of the anterior talofibular ligament was more profound from neutral to plantar flexion than that observed in 10° to 20° of dorsiflexion. When the deltoid ligament was sectioned, no tibial rotation was observed. This is consistent with the findings of

Michelson et al [47], whose report suggests a motion-coupling role for the deltoid ligament in addition to stabilization.

Rotation about a vertical axis occurs during walking [15, 36]. Rotatory stability is provided by tension in the collateral ligaments, by compression of the medial and lateral talar facets against their corresponding malleoli, and by the shape of the articular surfaces [22, 46, 64, 66]. Because of the truncated conical shape of the talus with its medially directed apex, the three separated lateral ligaments control the greater movement on the lateral side, whereas the deltoid ligament controls the lesser movement on the medial side. This has important implications for ligament balancing in total ankle replacement, as nonanatomic prosthetic design and/or inappropriate implantation may provoke medial ligament stress with consequent pain, posteromedial ossification and loss of range of motion [68], or lateral ligament insufficiency with consequent lateral ankle instability, respectively.

Stability in the loaded ankle depends on articular shape [22, 46, 64, 66]. Stormont et al [66] performed serial sectioning of the ankle ligaments, and subjected the ankle to physiologic torque and loads. The articular surface accounted for 30% of ankle stability in rotation and 100% of ankle stability in inversion and eversion. In a similar study, McCullough and Burge [46] found that increased rotatory forces are necessary to cause displacement with increased loading of the ankle. The congruity of the articular surface of the ankle joint thus creates an inherently stable articulation with loading, and no ligamentous restraints exist in inversion and eversion. The sole restraint of the joint under loaded conditions is provided by the articular surfaces. This has important implications in the design of total ankle prostheses, and may explain poor results with prosthetic designs that expose the ankle ligaments to eversion and inversion forces while the ankle is loaded [69].

During most activities, the soft tissues are the major torsional and anteroposterior stabilizers of the ankle [13, 14], while the ankle's articulating surface geometry is the major inversion/eversion stabilizer, with collateral ligaments playing a secondary role [46, 66]. If a prosthesis does not provide intrinsic inversion and eversion stability, an unstable ankle will result, as noted by Burge and Evans [9]. They used a spherical, meniscal bearing ankle design to define the role of the surfaces with respect to stabilization of the ankle. While eversion/inversion stability was fully provided by the prosthesis, they found an anteroposterior laxity of 7 mm. The authors concluded from this that the anteroposterior restraint (as provided by the normal tibial articular surface, which is concave in the sagittal plane) may be lost when the surface is replaced by a flat prosthetic surface. The more the geometry of the articular surfaces is changed from its physiological condition, the more the prosthesis depends upon the soft tissues for stability. A prosthesis should, therefore, be as anatomic as possible to mimic physiological joint motion and guarantee proper ligament balancing.

Analogously to total knee replacement, however, if the concave tibial surface is replaced by a flat surface, forward motion of the talus no longer results in tibiotalar separation and the stabilizing influence of joint load is absent [45]. A flat prosthetic surface has no protective effect on the ligaments and may expose them to forces that they cannot withstand. Stauffer et al [65] calculated an anteroposterior shear force of 70% body weight during walking. This study shows the importance of osseous and ligamentous anteroposterior restraint for the continuous neutralization of the aforementioned shear force. Restoration of correct soft-tissue tension is, then, mandatory with the use of unconstrained ankle prostheses, and this can only be achieved with anatomically shaped devices.

4.3 Bone Support at the Ankle

Proper bone support is fundamental to the success of any prosthetic arthroplasty. Lowery [40] found that the subchondral bone of the distal tibia has an elastic modulus in the order of 300 MPa to 450 MPa. After removal of the subchondral plate, compressive resistance was lowered by a range of 30% to 50%, and with sectioning of the subchondral bone 1 cm proximal to the subchondral plate, by a range of 70% to 90% (Fig. 4.9). In another laboratory study, Hvid et al [28] found talar bone to be 40% stronger than tibial bone (Fig. 4.10). Calderale et al [10] found that removing part of the

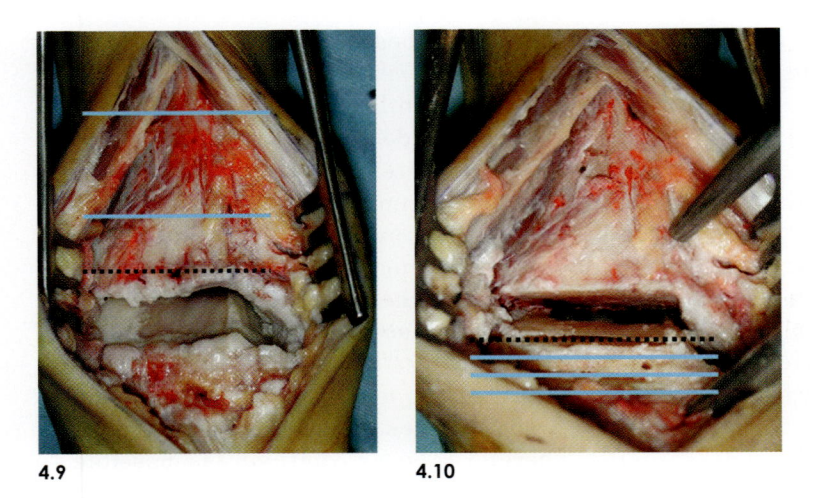

Fig. 4.9. Tibial bone compressive resistance.
The compressive resistance of bone greatly decreases as the site chosen for bony resection occurs higher on the distal tibia (see text)

Fig. 4.10. Talar bone compressive resistance.
The compressive resistance of bone decreases with the amount of bony resection on the talar body (see text)

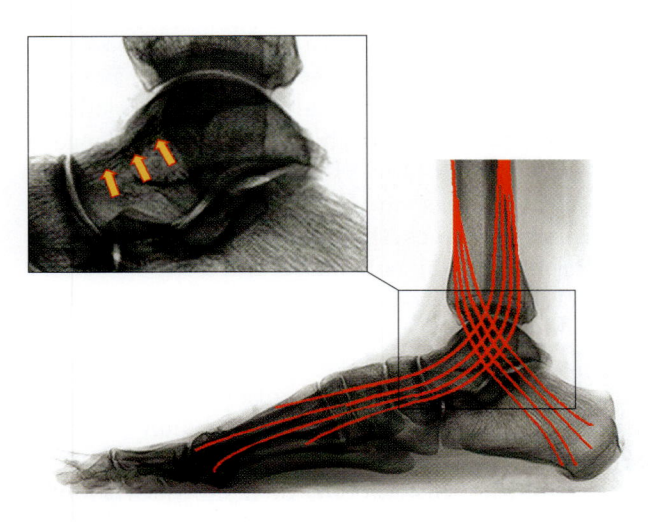

Fig. 4.11. Bony force trajectories.
The main trabecular lines through the foot and ankle (main force trajectories). There are important trabecular lines in the talar neck running close to the upper cortical shell. Removing part of the cortical shell of the talus places abnormal increased stress on the remaining weak talar cancellous bone (see text)

cortical shell of the talus placed abnormal increased stress on the remaining talar cancellous bone (Fig. 4.11). In other words, when part of the cortical shell of the talus is removed at the time of arthroplasty, the remaining bone must support a greater load than it did before the arthroplasty. Ideally, the talar component of the prosthetic should be anatomically sized, fully cover the talar body, and have a wide support on talar neck. It is, therefore, suggested that as much talar bone as possible be saved, particularly the anterior part of the talar body and talar neck. In general terms, to avoid collapse of the bone, minimal bone resection should be performed so that the stronger superficial subchondral bone is preserved. Conserving as much bone as possible at the time of surgery not only helps to ensure better support but also saves bone, which may be valuable should revision become necessary.

Hvid et al [28] also found an eccentricity of the area of maximal bone strength of the distal tibia that is posteromedial and not central (Fig. 4.12). This area of stiffer bone could act as a pivot point, with the risk of overloading the surrounding weaker anterolateral bone. To avoid "off center" forces on a prosthesis and possible collapse of the weak lateral tibia, proper alignment of the prosthesis and adequate ligament balancing of the ankle must be achieved. In particular, valgus malalignment should be corrected.

4.3 Bone Support at the Ankle

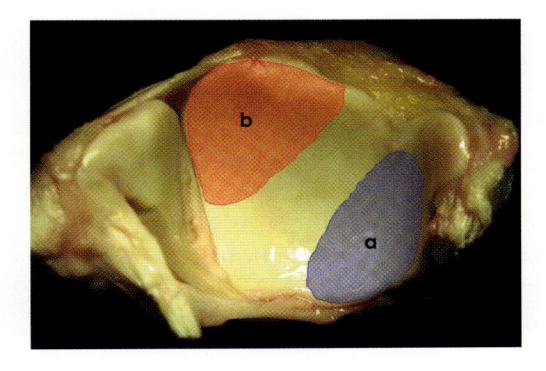

Fig. 4.12. Zones of superficial compressive resistance at tibial plafond.
Maximal bone strength (**a**) of the distal tibia is located posteromedially, whereas minimal bone strength (**b**) is located anterolaterally (see text)

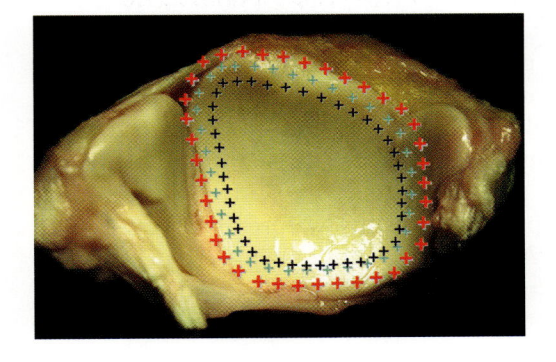

Fig. 4.13. Distribution of force transmission at tibial plafond.
Force transmission at the distal tibia occurs mainly eccentrically through the cortical rim, and there is almost no force transmission through the center of distal tibia

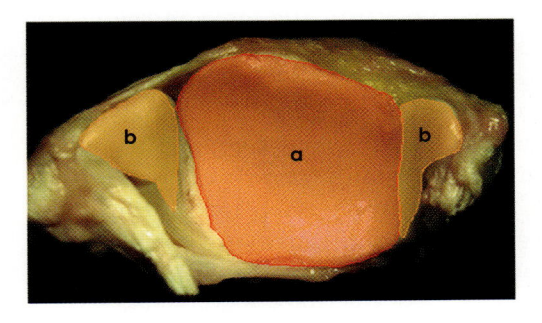

Fig. 4.14. Contact area at the ankle mortise.
A normal ankle has a surface contact area of approximately 12 cm², of which the tibiotalar contact area (**a**) accounts for approximately 7 cm², and the mediolateral contact areas (**b**) account for approximately 5 cm² (see text)

Recent studies (H. Trouillier, personal communication 2003) show that more than 90% of force transmission occurs within the cortical shell of the distal tibia (Fig. 4.13). Ideally, then, the tibial component should be anatomically sized, fully cover the tibial plafond, not weaken the cortical rim, and have a wide support on the cortical rim of the distal tibia.

Conserving as much bone as possible at the time of surgery not only helps to ensure better support but also saves bone, which may be valuable should revision become necessary. Total joint arthroplasties of the hip and knee have clearly demonstrated the fundamental importance of proper bone support, which is crucial for the long-term success of any arthroplasty. The reason for many failures was the excessive bone removal necessary for the insertion of a bulky prosthesis. Revision surgery after the removal of such implants was complicated by the very large amount of bone loss at the time of initial surgery. Fortunately, after a failed total knee or hip arthroplasty, it is often possible to revise the arthroplasty with long-stem implants, which makes it possible to bypass of the area of bone loss. In the ankle, however, a long-stem prosthesis is not an option for revision, particularly not on the talar side.

4.4 Contact Area and Forces at the Ankle

4.4.1 Contact Area

The complex geometry of the mortise and trochlea of the talus influences load characteristics [11, 6, 43, 44, 67]. Reports of whole ankle contact area vary from 1.5 cm^2 to 9.4 cm^2, depending on load and ankle position [73]. The tibiotalar area, however, accounts for only approximately 7 cm^2 [65] (Fig. 4.14). Controversies exist about changes in the contact area as a function of flexion position [6, 11, 44], which may be attributed to differences in load, position, and measurement technique [35]. Calhoun et al [11] found that contact surface area increased from plantar flexion to dorsiflexion, and that force per unit area decreased proportionately. They also observed that the medial and lateral facets had greatest contact with the malleoli in dorsiflexion. In another study, using a dynamic model, progressive lateral loading with concomitant medial unloading was observed during dorsiflexion and associated external rotation [49]. Further, for load-bearing human joints, it has been widely shown that a sufficiently sized area of congruent contact is the most desirable interface condition when using a deformable surface (for example, polyethylene) against metal [8, 45].

All of these findings implicate the need to achieve a physiological amount of joint contact area in total ankle replacement, with an appropriately aligned and properly balanced hindfoot.

4.4.2 Axial Load and Stress Forces of the Ankle

A vertical load on the ankle of 5.2 times body weight was found during gait [65]. In diseased ankles, the joint load decreased to approximately three times body weight; and the same values were noted in replaced ankles [65]. Anteroposterior and lateral shear forces during gait were estimated to reach levels of two and three times body weight, respectively. The vertical load that is transmitted to the trabecular bone at the prosthesis-bone interface may exceed the inherent trabecular bone strength in normal daily activities. With an interface area of 7 cm^2, the average compressive load per unit area at the interface during gait would be approximately 3.5 MPa in a patient of 700 N body weight. More strenuous physical activity could result in a much higher unit load, provoking a collapse of the cancellous bone surface of the tibia. By bone remodeling, the inherent strength of the bone is increased, however, it is estimated that bone strength must be at least three times higher than the aforementioned values to meet the requirements of daily physical activities if collapse is to be prevented.

Ground reaction, gravitational, ligament, and muscle forces produce a mixture of three-dimensional compressive, shear, and torsional loads in the ankle joint. Therefore, one may easily assume that force may not necessarily be directly perpendicular to the bone-implant interface, but more angular. This introduces shear forces in addition to those of direct compression. Furthermore, force vectors on a prosthesis are not necessarily central; instead, the point of application of many force vectors is often eccentric. Applied, this might show that when an eccentric force is placed on the medial side of the tibial prosthesis, there will be a downward force vector on the medial side, and a corresponding lift-off or compressive neutralizing force on the lateral side. This same phenomenon can also occur in the anteroposterior direction. The repeated contralateral force equalization might lead to microinstability and micromotion as well as loosening. Such micromotion can prevent bony ingrowth in a cementless prosthesis, especially in the early integration stage. It is believed that micromotion in excess of 0.15 mm will prevent bony ingrowth into a prosthetic implant [72]. Even after bony ingrowth has occurred, such continuous tilting stress may provoke failure of the bone-implant interface and consequent loosening of the implant, or contiguous constraint at the implant-polyethylene interface and consequent polyethylene wear. Implant design and hindfoot alignment must, therefore, accommodate the joint forces that are encountered during daily activities, especially walking and stair climbing.

Generally, the bigger the ankle prosthesis, the bigger the potential joint lever arms and moments and, thus, shear forces at the bone-implant interface, as created, for instance, by inversion/eversion torques (Fig. 4.15). Theoretically, the ideal ankle prosthesis should be small (necessitating minimal bone resection), as anatomic as possible (in order to mimic physiological joint motion and guarantee for proper ligament balancing), and consist of three components (to allow for unconstrained motion) [70]. The importance of using anatomically shaped components in total ankle arthroplasty, thereby avoiding excessive contact stress on the supporting bone, has been stated by Kempson et al [31] in an *in vivo* study. They found that after total ankle arthroplasty, ankle fractures occurred with 30% less force when a twisting motion was also applied.

The contact stress at the bone-implant interface also depends on contact area size: the bigger the contact area, the smaller the mean contact stress. With increased contact area, however, peak stresses can increase by eccentric loading (that is, edge loading) of the prosthesis, which contributes to prosthetic loosening. Based on the experience and personal opinion of the author, in order to minimize counterproductive joint contact stress, the ideal ankle prosthesis should have a large contact area between the contact surfaces, the point of load application should fall within the central third of the components, the ankle should be well aligned, and the ligaments should be well balanced.

4.5 Fixation of Total Ankle Prostheses

All current ankle arthroplasty designs rely on bone ingrowth for qualitative osseointegration and

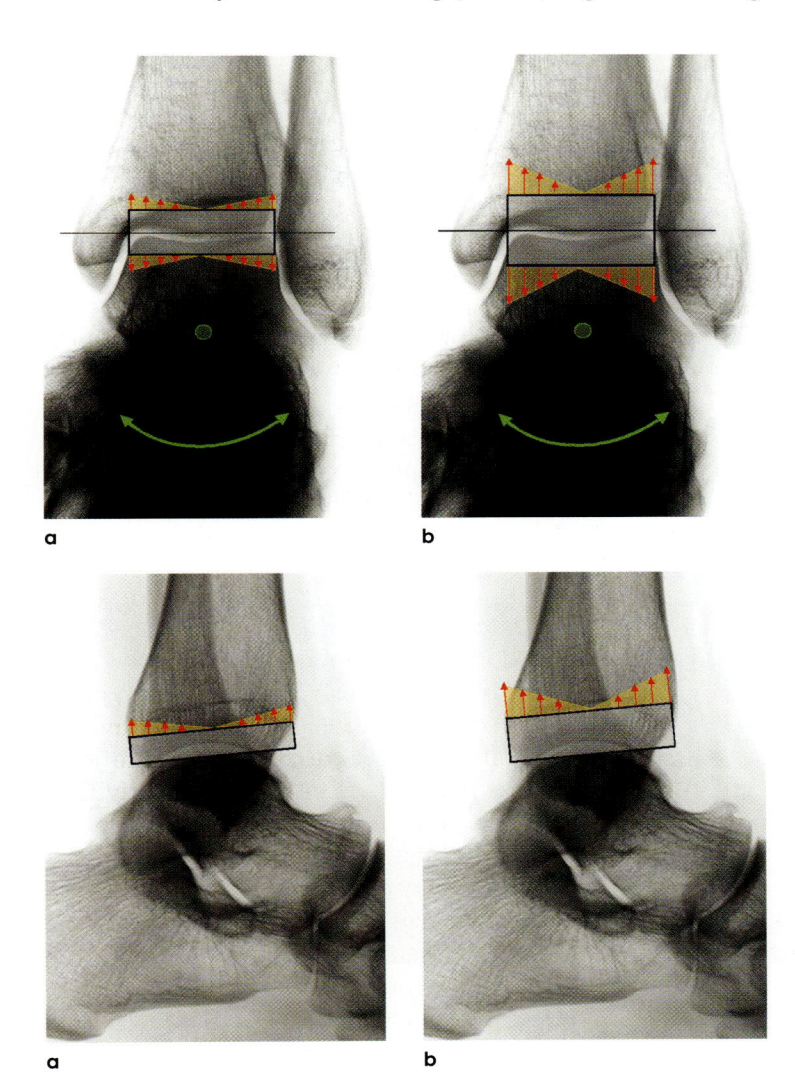

Fig. 4.15. Prosthetic thickness and shear forces at bone-implant interface.
These pictures show the influence of prosthetic size on created shear forces at the tibial bone-implant interface: (**a**) small prosthesis; (**b**) large prosthesis

implant stability. There are several major advantages to bone ingrowth (otherwise known as cementless implantation):
- Less bone resection is required because no space is required for fixation between the bone and the implant.
- The inserted prosthesis can be kept smaller than it would be with the additional cement mantle; and the smaller the prosthesis, the smaller the moments created at the bone-implant interface.
- Inadvertent cement displacement or intra-articular spillage (which could likely cause accelerated third-body wear) is avoided.
- Bone ingrowth approaches eliminate the damage to local delicate soft tissues that results from high levels of heat released by the exothermic process of curing acrylic cement.

Today, cementless or ingrowth prostheses incorporate a porous surface at the bone interface, a calcium hydroxyapatite coating, or a combination of both. This "biologic fixation" of an implant achieves the same strength as bone cement fixation by the fourth to 12th week [12], and there is additional ingrowth or remodeling of the bone area for periods of up to 24 months (Fig. 4.16). Shear forces in the anteroposterior and lateral directions should be avoided during the time of bone ingrowth and remodeling. Unsuccessful bone ingrowth results in fibrous ingrowth, which may increase the propensity of the components to migrate. Hydroxyapatite coating encourages molecular bonding between the crystals of the calcium hydroxyapatite and the bone bed. The time required for this bonding process appears to be shorter than that required for ingrowth into the sole porotic surface. In time, however, the hydroxyapatite coating is completely resorbed, leaving concerns regarding the long-term fixation of the components. Perhaps the most attractive current approach is the combined use of a porous surface with hydroxyapatite. Theoretically, this strategy allows for early fixation of the implant through hydroxyapatite bonding, followed later by secure ingrowth of bone within the porous, three-dimensional interstices.

Excessive force applied to the bone-implant interface is detrimental to the long-term stability of a prosthetic implant. Force is always measured per unit area. In fact, surface area represents a fundamental variable of the forces acting at the ankle. If a prosthesis is undersized, it is prone to subsidence in the remaining soft cancellous bone (see Fig. 4.13). Not only is the strongest bone removed at the time of the surgery, but the remaining bone surface often is not fully utilized for support. By expanding the prosthesis to encompass all available bone, the load is diminished per unit area.

The understructure of a prosthetic baseplate is important in resisting micromotion and shear, rotatory, and eccentric forces. Volz et al [72] studied tibial baseplate micromotion in the laboratory using four tibial baseplates of different designs. They implanted the baseplates into paired cadaveric tibias, subjected them to eccentric loads, and measured the resulting micromotion. They found that

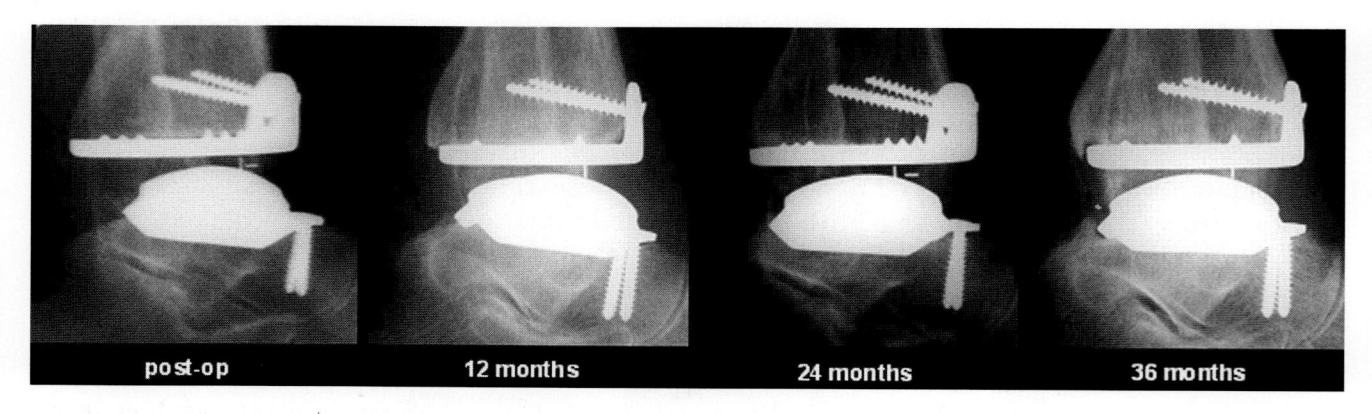

Fig. 4.16. Ingrowth and remodeling at the bone-implant interface.
At the distal tibia, the postoperative periprosthetic radiolucent line (see also Chap. 11: Complications of Total Ankle Arthroplasty) disappears and ingrowth and bone remodeling continue for up to 24 months

four peripherally placed screws with a central peg best resisted micromotion. Similar results were reported by others [18]. Many of today's prosthetic designs for total knee arthroplasties have a keel on the undersurface of the tibial baseplate. In the ankle, however, because of the anatomy and vascularization of the talus, the use of a keel is difficult, if not impossible, particularly on talar side. The problem with using a stem in the distal tibia is the need to make a window for its insertion. The creation of such a window may provoke a substantial weakening of the anterior tibial cortical architecture, thereby reducing its suitability to become the main support of the prosthetic tibial baseplate.

Finally, as reported previously, it is not only forces that are often eccentric, but also the strength of the bone support. The strongest bone is likely posteromedial in the distal tibia (see Fig. 4.12) [28]. This area of stiffer bone could act as a pivot point, with the risk of overloading the surrounding weaker anterolateral bone. A somewhat anterolaterally placed component could potentially aggravate this problem and increase the potential for failure.

4.6 Limitations of Polyethylene

The physical properties of polyethylene used for the mobile insert can vary according to the specific type of polyethylene used and because of a number of other variables. The contact stresses on five different total knee designs peaked between 20 MPa and 80 MPa [76]. By rounding or dishing the polyethylene tray, the peak contact stress was reduced from 55 MPa for a round-on-flat design, to 18 MPa for a design in which the polyethylene was more conforming [18]. Increasing the conformity reduces the peak contact stress on the polyethylene, but it also increases stresses that are transferred to the bone-prosthesis interface, and this can contribute to loosening. The durability of polyethylene is improved with increasing thickness [2, 3, 4]. While a minimum thickness of 4 mm to 6 mm is estimated to be needed for the hip, and 6 mm to 8 mm for the knee, minimum thickness standards for the ankle have not been determined at this time. Theoretically, thicker polyethylene components in the ankle may help to prevent polyethylene failures, but at the expense of increasing the lever arms of forces acting at the bone-implant interface, and of more generous bone cuts. The fundamental importance of bone conservation in the ankle, however, has been widely recognized, since the bone may be weak and the surface areas for support small [28]. Polyethylene requirements for the ankle are, therefore, contradictory to what is necessary for conserving bone strength.

There are also several potential risks related to polyethylene wear that may lead to a weakening and failure of the implanted total ankle arthroplasty. Problematic scenarios include:
— when the polyethylene does not fully conform in shape (congruency) with the metal tibial and talar components,
— when the polyethylene component extends past the surface of the metallic components,
— when there is an inappropriate capture mechanism on the tibial or talar component to guide the polyethylene component,
— when the ankle prosthesis has been implanted without being properly aligned and with a deficit in appropriate ligament balancing.

4.7 Component Design

There has been a relative paucity of basic scientific laboratory investigation of total ankle arthroplasty, and very little investigation into design criteria. In one of the few laboratory investigations of total ankle arthroplasty design, Falsig et al [19] evaluated stress transfer to the distal tibial trabecular bone for three different generic distal tibial prostheses: a polyethylene tibial component, a metal-backed polyethylene tibial component, and a long-stem metal-backed tibial component. An eccentric anterolateral load of 2'100 N (approximately three times body weight) was applied to the three prostheses. The addition of a metal backing reduced compressive stresses in the trabecular bone by 25%, from 20 N/mm^2 for an all-polyethylene tibial component to 15 N/mm^2 for a metal-backed component [19]. Shear stresses were also reduced. The long-stem implant resulted in an almost complete reduction of compressive stresses in the metaphysial trabecular bone because the

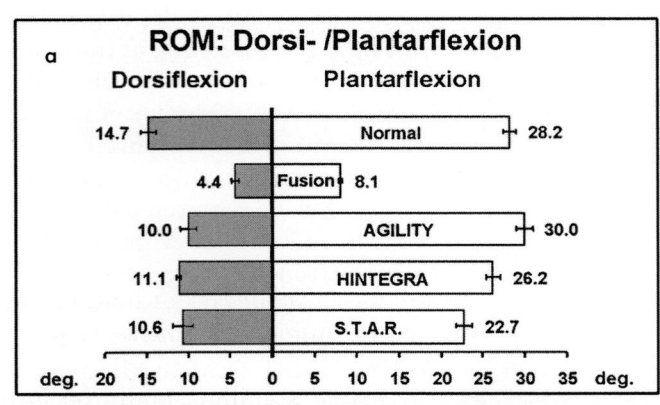

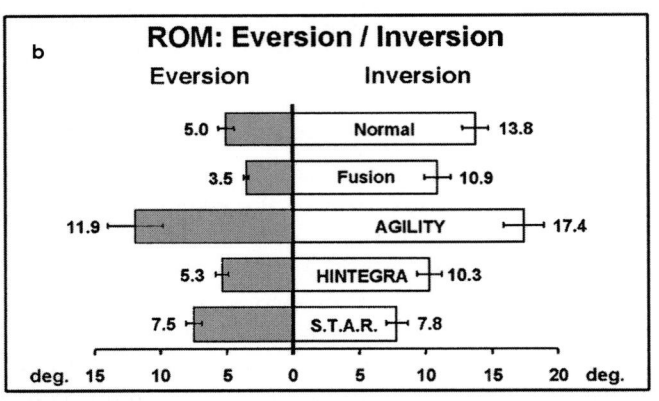

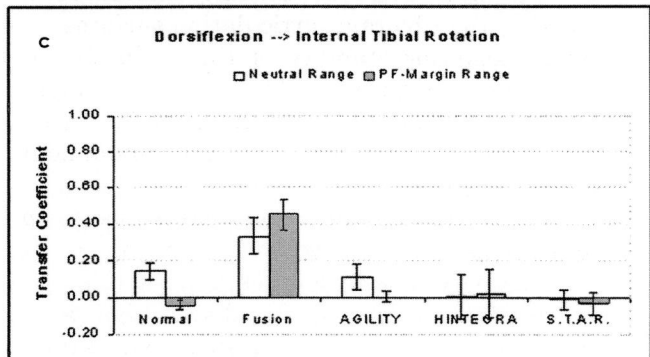

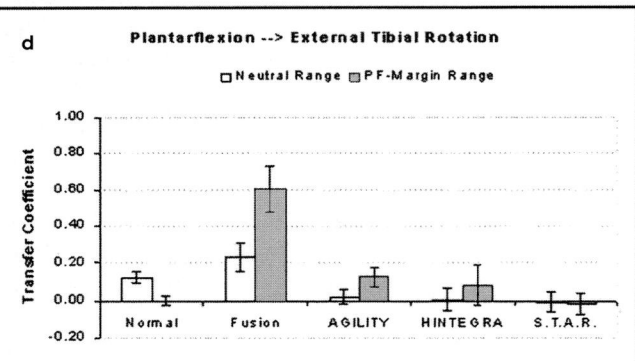

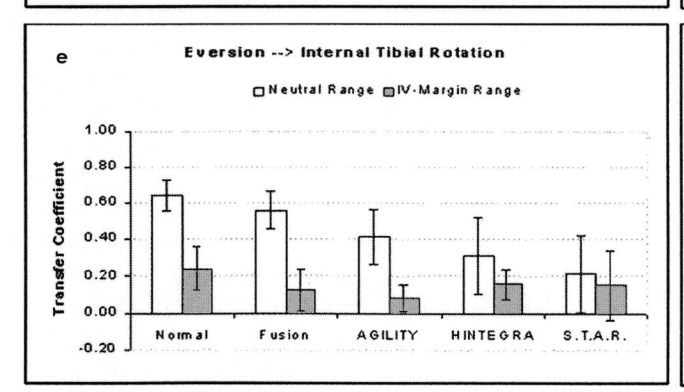

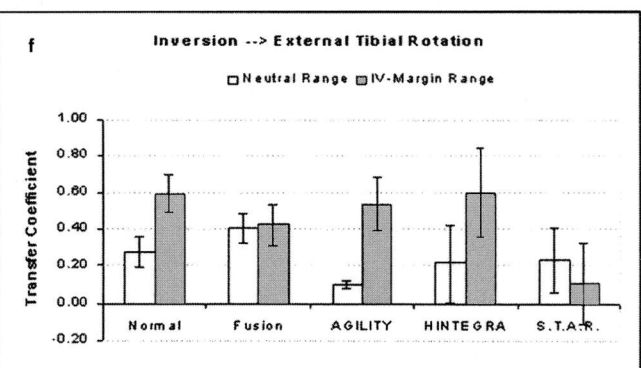

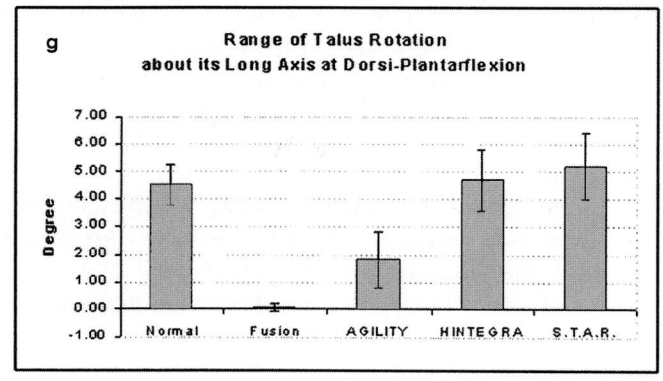

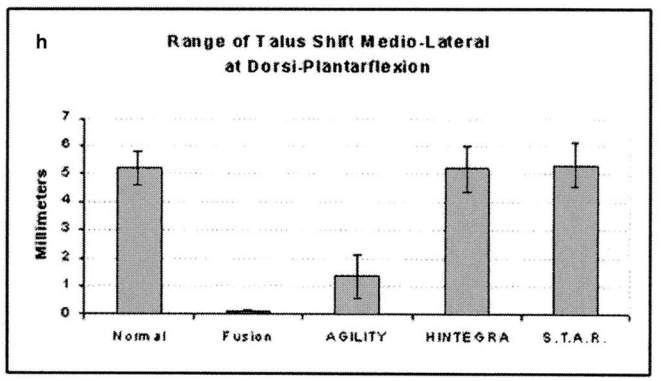

Chapter 4: Anatomic and Biomechanical Characteristics

a ROM: Dorsi- /Plantarflexion

	Dorsiflexion	Plantarflexion
Normal	14.7	28.2
Fusion	4.4	8.1
AGILITY	10.0	30.0
HINTEGRA	11.1	26.2
S.T.A.R.	10.6	22.7

b ROM: Eversion / Inversion

	Eversion	Inversion
Normal	5.0	13.8
Fusion	3.5	10.9
AGILITY	11.9	17.4
HINTEGRA	5.3	10.3
S.T.A.R.	7.5	7.8

c Dorsiflexion → Internal Tibial Rotation (Neutral Range, PF-Margin Range)

d Plantarflexion → External Tibial Rotation (Neutral Range, PF-Margin Range)

e Eversion → Internal Tibial Rotation (Neutral Range, IV-Margin Range)

f Inversion → External Tibial Rotation (Neutral Range, IV-Margin Range)

g Range of Talus Rotation about its Long Axis at Dorsi-Plantarflexion

h Range of Talus Shift Medio-Lateral at Dorsi-Plantarflexion

Fig. 4.17. Kinematic changes after fusion and total replacement of the ankle.
The first two graphs show the range of motion for the movement (**a**) dorsiflexion/plantar flexion, and (**b**) eversion/inversion (mean values with the plotted standard errors). Graphs **c**, **d**, **e** and **f** show the movement transfer between the foot and lower leg, as calculated by the transfer coefficient (that is, the ratio of output and input movement) in two areas of the movement pathway: neutral range (the area around neutral), and margin range (the area of greatest input). Graph **g** shows talar rotation about its anteroposterior axis during the maximal range of dorsiflexion/plantar flexion. Graph **h** shows lateral talar shift during the maximal range of dorsiflexion/plantar flexion. Shown are mean values with standard errors. ROM: range of motion.
(From Valderrabano V, Hintermann B, Nigg BM, Stefanyshyn D, Stergiou P (2003) Kinematic changes after fusion and total replacement of the ankle, part 2: movement transfer. Foot Ankle Int 24: 888–896; with permission)

stresses were transferred to the long stem, by-passing the distal tibia [19].

Recently, Valderrabano et al [69, 71] investigated, *in vitro*, the range of motion, movement transfer, and talar movement in the normal ankle, the fused ankle, and the replaced ankle (with three different ankle prostheses: S.T.A.R., HINTEGRA®, and AGILITY™). Motion at the ankle joint complex was restricted less by each of the three ankle prostheses than by ankle fusion [69]. The prostheses also changed the movement transfer within the ankle joint complex less than ankle fusion, especially during dorsiflexion/plantar flexion of the foot (Fig. 4.17) [70]. The two-component ankle (AGILITY™) restricted talar motion within the ankle mortise, whereas (except for medial motion) the three-component ankles (HINTEGRA® and S.T.A.R.) seemed to allow talar motion comparable to that in the normal ankle. Such a restriction of talar motion is suggested to result in an increase of stress forces within and around the prosthesis, which may ultimately lead to polyethylene wear and potential loosening at the bone-implant interfaces. The authors therefore concluded that the kinematics of the replaced ankle are closer to those of the normal ankle than is the case for the fused ankle. A successful design for total ankle arthroplasty should be shaped as anatomically as possible, and provide a physiological range of motion at the ankle joint, full transmission of movement transfer between foot and lower leg, and unconstrained talar motion within the ankle mortise.

4.8 Conclusions

The following are the main conclusions obtained from the literature for successful total ankle replacement.

- A total ankle prosthesis should be as anatomic as possible in order to mimic the unique requirements of the ankle.
- Eversion and inversion stability should be provided by the tibiotalar articulating surfaces.
- Anteroposterior stability of the replaced ankle joint should be provided by tibiotalar ligaments. Proper ligament balancing should be achieved by precise implantation technique and anatomic surfaces.
- Bone resection should be minimal to ensure optimal support and to save bone, which is valuable should revision become necessary.
- Force transmission of the distal tibia mainly occurs through its cortical shell. The anterior cortical shell should, therefore, not be weakened, and the whole tibial size should be used for cortical bony support of the tibial component to prevent component subsidence while weight-bearing.
- To minimize contact stress and to avoid edge loading, the ankle prosthesis should have a large contact area between the surfaces, the point of load application should fall within the central third of the components, the ankle should be well aligned, and the ligaments should be well balanced.
- To decrease the potential risks for polyethylene wear, the polyethylene should be perfectly congruent with the metal tibial and talar components, it should include an effective capture mechanism on the tibial or talar component to guide the polyethylene inlay, and it should not extend past the surface of the metallic components.

The success of ankle arthroplasty may depend on how successfully prosthetic designs can mimic the normal kinematics and kinetics of the ankle joint (Table 4.1). Several studies have shown that total ankle arthroplasty is closer to the normal ankle than is ankle arthrodesis in terms of range of motion,

Table 4.1. Goals for the design of a total ankle arthroplasty*

Goal 1	Minimize bone removal on both sides of the joint.
Goal 2	Maximize the surface area for support of the prosthesis.
Goal 3	Maximize the surface area for stabilization of the prosthesis, but without excessive bone loss and without an excessive bone stem.
Goal 4	If polyethylene is used, allow sufficient thickness of polyethylene as well as a conforming geometry.
Goal 5	Establish the proper balance between constraint and freedom.
Goal 6	Use a bearing surface that minimizes wear.
Goal 7	Use a firm, expanded surface-area locking mechanism for ankles that use a fixed, nonmobile polyethylene.
Goal 8	Improve instrumentation to help ensure proper alignment to minimize shear and eccentric forces.

* Adapted from Gill LH (2002) Principles of joint arthroplasty as applied to the ankle. AAOS Instruct. Course Lect, Vol. 51, pp 117–128 [20]

movement transfer between the foot and lower leg, and talus movement within the ankle mortise. The closer total ankle arthroplasty design is to the bony anatomy of the normal ankle, and the more compact the components within the prosthetic system, the closer the kinematics were shown to be replicated with respect to normal joints. Nevertheless, further biomechanical research is necessary in the field.

References

[1] Barnett CH, Napier JR (1952) The axis of rotation at the ankle joint in man. Its influence upon the form of the talus and mobility of the fibula. J Anatomy 86: 1–9
[2] Bartel DL, Bicknell VL, Wright TM (1986) The effect of conformity, thickness, and material on stresses in ultra-high molecular weight components for total joint replacement. J Bone Joint Surg Am 68: 1041–1051
[3] Bartel DL, Burstein AH, Toda MD, Edwards DL (1985) The effect of conformity and plastic thickness on contact stresses in metal-backed plastic implants. J Biomech Eng 107: 193–199
[4] Bartel DL, Rawlinson JJ, Burstein AH, Ranawat CS, Flynn WF, Jr. (1995) Stresses in polyethylene components of contemporary total knee replacements. Clin Orthop 317: 76–82
[5] Baumhauer JF, Alosa DM, Renstroem PA, Trevino S, Beynnon B (1995) A prospective study of ankle injury risk factors. Am J Sports Med 23: 564–570
[6] Beaudoin AJ, Fiore WR, Krause WR (1991) Effect of isolated talocalcaneal fusion on contact in the ankle and talonavicular joints. Foot Ankle 12: 19–25
[7] Boss AP, Hintermann B (2002) Anatomical study of the medial ankle ligament complex. Foot Ankle Int 23: 547–553
[8] Buechel FF, Pappas MJ, Iorio LJ (1988) New Jersey low contact stress total ankle replacement: biomechanical rationale and review of 23 cementless cases. Foot Ankle 8: 279–290
[9] Burge PD, Evans M (1986) Effect of surface replacement arthroplasty on stability of the ankle. Foot Ankle 7: 10–17
[10] Calderale PM, Garro A, Barbiero R, Fasolio G, Pipino F (1983) Biomechanical design of the total ankle prosthesis. Eng Med 12: 69–80
[11] Calhoun JH, Li F, Ledbetter BR, Viegas SF (1994) A comprehensive study of pressure distribution in the ankle joint with inversion and eversion. Foot Ankle Int 15: 125–133
[12] Cameron HU, Pilliar RM, Macnab I (1976) The rate of bone ingrowth into porous metal. J Biomed Mater Res 10: 295–302
[13] Cass J, Morrey EY, Chao EY (1984) Three-dimensional kinematics of ankle instability following serial sectioning of lateral collateral ligaments. Foot Ankle 5: 142–149
[14] Cass JR, Settles H (1994) Ankle instability: in vitro kinematics in response to axial load. Foot Ankle Int 15: 134–140
[15] Close JR (1956) Some applications of the functional anatomy of the ankle joint. J Bone Joint Surg Am 38: 761–781
[16] Colville MR, Marder RA, Boyle JJ, Zarins B (1990) Strain measurement in lateral ankle ligaments. Am J Sports Med 18: 196–200
[17] Deland JT, Morris GD, Sung IH (2000) Biomechanics of the ankle joint. A perspective on total ankle replacement. Foot Ankle Clin 5: 747–759
[18] Ewald FC, Walker PS (1988) The current status of total knee replacement. Rheum Dis Clin North Am 14: 579–590
[19] Falsig J, Hvid I, Jensen N (1986) Finite element stress analysis of some ankle joint prostheses. Clin Biomech 1: 71–76
[20] Gill LH (2002) Principles of joint arthroplasty as applied to the ankle. AAOS Instructional Course Lect, chap 13, pp 117–128
[21] Grath G (1960) Widening of the ankle mortise. A clinical and experimental study. Acta Orthop Scand 263 (Suppl): 1–88
[22] Harper MC (1987) Deltoid ligament: an anatomical evaluation of function. Foot Ankle 8: 19–22
[23] Hicks JH (1953) The mechanics of the foot. 1. The joints. J Anatomy 87: 345–357
[24] Hintermann B, Nigg BM (1995) In vitro kinematics of the loaded ankle/foot complex in response to dorsi-/plantar flexion. Foot Ankle Int 16: 514–518
[25] Hintermann B, Nigg BM, Sommer C, Cole GK (1994) Transfer of movement between calcaneus and tibia in vitro. Clin Biomech 9: 349–355
[26] Hintermann B, Sommer C, Nigg BM (1995) The influence of ligament transection on tibial and calcaneal rotation with loading and dorsi-/plantar flexion. Foot Ankle Int 9: 567–571

References

[27] Hollis JM, Blasier RD, Flahiff CM (1995) Simulated lateral ankle ligamentous injury. Change in ankle stability. Am J Sports Med 23: 672–677

[28] Hvid I, Rasmussen O, Jensen NC, Nielsen S (1985) Trabecular bone strength profiles at the ankle joint. Clin Orthop 199: 306–312

[29] Inman VT (1991) The joints of the ankle, 2nd ed. Williams & Wilkins, Baltimore, pp 31–74

[30] Johnson EE, Markolf KL (1983) The contribution of the anterior talofibular ligament to the ankle laxity. J Bone Joint Surg Am 65: 81–88

[31] Kempson GE, Freeman MA, Tuk MA (1975) Engineering considerations in the design of an ankle joint. Biomed Eng 10: 166–180

[32] Knupp M, Magerkurth O, Ledermann HP, Hintermann B: The surgical tibiotalar angle – a radiological study. Foot Ankle Int (submitted)

[33] Leardini A (2001) Geometry and mechanics of the human ankle complex and ankle prosthesis design. Clin Biomech 16: 706–709

[34] Leardini A, O'Connor JJ, Catani F, Giannini S (1999) A geometric model of the human ankle joint. J Biomech 32: 585–591

[35] Leardini A, O'Connor JJ, Catani F, Giannini S (2000) The role of the passive structures in the mobility and stability of the human ankle joint: a literature review. Foot Ankle Int 21: 602–615

[36] Levens AS, Berkeley CE, Inman VT, Blosser JA (1948) Transverse rotation of the segments of the lower extremity in locomotion. J Bone Joint Surg Am 30: 859–872

[37] Lewis G (1994) The ankle joint prosthetic replacement: clinical performance and research challenges. Foot Ankle Int 15: 471–476

[38] Lindsjo U, Danckwardt-Lilliestrom G, Sahlstedt B (1985) Measurement of the motion range in the loaded ankle. Clin Orthop 199: 68–71

[39] Locke M, Perry J, Campbell J (1984) Ankle and subtalar motion during gait in arthritic patients. Phys Ther 64: 504–509

[40] Lowery RB (1995) Fractures of the talus and os calcis. Opin Orthop 6: 25–34

[41] Lundberg A (1989) Kinematics of the ankle and foot. *In vitro* stereophotogrammetry. Acta Orthop Scand 60 (Suppl 233): 1–24

[42] Lundberg A, Goldie I, Kalin B, Selvik G (1989) Kinematics of the ankle/foot complex, part 1: Plantar flexion and dorsiflexion. Foot Ankle 9: 194–200

[43] Lundberg A, Svensson OK, Nemeth G, Selvik G (1989) The axis of rotation of the ankle joint. J Bone Joint Surg Br 71: 94–99

[44] Macko VW, Matthews LS, Zwirkoski P (1991) The joint-contact area of the ankle. J Bone Joint Surg Br 73: 347–351

[45] Markolf KL, Barger WL, Shoemaker SC, Amstutz HC (1981) The role of joint load in knee stability. J Bone Joint Surg Am 63: 570–585

[46] McCullough CJ, Burge PD (1980) Rotatory stability of the load-bearing ankle. An experimental study. J Bone Joint Surg Br 62: 460–464

[47] Michelson JD, Clarke HJ, Jinnah RH (1990) The effect of loading on tibiotalar alignment in cadaver ankles. Foot Ankle 10: 280–284

[48] Michelson JD, Hamel AJ, Buczek FL, Sharkey NA (2002) Kinematic behavior of the ankle following malleolar fracture repair in a high-fidelity cadaver model. J Bone Joint Surg Am 84: 2029–2038

[49] Michelson JD, Helgemo SLJ (1995) Kinematics of the axially loaded ankle. Foot Ankle Int 16: 577–582

[50] Michelson JD, Schmidt GR, Mizel MS (2000) Kinematics of a total arthroplasty of the ankle: comparison to normal ankle motion. Foot Ankle Int 21: 278–284

[51] Milner CE, Soames RW (1998) Anatomy of the collateral ligaments of the human ankle joint. Foot Ankle Int 19: 757–760

[52] Milner CE, Soames RW (1998) The medial collateral ligaments of the human ankle joint: anatomical variations. Foot Ankle Int 19: 289–292

[53] Murray MP, Drought AB, Kory RC (1964) Walking patterns of normal men. J Bone Joint Surg Am 46: 335–349

[54] Rasmussen O, Kroman-Andersen C, Boe S (1983) Deltoid ligament: functional analysis of the medial collateral ligamentous apparatus of the ankle joint. Acta Orthop Scand 54: 36–44

[55] Rasmussen O, Tovberg-Jensen I (1982) Mobility of the ankle joint: recording of rotatory movements in the talocrural joint *in vitro* with and without the lateral collateral ligaments of the ankle. Acta Orthop Scand 53: 155–160

[56] Renstrom P, Wertz M, Incavo S, Pope M, Ostgaard HC, Arms S, Haugh L (1988) Strain in the lateral ligaments of the ankle. Foot Ankle 9: 59–63

[57] Roaas A, Andersson GB (1982) Normal range of motion of the hip, knee and ankle joints in male subjects, 30–40 years of age. Acta Orthop Scand 53: 205–208

[58] Sammarco GJ, Burstein AH, Frankel VH (1973) Biomechanics of the ankle: a kinematic study. Ortho Clin North Am 4: 75–96

[59] Sammarco J (1977) Biomechanics of the ankle: surface velocity and instant center of rotation in the sagittal plane. Am J Sports Med 5: 231–234

[60] Sands A, Early J, Sidles J, Sangeorzan BJ (1995) Uniaxial description of hindfoot angular motion before and after calcaneocuboid fusion. Orthop Trans 19: 936–937

[61] Sangeorzan BJ, Sidles J (1995) Hinge-like motion of the ankle and subtalar articulations. Orthop Trans 19: 331–332

[62] Sarrafian SK (1994) Anatomy of foot and ankle, 2nd ed. Lippincott, Philadelphia, pp 239–240

[63] Siegler S, Chen J, Schneck CD (1988) The three-dimensional kinematics and flexibility characteristics of the human ankle and subtalar joint. J Biomech Eng 110: 364–373

[64] Sommer C, Hintermann B, Nigg BM, Bogert van den AJ (1996) Influence of ankle ligaments on tibial rotation: an *in vitro* study. Foot Ankle Int 17: 79–84

[65] Stauffer RN, Chao EY, Brewster RC (1977) Force and motion analysis of the normal, diseased, and prosthetic ankle joint. Clin Orthop 127: 189–196

[66] Stormont DM, Morrey BF, An KN, Cass JR (1985) Stability of the loaded ankle. Am J Sports Med 13: 295–300
[67] Tarr RR, Resnick CT, Wagner KS (1985) Changes in tibiotalar joint contact areas following experimentally induced tibial angular deformities. Clin Orthop 199: 72–80
[68] Valderrabano V, Hintermann B, Dick W (2004) Scandinavian total ankle replacement: a 3.7-year average follow-up of 65 patients. Clin Orthop 424: 47–56
[69] Valderrabano V, Hintermann B, Nigg BM, Stefanyshyn D, Stergiou P (2003) Kinematic changes after fusion and total replacement of the ankle, part 1: range of motion. Foot Ankle Int 24: 881–887
[70] Valderrabano V, Hintermann B, Nigg BM, Stefanyshyn D, Stergiou P (2003) Kinematic changes after fusion and total replacement of the ankle, part 2: movement transfer. Foot Ankle Int 24: 888–896
[71] Valderrabano V, Hintermann B, Nigg BM, Stefanyshyn D, Stergiou P (2003) Kinematic changes after fusion and total replacement of the ankle, part 3: talar movement. Foot Ankle Int 24: 897–900
[72] Volz RG, Nisbet JK, Lee RW, McMurtry MG (1988) The mechanical stability of various noncemented tibial components. Clin Orthop 226: 38–42
[73] Ward KA, Soames RW (1997) Contact patterns at the tarsal joints. Clin Biomech 12: 496–501
[74] Weseley MS, Koval R, Kleiger B (1969) Roentgen measurement of ankle flexion-extension motion. Clin Orthop 65: 167–174
[75] Wright DG, Desai SM, Henderson WH (1964) Action of the subtalar and ankle-joint complex during the stance phase of walking. J Bone Joint Surg Am 46: 361–382
[76] Wright TM, Bartel DL (1968) The problem of surface damage in polyethylene total knee components. Clin Orthop 205: 67–74

Chapter 5

HISTORY OF TOTAL ANKLE ARTHROPLASTY

The search for a workable ankle design has taken many different approaches. Early results with total ankle replacement were disappointing, and had no more satisfactory outcomes than did ankle arthrodeses. Durable fixation of components was a major concern in each of the total ankle designs introduced in the 1970s and 80s, and this brought the method as such into disrepute. Indeed, it was questioned whether the ankle joint could be replaced at all [45].

The past decade, however, has brought renewed interest in ankle replacement, and a few new designs appear to show promising results, not only in inflammatory arthritis but also in degenerative and post-traumatic osteoarthrosis [17, 50, 74, 96]. This renewed interest may derive partly from dissatisfaction with ankle arthrodesis, as well as from the success of total hip and knee arthroplasty [23, 81, 99].

Ankle replacement has taken longer to develop than hip and knee replacement, because of difficulties related to the:
– smaller size of the joint [80],
– higher resultant moment [79],
– high compressive force [95, 113],
– potential malalignment and instability [30, 99],
– soft-tissue contractures [37, 52],
– presence of end-stage arthritis in generally younger and more active patients [52],
– disregard for anatomic component shape and physiological ankle biomechanics [52].

5.1 Classification of Total Ankle Arthroplasties

As outlined in Table 5.1, total ankle arthroplasties can be classified according to the following six factors, which will be discussed in this chapter:
– fixation type,
– number of components,
– constraint type,
– congruency/conformity type,
– component shape,
– bearing type.

The main classification is fixation type: either cemented or uncemented. Most of the first-generation ankle designs were cemented, and resulted in high revision and failure rates. Based on this experience, modern designs normally use noncemented methods of fixation.

Many different approaches to total ankle arthroplasty have been tried in the past, and more than 25 different designs were developed during the 1970s and 80s (Table 5.2). All but two of these

Table 5.1. Classification of total ankle arthroplasty

Classification	Type	Specification
Fixation	Cemented Uncemented	
Number of components	Two components Three components	
Constraint	Constrained Semiconstrained Nonconstrained	
Congruency/conformity	Incongruent	Trochlear Bispherical Concave/convex Convex/convex
	Congruent	Spherical Spheroidal Cylindrical Sliding/cylindrical Conical
Component shape	Non-anatomic Anatomic	
Bearing	Fixed/incorporated Mobile	

early designs (New Jersey LCS [17], and S.T.A.R. [69, 73]) featured two components. Two-component designs can be classified as *constrained, semiconstrained,* and *nonconstrained*. Early constrained designs supplemented ligamentous ankle support [90], whereas the semiconstrained [2, 96] and nonconstrained designs required ligament stability but permitted increased axial rotation [17, 52, 53, 70]. Based on the shapes of the surfaces, two-component designs can also be categorized as *incongruent* (which includes trochlear, bispherical, concave/convex, and convex/convex types), and congruent (which includes spherical, spheroidal, conical, cylindrical, and sliding-cylindrical types) [8, 36, 94]. Spherical types allowed motion in all directions [19, 78], spheroidal or conical types allowed inversion and eversion [92, 128], and cylindrical and even more

Table 5.2. List of known ankle designs*

Name	Inventor	Type	Year	Design paper(s)	Clinical outcome paper(s)
Lord	Lord	UNCO	1970	83	84
Smith	Smith	UNCO	1972	63, 129	1, 26, 28, 33, 63, 64, 126
ICLH	Freeman et al	CONS	1972	62, 115	7, 9, 31, 34, 48, 49, 60
St. Georg	Buchholz et al	SEMI	1973	11, 32	26, 47, 60, 120
Newton	Newton	UNCO	1973	90	92
Link HD		SEMI	1974		
Schlein	Schlein	UNCO	1974		
CONAXIAL	Beck, Steffee	CONS	1974		135
Lennox		SEMI	1975		
Giannastras, Sammarco	Giannastras, Sammarco	CONS	1975		
IRVINE	Waugh	UNCO	1975	128	33
TPR	Thompson et al	SEMI	1976		25, 26, 57, 58, 60, 102, 105, 134
PCA	Scholz	CONS	1976	107	108
Mayo 1	Stauffer	CONS	1976	110, 113	78, 111, 112, 114, 121
OREGON	Groth, Fagan	CONS	1977	44	42
Balgrist	Schreiber, Zollinger, Dexel	CONS	1977	109	
New Jersey LCS	Buechel, Pappas	3COM	1978	94	12, 15, 16, 17
Demottaz	Demottaz	CONS	1979		27
Wang	Wang	CONS	1980		127
TNK	Takakura	CONS	1980	116	117
S.T.A.R. 1	Kofoed	SEMI	1981	69	70, 74
Pipino/Calderale	Pipino, Calderale	CONS	1983	18	
AGILITY™	Alvine	SEMI	1984	2	4, 96, 97, 100, 101
Bath-Wessex	Bath, Wessex	UNCO	1984	86	19, 21, 64, 126
Mayo 2	Keblish	SEMI	1989	61	66, 67
Buechel-Pappas™	Buechel, Pappas	3COM	1989		14, 16, 56, 82, 97, 133, 134
S.T.A.R. 2	Kofoed	3COM	1990	73	5, 24, 35, 38, 50, 55, 57, 72, 75, 76, 89, 93, 97, 104, 105, 122, 131, 132, 133, 134
ESKA	Rudigier	3COM	1990	98	98
AKILE	Chauveaux	3COM	1995	22	
Sammarco	Sammarco	3COM	1996		
FOURNOL		3COM	1997		
ALBATROS		3COM	1997		
SALTO®	Judet et al	3COM	1998	59	10
Ramses	Mendolia et al	3COM	1998	88	87
AES	Asencio et al	3COM	1998	6	
ALPHA-NORM	Tillmann	3COM	1999		
HINTEGRA®	Hintermann et al	3COM	2000	123, 124, 125	51, 53, 54

CONS = constrained; SEMI = semiconstrained; UNCO = unconstrained; 3COM = three components

* Adapted from Giannini S, Leardini A, O'Connor JJ (2000) Total ankle replacement: review of the designs and of the current status. Foot Ankle Surg 6: 77–88 [36] (with permission)

5.2 First-Generation Total Ankle Arthroplasty – Cemented Type

so conical types resembled the human ankle joint [11, 28, 94, 114, 117]. Noncongruent designs demonstrated early failures [13].

Modern total ankle arthroplasty implants have varied substantially from the early constrained, semiconstrained [2, 3, 96], nonconstrained [13, 16, 17, 53, 70, 74], and noncongruent designs described above [13]. The new implants feature congruent designs that tend to provide acceptable wear characteristics and good pressure distribution [52, 70]. Minimal resection of the talar dome and distal tibia are advocated to preserve strong metaphysial bone [17, 43, 52, 53, 73, 91, 117, 122].

There are two design philosophies concerning bearing type: fixed or incorporated bearings and mobile bearings. While fixed-bearing ankles have only one articulation between the tibial and talar components, mobile-bearing ankles are characterized by a moving polyethylene bearing that separates the convex talar component from the flat tibial component. This results in two separate articulation surfaces.

5.2 First-Generation Total Ankle Arthroplasty – Cemented Type

In the early days of total ankle arthroplasty, ankle prostheses were implanted with cement, reflecting the tendency of joint arthroplasty in general. Cement fixation produced poor results, however, and today the preference is to perform total ankle arthroplasty without cement.

5.2.1 Pioneers in Total Ankle Arthroplasty

The first total ankle arthroplasty was performed in 1970 by Lord and Marrott (Table 5.2) [83]. The tibial component of this prosthesis had a long stem (similar to a femoral prosthesis), coupled with a polyethylene talar component that replaced the body of the talus. Subtalar fusion was necessary at the time of this surgery. After 10 years, 12 of the 25 Lord arthroplasties had failed, and only seven results could be considered satisfactory [84]. The procedure was abandoned.

The St. Georg prosthesis was used in Sweden in 1973, but after the insertion of eight implants, the failure rate was so high that the procedure was also abandoned [11, 32]. The Imperial College of London Hospital (ICLH) implant was designed to prevent medial and lateral subluxation of the talar component by the presence of a 3-mm elevation to the medial and lateral walls of the tibial component (Fig. 5.1) [3, 62]. The implant was plagued by clearance problems between the malleoli and the talus, and this, despite many revisions, continued to be a source of pain in many patients [9, 31, 34, 49, 60, 102]. While most early ankle designs were of the congruous type, the Newton ankle prosthesis had an incongruous surface [90]. This resulted in very high polyethylene wear and the subsequent discontinuation of the implant [92].

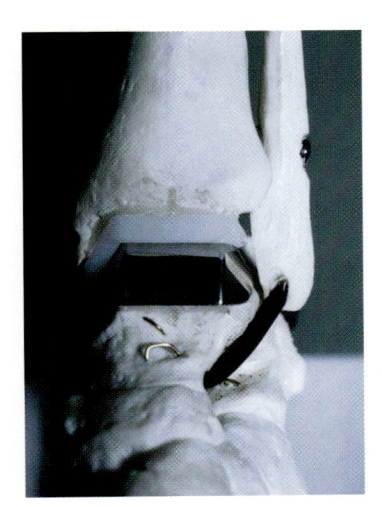

Fig. 5.1. The ICLH (Imperial College of London Hospital) total ankle.
The ICLH total ankle included a 3-mm elevation to the medial and lateral walls of the tibial component *(Courtesy of Dr. A. Cracchiolo, Los Angeles, CA, USA)*

Table 5.3. Satisfaction, loosening, and revision rates after total ankle replacements [a]

Author(s)	Prosthesis	Period of Study	Year of Publication	No. of Ankles	Diagnosis SA [%]	PA [%]	OA [%]	Average Follow-up [mo]	Satisfaction Rate [%]	Loosening Rate [%]	Revision Rate [%]
Stauffer [112, 114]	Mayo	1974–1977	1979	102	42	0	58	23	73	5	26
Dini and Bassett [28]	Smith	1974–1977	1980	21	14	0	76	27	46	14	†
Lord and Marrotte [84]	Lord	1970–1971	1980	25	†	†	†	60	28	48	†
Goldie and Herberts [39, 49]	ICLH	†	1981	18	72	0	28	36	60	39	†
Newton [92]	Newton	1973–1978	1982	50	20	12	68	36	57	16	28
Kaukonen and Raunio [60]	TPR	1976–1980	1983	28	100	0	0	21	93	18	0
Lachiewicz et al [78]	Mayo	1976–1981	1984	14	76	6	18	39	100	43	0
Bolton-Maggs et al [9]	ICLH	1972–1981	1985	41	†	†	†	66	31	32	31
Kirkup [63]	Smith	1975–1979	1985	24	82	5	13	84	61	39	23
Helm and Stevens [48]	ICLH	†	1986	19	100	0	0	54	69	58	†
Buechel et al [17]	New Jersey LCS	1981–1984	1988	23	26	22	52	35	85	†	4
Kumar [77]	TPR	†	1988	37	†	†	†	60	52	26	†
Unger et al [121]	Mayo	1976–1984	1988	23	100	0	0	66	65	93	4
Takakura et al [117]	TNK (cemented)	1975–1987	1990	30	33	6	61	97	27	85	17
	TNK (uncemented)	1979–1987	1990	39	31	10	59	49	67	23	3
Endrich and Terbrüggen [31]	ICLH	1982–1989	1991	10	0	0	100	54	60	20	40
Jensen and Kroner [58]	TPR	1980–1987	1992	23	90	5	5	59	69	52	9
Teigland [118]	TPR	1981–1986	1992	66	94	0	6	60	83	5	2
Wynn and Wilde [135]	CONAXIAL	1975–1977	1992	36	50	11	39	131	8	90 [b]	36
Carlsson et al [19, 20]	Bath-Wessex	1984–1996	1994	52	100	0	0	60	81	67	†
Hay and Smith [47]	St. Georg	1977–1983	1994	15	53	20	27	120	13	87	33
Kitaoka et al [67]	Mayo	1974–1988	1994	204	61	7	32	108	†	† [c]	30 [c]
Kofoed [70]	S.T.A.R. [d]	1981–1985	1995	28	46	25	29	136	†	18	25 [e]
Kofoed and Danborg [73]	S.T.A.R.	1991–1994	1995	20	0	10	90	30	90	0	5
Kitaoka and Patzer [66]	Mayo	1974–1988	1996	160	60	5	35	108	19	65	39
Tillmann and Schaar [119]	TPR	1983–1996	1997	67	67	0	0	62	94	31	25
Doets [29]	Buechel-Pappas™	1988–1994	1998	27	96	0	4	60	†	5	15
Pyevich et al [96]	AGILITY™	1984–1993	1998	86	26	29	45	57	92	19	6
Hansen [46]	AGILITY™	†	1998	86	†	†	†	55	95	13	†
Mendolia [87]	Ramses	1990–1995	1998	38	23	20	57	50	74	8	13
Funke et al [35]	S.T.A.R.	1996–1997	1998	6	33	33	33	6	83	0	0
Huber et al [55]	S.T.A.R.	1995–1997	1998	23	4	44	52	15	83	†	†
Kofoed and Sørensen [74, 103]	S.T.A.R. [f]	1981–1989	1998	52	52	19	29	108	†	†	21 [g]
Kofoed [71]	S.T.A.R. (cemented)	1986–1989	1998	36	53	0	47	84	†	†	20
	S.T.A.R. (uncemented)	1990–1996	1998	40	36	0	54	84	†	†	8
Kofoed [72]	S.T.A.R.	1990–1996	1998	31	0	0	100	50	†	0	3 [h]
Schill et al [105, 106]	TPR	1984–1993	1998	27	85	0	15	102	75	53	7
Schill et al [105, 106]	S.T.A.R.	1991–1996	1998	22	73	0	27	37	95	0	9
Schernberg [104]	S.T.A.R.	1990–1996	1998	131	68	11	52	29	88	†	10
Wood [131]	S.T.A.R.	†	1998	19	100	0	0	36	†	0	†
Rippstein [97]	Buechel-Pappas	1999–2002	1998	20	20	0	80	15	†	0	†
Voegeli [126]	Smith (n=13) Bath-Wessex (n=27)	1975–1992	1998	40	20	35	45	†	40	†	35
Kostli et al [76]	S.T.A.R.	1995–1996	1999	21	9	48	43	21	86	5	9
Nogarin et al [93]	S.T.A.R.	1994–1998	1999	13	21	10	69	34	70	10	10
Hintermann [50]	S.T.A.R.	1996–1998	1999	50	22	9	69	20	91	0	15
Wood [134]	S.T.A.R.	1993–1995	2000	7	100	0	0	66	†	12	7
Wood et al [134]	TPR	1991–1992	2000	7	100	0	0	87	14	57	29
Carlsson et al [21]	Bath-Wessex	1984–1996	2001	72	100	0	0	132	39	59	58 [i]
Rudigier et al [98]	ESKA	1990–1995	2001	40	28	0	72	38	†	8	10
Buechel et al [14]	Buechel-Pappas	1991–1998	2002	50	14	20	66	60	88	15	7
Buechel et al [14, 16]	New Jersey LCS	1981–1988	2002	40	23	0	77	120	85	46	18
Hintermann et al [51]	HINTEGRA®	2000–2001	2002 [j]	32	6	31	63	16	97	13	22
Anderson et al [5]	S.T.A.R.	1993–1999	2003	51	55	25	20	52	79	29	39
Wood and Deakin [130]	S.T.A.R.	1993–2000	2003	200	60	17	13	46	73	7	11 [k]

Author(s)	Prosthesis	Period of Study	Year of Publication	No. of Ankles	Diagnosis SA [%]	PA [%]	OA [%]	Average Follow-up [mo]	Satisfaction Rate [%]	Loosening Rate [%]	Revision Rate [%]
Hintermann and Valderrabano [52]	HINTEGRA®	2000–2002	2003	96	9	21	70	18	53	2	4
Bonnin et al [10]	SALTO®	1997–2000	2004	98	29	0	69	35	†	2	6
Valderrabano et al [122]	S.T.A.R.	1996–1999	2004	68	16	13	71	44	97	13	34
Hintermann et al [53]	HINTEGRA®	2000–2003	2004	122	12	13	75	28	84	2	7

SA = systemic arthritis, PA = post-traumatic arthritis, OA = osteoarthrosis
† Data not reported
a Listed chronologically by year of publication
b Loosening rate at two years, 27%; at five years, 60%; and at 10 years, 90%
c Estimated survival rate at five years, 79%; at 10 years, 65%; and at 15 years, 61%
d Noncommercial, cemented ankle prosthesis of two components
e Estimated survival rate at 12 years, 70%
f Noncommercial, cemented ankle prosthesis of two components (25 ankles) and three components (27 ankles)
g Estimated survival rate at 10 years, 73% (osteoarthrosis group) and 76% (rheumatoid arthritis group)
h Estimated survival rate at seven years, 97%
i Estimated survival rate at five years, 83%; at 10 years 66%
j Including the pilot series (12 ankles) with a hydroxyapatite single coat
k Estimated survival rate at five years, 93%

5.2.2 Short-Term Results

The early reports of total ankle arthroplasty were actually quite good (Table 5.3). Waugh et al [128] in an initial review of 20 ankles treated with the IRVINE total ankle reported that "the immediate results on 20 ankles are most encouraging." Stauffer [111], at the Mayo clinic, reported on 63 ankles reviewed at an average of six months post-operatively. There were 52 excellent (83%), 6 fair (10%), and 5 poor (7%) results. Subsequently, Stauffer [112, 114] reported results in 102 ankles (94 patients) at a longer follow-up of 23 months. There were 43 excellent (43%) and 29 good (29%) results, with an overall satisfaction rate of 73%. The clinical results in patients with rheumatoid arthritis and in older persons with post-traumatic degenerative disease were better than in younger, more active patients. Newton [92], in 1982, reported on 50 patients at an average follow-up of 36 months that "predictably good results" could be obtained in selected patients. He noted that 24 of 34 patients with osteoarthrosis were "extremely happy," and that patients with rheumatoid arthritis did well when they had not required long-term steroid use (because of its secondary deleterious effects on bone quality). Lachiewicz et al [78], at The Hospital for Special Surgery, reported excellent results and a high level of patient satisfaction at an average follow-up of 39 months in 15 rheumatoid arthritis patients who had undergone total ankle replacement (14 ankles with Mayo prosthesis; one ankle with St. Georg prosthesis).

5.2.3 Mid- to Long-Term Results

The early encouraging results with total ankle arthroplasty were, however, followed by high failure rates and complications at long-term follow-up (Table 5.3). Unger et al [121] reviewed results after an average of 5.6 years on a series of 23 ankles (17 patients), including the 15 ankles of Lachewicz's previously reported series. Unger found significant deterioration of the clinical results and a 93% rate of loosening. Kitaoka et al [67], in a subsequent follow-up study of Stauffer and Segal's series [114], reported failure rates of 21%, 35%, and 39% at five, 10, and 15 years, respectively (Fig. 5.2).

Several other studies reported less favorable results for the constrained group of implants. After five years, 60% of CONAXIAL Beck-Steffee prostheses showed loosening, and after 10 years the rate increased to 90% [135]. In 62 ankles using the ICLH design, 100% of patients had some form of complication after 5.5 years, and only 11 patients showed no evidence of loosening and subsidence [9].

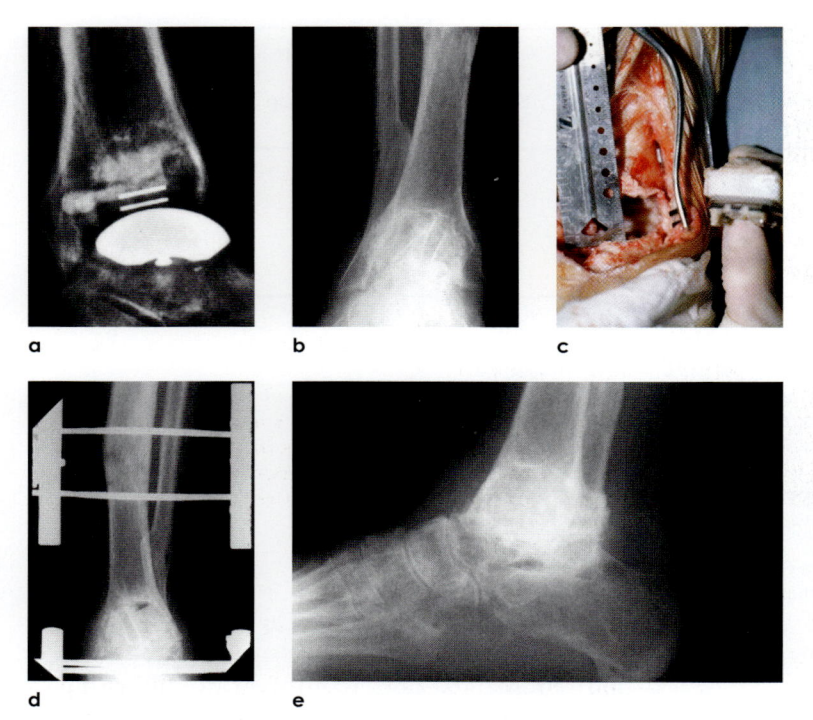

Fig. 5.2. Loosening of a cemented, two-component prosthesis.
Loosening of a two-component, cylindrical prosthesis (Mayo ankle) after two years (**a, b**). The removal of this loose ankle prosthesis shows the gap that required filling for a fusion (**c**). An external fixator and copious amounts of iliac crest strut grafts were used for the fusion (**d**). View (**e**) shows the successful fusions
(Courtesy of Dr. A. Cracchiolo, Los Angeles, CA, USA)

Nonconstrained designs with incongruent articular surfaces, such as the Smith ankle, showed only slightly better results, with loosening rates from 14% to 29% after a follow-up of 27 months [28] and 84 months [63], respectively. Furthermore, inherently poor wear, deformation resistance, and poor stability have been reported with this type of replacement [36].

5.2.4 Specific Problems with Early Use of Total Ankle Implants

Multiple problems were encountered during the early use of total ankle implants.

Appropriate surgical instruments were often lacking or poorly designed, and this resulted in poor or inaccurate positioning of the implants (Fig. 5.3). Methyl methacrylate was used for fixation, and multiple difficulties were encountered both in cementing techniques and in retrieving cement from behind the implant. Fractures of both malleoli occurred because of inaccurate sizing and poor instrumentation [9, 17]. Excessive bone removal resulted in the implant being seated on soft cancellous bone that could not support the bone-cement interface. In addition, trabecular bone strength at the resected surface was insufficient to support body weight, and this resulted in subsidence of the implant into the distal tibial metaphysis and the talar body. Finally, excessive traction in the skin during surgery resulted in a high incidence of skin complications [9].

Constrained designs have been associated with early component loosening [9, 28, 43, 67, 121, 135]. In an extensive review of the literature on first-generation cemented total ankle replacement, Kitaoka and Patzer [66] found only three studies that reported results with more than five-year follow-up [9, 117, 121], and in these studies, a 12% complication rate and 41% revision rate were observed. Other reported complications associated with constraint implants included subsidence (varying from 71% to 90%) [91, 135], wound dehiscence [9], infection [13, 17, 65], malleolar fracture [9, 17], malleolar abutment [28, 102], and subluxation of components [13, 17]. Based on their experience with cemented ankle prostheses, Bolton-Maggs et al [9] pessimistically stated that "it is only a matter of time before all prostheses fail and require arthrodesis," and noted that 73% of the patients they evaluated did not have adequate pain relief after total ankle arthroplasty.

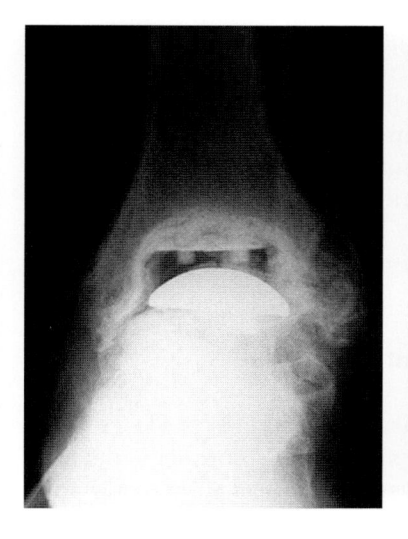

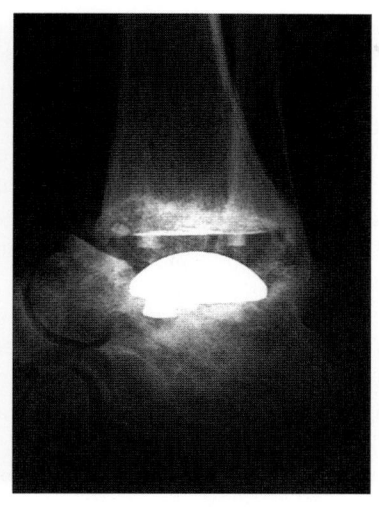

Fig. 5.3. Subsidence with a cemented, two-component prosthesis.
Subsidence and loosening of a two-component, spherical prosthesis after 4.5 years (male, 63 years old). This Bath-Wessex ankle uses methyl methacrylate for fixation of the two components (tibial component, polyethylene; talar component, metallic)

Newton [92] rationalized that "amputation was not truly a complication of total ankle replacement, but rather the last method of relieving pain."

Most of the two-component prostheses had insufficient surface area to distribute load and force adequately at the bone-implant interface. Because of their high failure rate [9, 12, 15, 66, 67, 117, 135], and because of the difficult salvage procedures necessary after failure [65, 43], enthusiasm for total ankle replacement waned, and all of the early two-component designs disappeared from the market.

5.3 Second-Generation Total Ankle Arthroplasty – Uncemented Type

Interest in total ankle arthroplasty has been revived in the advent of uncemented or biologic fixation [73, 117], more congruent prosthetic designs, the introduction of three-component designs, the development of anatomically shaped components, and improved surgical instrumentation.

5.3.1 Basic Biomechanical Considerations in New Prosthetic Designs

There are two design philosophies in second-generation total ankle arthroplasty: constraint type and conformity/congruency type. In order to understand these philosophies, the following terms must be defined:
– *Constraint* is the resistance of an implant to a particular degree of freedom, such as anteroposterior translation or axial rotation. Excessive constraint leads to high shear forces at the bone-implant interface and thus to early component loosening. Reducing constraint minimizes the transmission of shear forces at the bone-implant interface.
– *Conformity and congruency* are geometric measures of closeness of fit of the articulation. Fully conforming or congruent prostheses have articular surfaces with the same sagittal radii of curvature, which results in full articular contact. Fully conforming or congruent articulations typically have low wear rates because the polyethylene contact stress remains below its fatigue threshold for delamination and pitting. Partially conforming or incongruent articulations have a wide range of articular surfaces, from round-on-flat designs to articulations with radii of curvature that vary by only a few millimeters.

The "constraint-conformity/congruency conflict" becomes obvious in fixed-bearing designs that have fully conforming articulations. Such designs create high axial constraint, which results in excessive axial loosening torque. Mobile-bearing implants attempt to overcome this constraint-conformity conflict by offering two separate, fully conforming or congruent articulations that function together to reduce axial and shear constraint at the bone-implant interfaces.

Theoretically, to reduce constraint, fixed-bearing ankles can be only partially conforming. As a result, they have higher wear rates because polyethylene contact stresses are increased. With less conformity, wear is typically greater. This is particularly true when the prosthesis is not perfectly balanced. In such a case, edge loading may occur, leading to high contact stress on thin polyethylene.

The two-component TNK and AGILITY™ implants have fixed bearings. They decrease stress at the bone-implant interface by being less conforming than first-generation designs. For example:
- The TNK design attempts to solve fixation difficulties by means of hydroxyapatite-coated ceramic and a tibial component screw.
- The AGILITY™ design includes a syndesmotic fusion to prevent tibial component subsidence, and also resurfaces the medial and lateral ankle to enhance fixation and alignment.

Theoretically, wear in these partially conforming articulations manifests primarily as delamination and pitting, with some secondary abrasion.

Three-component implants (such as S.T.A.R., Buechel-Pappas™, HINTEGRA®, and SALTO®) have mobile bearings with full conformity and minimal constraint. They are designed to reduce load transfer to the bone-implant interface and to decrease polyethylene contact stress while maintaining ankle kinematics. All of these designs require only minimal bone resection and simply resurface the talus. Theoretically, wear in these fully conforming articulations occurs primarily by abrasion.

5.3.2 Two-Component Designs

The TNK design (Nara, Japan) [116] is a fixed-bearing prosthesis and, since 1980, has been made of ceramic and employed without cement [116, 117]. Bony fixation methods include hydroxyapatite-coated beads and a tibial screw. The ceramic concave talus articulates with a flat polyethylene tray that includes a flange to resurface the medial recess. The polyethylene tray is secured to the ceramic tibial tray.

The AGILITY™ design (DePuy, Warsaw, IN, USA) [2] represents another approach to total ankle arthroplasty prostheses that permits semi-constrained movement (Fig. 5.4). It is a two-component design with a wider tibial inferior articular surface than talar component. This congruency

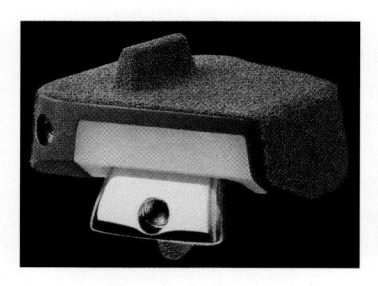

Fig. 5.4. The AGILITY™ total ankle prosthesis.
The AGILITY™ ankle is a two-component prosthesis for uncemented fixation (see text).
(From AGILITY™ Total Ankle System, DePuy Orthopaedics, Warsaw, IN, USA, with permission)

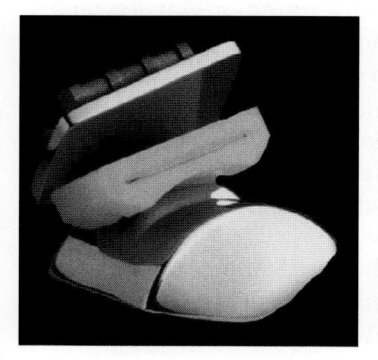

Fig. 5.5. The S.T.A.R. total ankle prosthesis.
The S.T.A.R. (Scandinavian Total Ankle Replacement) ankle is a three-component prosthesis for uncemented fixation (see text). *(From S.T.A.R. Scandinavian Total Ankle Replacement, Waldemar Link in Hamburg, Germany, with permission)*

mismatch allows some gliding and rotational motion. In an effort to further expand the weight-bearing surfaces, the tibial component was completely redesigned. The porous-coated, obliquely rectangular tibial component allows the implant to bridge the tibiofibular syndesmosis and bear weight through the fibula into the prosthesis. Support is achieved by bridging the lateral cortex of the tibia and the medial cortex of the fibula, and also by fusing the tibiofibular syndesmosis. The talar component was designed to be semiconstrained in nature and to be wider anteriorly than posteriorly to provide more stability in the stance phase of gait. It is placed perpendicular to the polyethylene tibial surface. A total of 60° of motion was built into this implant.

5.3.3 Three-Component Designs

The Buechel-Pappas™ Total Ankle Replacement is a mobile-bearing, fully conforming, titanium, porous-coated, cementless design developed from the New Jersey LCS (LCS: low contact stress) ankle (Endotec, South Orange, NJ, USA) [94]. It is designed to give a total of 65° of motion. The talar component uses a sulcus that allows some inversion and eversion without producing edge loading.

The initial design of the S.T.A.R. (Scandinavian Total Ankle Replacement) ankle was a cemented, fixed-bearing, two-component design (S.T.A.R. 1). It was later revised to become a cemented, three-component, mobile-bearing design (S.T.A.R. 2). The current S.T.A.R. implant is a cementless, minimally axially constrained, fully conforming, and mobile-bearing implant (Fig. 5.5).

The ESKA ankle was introduced by Rudigier et al [98] in 1990. The design was an attempt to meet the cancellous trabeculae of the distal tibia and the talus as perpendicularly as possible, thus weakening the load-bearing cancellous bone as minimally as possible. As was the case for the earlier St. Georg design, the ESKA total ankle requires a lateral approach by fibular osteotomy.

More recently, several other ankle designs have appeared on the market. These will be discussed in more detail in Chap. 6: Current Designs of Total Ankle Prostheses.

5.3.4 First Results

Takakura et al [117] reported on a series of 69 ankles (63 patients) after replacement with the TNK prosthesis. Sixty patients were replaced with cement, and nine were replaced without cement. After a follow-up period of 8.1 years for the cemented cases and 4.1 years for the uncemented cases, 27% of the cemented cases and 67% of the uncemented cases were satisfactory [117]. Loosening and migration were observed in as many as 85% of the cemented ankles, whereas only 23% evidenced loosening and migration in the uncemented group. Six ankles, all in the cemented group, needed revision. Based on this and other similar studies, the author concludes that total ankle arthroplasty should no longer be performed with cement.

A recent clinical paper [96] reported on the AGILITY™ ankle, a two-component, semiconstrained, and not fully congruent design. Of the first 100 patients who received this unique ankle replacement, the following results were reported after 4.8 years [96]: five major complications involving three talar component revisions, one tibial component revision, and one total ankle resection with arthrodesis. At follow-up, 54% of patients had no pain, 29% had mild pain, 16% had moderate pain, and no patients had severe pain. There were, however, 19 cases of component migration, with 12 tibial and talar components showing radiographic migration. The best reported survival rate of two-component prostheses was the Takakura ankle, with 85% at 10 years [117], but this was based on an analysis of only 25 patients.

Results from current three-component, semi- or nonconstrained designs are more satisfactory. Intermediate results using the Buechel-Pappas™ cementless total ankle arthroplasty showed the following 12 complications in 30 of 38 ankles after 4.5 years: six wound healing problems, two cases of subtalar degenerative joint disease (secondary to osteonecrosis and component collapse), two revisions (one talar and one tibial component), one arthrodesis for pain, and one malleolar nonunion [82]. At follow-up, five patients had no pain, 11 patients reported slight pain, and eight patients reported moderate pain. Buechel and Pappas reported a 94.75% survival rate at 10 years in their most recent study [16], but the confidence interval is not known.

For the S.T.A.R. ankle, a recent long-term study of 52 patients with osteoarthrosis and rheumatoid arthritis reported a survival rate at 10 years of 72.7% and 75.5%, respectively, with a confidence interval as large as 50% [74]. Six ankles in the osteoarthrosis group and five in the rheumatoid arthritis group required revision or arthrodesis. In this study, however, all ankles were fixed by methyl methacrylate. The intermediate results of the noncemented S.T.A.R. ankle, by contrast, have been much more encouraging. At 3.5 years, only one of 35 ankles required revision for malalignment, and none showed evidence of component loosening or subsidence [73].

5.3.5 Critical Issues in Second-Generation Total Ankle Replacement

While all current ankle arthroplasty designs rely on bone ingrowth for implant stability, various differences exist in the number of articulations that are resurfaced, and the size and geometry of the contact area between bone and implant (Table 5.4). Currently, it is not known which patients are best treated by replacing the superior tibiotalar articulation alone, and which require replacement of all three joints: superior tibiotalar, talofibular, and medial tibiotalar. In general, increasing the number of replaced articulations leads to more involved surgeries.

Another major issue is how closely the implants can mimic the biomechanics of the ankle joint. With regard to those designs that have been more successful in early follow-up, it is possible to note some consistencies. These prostheses are semiconstrained or nonconstrained, allowing for change in axis motion. This is important not only in normal movement of the ankle, but also because it allows for some deviation in the placement of the implants. Appropriate balancing of the ankle ligaments is (particularly in three-component, mobile-bearing systems) mandatory in order to achieve stability and alignment of the replaced ankle. This, in turn, depends primarily upon how closely the implants can mimic the anatomy of a normal ankle. In an attempt to make the shapes of the prosthetic articular surfaces compatible with the geometry of the ligamentous structures, there is, not surprisingly, a tendency towards tronconically and therefore more anatomically shaped talar components (Table 5.4). This allows the articular surfaces to slide and roll on each other without changing the helical axis of the ankle joint [85]. It also allows the ligaments to

Table 5.4. Characteristics of current ankle designs*

Device (Date)	Components	Talus Form	Talus Fixation	Tibia Form	Tibia Fixation	Resurfacing Medial	Resurfacing Lateral	Rotational Displacement	Medial-Lateral Displacement	Anterior-Posterior Displacement	Eversion-Inversion
AES (1998)	3	Cylindrical	Fin	Flat	Stem	No	No	∞	∞	∞	<10°
AGILITY™ (1984)	2	Non-anatomic	Fin	Non-anatomic	Fin	Yes	Yes	Some	4.5 mm	0	∞
Buechel-Pappas (1989)	3	Cylindrical	Fin	Flat	Stem	No	No	∞	∞	∞	<10°
ESKA (1990)	3	Cylindrical	Fin	Flat	Fin	Yes	Yes	∞	∞	∞	<10°
HINTEGRA® (2000)	3	Conical	Press fit/ 2 pegs 2 screws	Flat	2 screws	Yes	Yes	∞	∞	∞	0
Ramses (1998)	3	Spherical	Peg	Flat	2 pegs	Res.	Res.	∞	0	∞	∞
SALTO® (1998)	3	Conical	Screwed peg	Flat	Fin	No	(Yes)	∞	∞	∞	<10°
S.T.A.R. (1981)	3	Cylindrical	Fin	Flat	2 bars	Yes	Yes	∞	∞	∞	0
TNK (1980)	2	Cylindrical	Fin	Spheroidal	Fin	Yes	No	0	0 medial ∞ lateral	0	0

* Alphabetical order
Res. = resected
∞ = nonlimited

rotate about their origins and insertions on the bones without resistance, and therefore without tissue deformation (for example, surface indentation or ligament stretch) [36].

New anatomic surgical approaches have been developed to overcome some of the difficulties associated with inserting implants and removing cement, including: medial and posterior approach [34], anterior transverse incision [68], posterior approach with calcaneal osteotomy along the Achilles tendon [102], anterolateral incision [11], lateral approach with fibular osteotomy [98, 117], anterolateral approach [63] and various types of anterior approaches [74, 108]. Although most current ankle designs prefer an anterior approach through a vertical incision, further studies may be necessary to define the most reliable approach in terms of minimizing damage to the soft-tissue envelope around the ankle joint.

The arthritic process of the ankle often produces mechanical malalignment, soft-tissue contracture, and/or instability. Unlike total knee arthroplasty, the surgical principles for achieving proper alignment and soft-tissue balance in total ankle arthroplasty are not well established [52]. What is understood is that failure to obtain a plantigrade, neutrally aligned, stable, weight-bearing hindfoot generally results in poor outcomes [30, 40, 41, 52].

5.4 Conclusions

Total ankle replacement designs can be classified according to the following six factors: fixation type (either cemented or uncemented), number of components (either two or three components), constraint type (either constrained or unconstrained), conformity or congruency type (either incongruent or congruent), component shape (non-anatomic or anatomic), and bearing type (either fixed or mobile).

Following the first total ankle arthroplasty in 1970 by Lord and Marrott, more than 25 different types of ankle arthroplasties were developed. Most of these first-generation ankle designs (pre-1990) resulted in high revision and failure rates because of constraint behavior, incongruous surfaces, cement fixation, non-anatomically shaped components, and inadequate surgical instrumentation.

The second generation of total ankle replacement implants has shown encouraging intermediate results. These implants all have some untested features, however, including their bearing surfaces and fixation methods, and the optimal articulation configuration is currently not known. Mobile-bearing and anatomically shaped designs theoretically offer less wear and loosening because of full conformity and minimal constraint. Fixed-bearing designs avoid bearing dislocation and the potential for added wear from a second articulation.

Most features of the current designs could certainly be improved. Further progress may also result from improved instrumentation and surgical techniques. Therefore, objective and controlled research is needed to replace the past more anecdotal experience with total ankle replacement.

References

[1] Alexakis P, Smith RC, Wellish M (1977) Indications for ankle fusion versus total ankle replacement versus pantalar fusion. Orthop Trans 1: 87
[2] Alvine FG (1991) Total ankle arthroplasty: new concepts and approaches. Contemp Orthop 22: 397–403
[3] Alvine FG (2000) Total ankle arthroplasty. In: Foot and ankle disorders (Myerson MS, ed), chap 45. Saunders, Philadelphia, pp 1085–1102
[4] Alvine FG (2002) The AGILITY ankle replacement: the good and the bad. Foot Ankle Clin 7: 737–754
[5] Anderson T, Montgomery F, Carlsson A (2003) Uncemented S.T.A.R. total ankle prosthesis. Three to eight-year follow-up of fifty-one consecutive ankles. J Bone Joint Surg Am 85: 1321–1329
[6] Asencio J (2001) The AES total ankle. In: Proc. Int. Day of Foot and Ankle Surgery, Nimes, France
[7] Bamert P (1978) Endoprosthesis in the region of the ankle with special reference to the ICLH prosthesis. Ther Umsch 35: 342–349
[8] Bauer G, Eberhardt O, Rosenbaum D, Claes L (1996) Total ankle replacement. Review and critical analysis of the current status. Foot Ankle Surg 2: 119–126
[9] Bolton-Maggs BG, Sudlow RA, Freeman MA (1985) Total ankle arthroplasty. A long-term review of the London Hospital experience. J Bone Joint Surg Br 67: 785–790
[10] Bonnin M, Judet T, Colombier J, Piriou P, Gravaleau N, Buscayret F (2004) Mid-term results of the first 98 consecutive SALTO total ankle arthroplasties. In: Proc. AAOS Congress, San Francisco, USA
[11] Buchholz HW, Engelbrecht E, Siegel A (1973) Complete ankle joint endoprosthesis type "St. Georg." Chirurg 44: 241–244

[12] Buechel FF (1979) Complications of 292 total ankle replacements. In: Proc. 9th Annual Meeting of the American Orthopaedic Foot and Ankle Society, San Francisco, USA

[13] Buechel FF (1991) Total ankle replacement: state of the art. In: Disorders of the foot and ankle (Jahss MH, ed). Saunders, Philadelphia, pp 2671–2687

[14] Buechel FF, Buechel FF, Pappas MJ (2002) Eighteen-year evaluation of cementless meniscal bearing total ankle replacements. AAOS Instruct. Course Lect., chap 16, pp 143–151

[15] Buechel FF, Pappas MJ (1980) Failure mode of cylindrical total ankle replacement. In: Proc. 10th Annual Meeting of the American Orthopaedic Foot and Ankle Society, Atlanta, USA

[16] Buechel FF, Pappas MJ (1992) Survivorship and clinical evaluation of cementless, meniscal-bearing total ankle replacements. Semin Arthroplasty 3: 43–50

[17] Buechel FF, Pappas MJ, Iorio LJ (1988) New Jersey low contact stress total ankle replacement: biomechanical rationale and review of 23 cementless cases. Foot Ankle 8: 279–290

[18] Calderale PM, Garro A, Barbiero R, Fasolio G, Pipino F (1983) Biomechanical design of the total ankle prosthesis. Eng Med 12: 69–80

[19] Carlsson AS, Henricson AS, Linder L (1994) A survival analysis of 52 Bath-Wessex ankle replacements. Foot 4: 34–40

[20] Carlsson AS, Henricson AS, Linder L, Nilsson JA (1998) Medium-term results in rheumatoid arthritis with the Bath and Wessex ankle prosthesis. In: Current status of ankle arthroplasty (Kofoed H, ed), chap 18. Springer, Berlin, pp 86–89

[21] Carlsson AS, Henricson AS, Linder L, Nilsson JA, Redlund-Johnell I (2001) A 10-year survival analysis of 69 Bath and Wessex ankle replacements. Foot Ankle Surg 7: 39–44

[22] Chauveaux D, Laffenetre O, Liquois F (2002) The AKILE C.L.L. ankle. In: Proc. of the Int. Day of Foot and Ankle Surgery, Nîmes, France

[23] Coester LM, Saltzman CL, Leupold J, Pontarelli W (2001) Long-term results following ankle arthrodesis for post-traumatic arthritis. J Bone Joint Surg Am 83: 219–228

[24] Coughlin MJ (2002) The Scandinavian total ankle replacement prosthesis. AAOS Instruct. Course Lect., chap 15, pp 135–142

[25] Das AKJR (1988) Total ankle arthroplasty. A review of 37 cases. J Ten Med Assoc 81: 682–685

[26] De Bastiani G, Vecchini L (1981) Arthroprosthesis of the ankle joint. Ital J Orthop Traumatol 7: 31–39

[27] Demottaz JD, Mazur JM, Thomas WH, Sledge CB, Simon SR (1979) Clinical study of total ankle replacement with gait analysis. A preliminary report. J Bone Joint Surg Am 61: 976–988

[28] Dini A, Bassett III FH (1980) Evaluation of the early result of Smith total ankle replacement. Clin Orthop 146: 228–230

[29] Doets HC (1998): The low contact stress Buechel-Pappas total ankle prosthesis. In: Current status of ankle arthroplasty, (Kofoed H, ed), chap 6. Springer, Berlin, pp 29–33

[30] Easley ME, Vertullo CJ, Urban WC, Nunley JA (2002) Total ankle arthroplasty. J Am Acad Orthop Surg 10: 157–167

[31] Endrich B, Terbruggen D (1991) Endoprosthesis of the ankle joint. Indications and long-term results. Unfallchirurg 94: 525–530

[32] Engelbrecht E (1975) Ankle-joint endoprosthesis model "St. George." Z Orthop Grenzgeb 113: 546–548

[33] Evanski PM, Waugh TR (1977) Management of arthritis of the ankle. An alternative to arthrodesis. Clin Orthop 122: 110–115

[34] Freeman MA, Kempson GE, Tuke MA (1979) Total replacement of the ankle with the ICLH prosthesis. Int Orthop 2: 237–331

[35] Funke E, Rippstein P, Munzinger U (1988) First experience and early results with an uncemented total ankle arthroplasty. In: Current status of ankle arthroplasty (Kofoed H, ed), chap 17. Springer, Berlin, pp 83–85

[36] Giannini S, Leardini A, O'Connor JJ (2000) Total ankle replacement: review of the designs and of the current status. Foot Ankle Surg 6: 77–88

[37] Gill LH (2002) Principles of joint arthroplasty as applied to the ankle. AAOS Instruct. Course Lect., chap 13, pp 117–128

[38] Gittins J, Mann RA (2002) The history of the STAR total ankle arthroplasty. Foot Ankle Clin 7: 809–817

[39] Goldie I, Herberts P (1981) Prosthetic replacement of the ankle joint. Reconstr Surg Traumatol 18: 205–210

[40] Gould JS, Alvine FG, Mann RA, Sanders RW, Walling AK (2000) Total ankle replacement: a surgical discussion. Part I. Replacement systems, indications, and contraindications. Am J Orthop 29: 604–609

[41] Gould JS, Alvine FG, Mann RA, Sanders RW, Walling AK (2000) Total ankle replacement: a surgical discussion. Part II. The clinical and surgical experience. Am J Orthop 29: 675–682

[42] Groth HE (1983) Total ankle replacement with the Oregon ankle: evaluation of 44 patients followed two to seven years. Orthop Trans 7: 488–489

[43] Groth HE, Fitch HF (1987) Salvage procedures for complications of total ankle arthroplasty. Clin Orthop 224: 244–250

[44] Groth HE, Shen GS, Fagan PJ (1977) The Oregon ankle: a total ankle designed to replace all three articular surfaces. Orthop Trans 1: 86

[45] Hamblen DL (1985) Editorial. Can the ankle joint be replaced? J Bone Joint Surg Br 67: 689–690

[46] Hansen ST, Jr. (1998) Cementless ankle arthroplasty in the United States of America. In: Current status of ankle arthroplasty (Kofoed H, ed), chap 8. Springer, Berlin, pp 37–40

[47] Hay SM, Smith TW (1994) Total ankle arthroplasty: a long-term review. Foot 4: 1–5

[48] Helm R, Stevens J (1986) Long-term results of total ankle replacement. J Arthroplasty 1: 271–277

References

[49] Herberts P, Goldie IF, Korner L, Larsson U, Lindborg G, Zachrisson BE (1982) Endoprosthetic arthroplasty of the ankle joint. A clinical and radiological follow-up. Acta Orthop Scand 53: 687–696

[50] Hintermann B (1999) The S.T.A.R. ankle. Short- to midterm experience. Orthopäde 28: 792–803

[51] Hintermann B, Klinke M, Valderrabano V (2002) Preliminary results of a new ankle design. Med Chir Pied 18: 158–165

[52] Hintermann B, Valderrabano V (2003) Total ankle replacement. Foot Ankle Clin 8: 375–405

[53] Hintermann B, Valderrabano V, Dereymaeker G, Dick W (2004) The HINTEGRA ankle: rationale and short-term results of 122 consecutive ankles. Clin Orthop 424: 57–68

[54] Hintermann B, Valderrabano V, Klinke M (2004) First results with the HINTEGRA total ankle prosthesis. Foot Ankle Surg (in press)

[55] Huber H, Kellenberger R, Huber M (1998) Scandinavian total ankle replacement (LINK S.T.A.R.). In: Current status of ankle arthroplasty (Kofoed H, ed), chap 22. Springer, Berlin, pp 106–110

[56] Jarde O, Gabrion A, Meire P, Trinquier-Lautard JL, Vives P (1997) Complications and failures of a total ankle prosthesis. Apropos of 21 cases. Rev Chir Orthop Reparatrice Appar Mot 83: 645–651

[57] Jari S, Wood P (2002) A comparison of the outcome following two different total ankle replacement systems in rheumatoid arthritis. In: Proc. Annual Congress of the British Orthopaedic Association, Cardiff, UK

[58] Jensen NC, Kroner K (1992) Total joint replacement: a clinical follow-up. Orthopaedics 15: 236–239

[59] Judet T, Colombier JA, Bonnin M, Piriou P, Siguier T, Elis JB (2001) The SALTO total ankle. In: Proc. of the Int. Day of Foot and Ankle Surgery, Nîmes, France

[60] Kaukonen JP, Raunio P (1983) Total ankle replacement in rheumatoid arthritis: a preliminary review of 28 arthroplasties in 24 patients. Ann Chir Gyn 72: 196–199

[61] Keblish A (1990) Porous coat New Jersey Ankle. Technical Report 1990.

[62] Kempson GE, Freeman MA, Tuk MA (1975) Engineering considerations in the design of an ankle joint. Biomed Eng 10: 166–180

[63] Kirkup J (1985) Richard Smith ankle arthroplasty. J R Soc Med 78: 301–304

[64] Kirkup J (1990) Rheumatoid arthritis and ankle surgery. Ann Rheum Dis 49 Suppl 2: 837–844

[65] Kitaoka HB (1991) Salvage of nonunion following ankle arthrodesis for failed total ankle arthroplasty. Clin Orthop 268: 37–43

[66] Kitaoka HB, Patzer GL (1996) Clinical results of the Mayo total ankle arthroplasty. J Bone Joint Surg Am 78: 1658–1664

[67] Kitaoka HB, Patzer GL, Strup DMI, Wallrichs SI (1994) Survivorship analysis of the Mayo total ankle arthroplasty. J Bone Joint Surg Am 76: 974–979

[68] Kitaoka HB, Romness DW (1992) Arthrodesis for failed ankle arthroplasty. J Arthroplasty 7: 277–284

[69] Kofoed H (1986) A new total ankle joint prosthesis. In: Material sciences and implant orthopaedic surgery (Kossowsky R, Kossowsky N, eds). Martinus-Nijhoff, Dordrecht, pp 75–84

[70] Kofoed H (1995) Cylindrical cemented ankle arthroplasty: a prospective series with long-term follow-up. Foot Ankle Int 16: 474–479

[71] Kofoed H (1998) Comparison of cemented and cementless ankle arthroplasty. In: Current status of ankle arthroplasty (Kofoed H, ed), chap 10. Springer, Berlin, pp 47–49

[72] Kofoed H (1998) Medium-term results of cementless Scandinavian total ankle replacement prosthesis (LINK S.T.A.R.) for osteoarthrosis. In: Current status of ankle arthroplasty (Kofoed H, ed), chap 24. Springer, Berlin, pp 116–120

[73] Kofoed H, Danborg L (1995) Biological fixation of ankle arthroplasty. Foot 5: 27–31

[74] Kofoed H, Sorensen TS (1998) Ankle arthroplasty for rheumatoid arthritis and osteoarthritis: prospective long-term study of cemented replacements. J Bone Joint Surg Br 80: 328–332

[75] Kofoed H, Stürup J (1994) Comparison of ankle arthroplasty and arthrodesis. A prospective series with long-term follow-up. Foot 4: 6–9

[76] Kostli A, Huber M, Huber H (1999) Short-term follow-up of a series of 21 uncemented total ankle prostheses. Swiss Surg 5: 265–270

[77] Kumar DJR (1988) Total ankle arthroplasty: A review of 37 cases. J Tenn Med Assoc 81: 682–685

[78] Lachiewicz PF, Inglis AE, Ranawat CS (1984) Total ankle replacement in rheumatoid arthritis. J Bone Joint Surg Am 66: 340–343

[79] Leardini A (2001) Geometry and mechanics of the human ankle complex and ankle prosthesis design. Clin Biomech 16: 706–709

[80] Leardini A, O'Connor JJ, Catani F, Giannini S (1999) A geometric model of the human ankle joint. J Biomech 32: 585–591

[81] Lewis G (1994) The ankle joint prosthetic replacement: clinical performance and research challenges. Foot Ankle Int 15: 471–476

[82] Lin S, Drzala M (1998) Independent evaluation of Buechel-Pappas 2nd generation cementless total ankle arthroplasty; Intermediate-term results. In: Proc. American Orthopaedic Foot and Ankle Society Specialty Day Meeting, New Orleans, USA

[83] Lord G, Marotte JH (1973) Total ankle prosthesis. Technique and 1st results. Apropos of 12 cases. Rev Chir Orthop Reparatrice Appar Mot 59: 139–151

[84] Lord G, Marotte JH (1980) Total ankle replacement. Rev Chir Orthop Reparatrice Appar Mot 66: 527–530

[85] Lundberg A, Svensson OK, Nemeth G, Selvik G (1989) The axis of rotation of the ankle joint. J Bone Joint Surg Br 71: 94–99

[86] Marsh CH, Kirkup JR, Regan MW (1987) The Bath and Wessex ankle arthroplasty. J Bone Joint Surg Br 69: 153–154

[87] Mendolia G (1998) Ankle arthroplasty – the Ramses prosthesis. Current status of ankle arthroplasty (Kofoed H, ed), chap 21. Springer, Berlin, pp 99–105
[88] Mendolia G (2000) The ramses ankle – concept and realization. In: Proc. Int. Day of Foot and Ankle Surgery, Nîmes, France
[89] Natens P, Matricali GA, Dereymaeker G (2002) Pellenburg results after seven years experience with the S.T.A.R. uncemented total ankle prosthesis. The Pellenburg Orthopaedic Yearbook, pp 46–53
[90] Newton SE (1979) An artificial ankle joint. Clin Orthop 142: 141–145
[91] Newton SE (1982) Total ankle arthroplasty. In: Disorders of the foot and ankle (Jahss MH, ed). Saunders, Philadelphia, pp 816–825
[92] Newton SE (1982) Total ankle arthroplasty. Clinical study of fifty cases. J Bone Joint Surg Am 64: 104–111
[93] Nogarin L, Rebeccato A, Santini S, Salmaso GP (1999) S.T.A.R. total ankle 90: our experience. Ital J Orthop Traumatol 25: 183–191
[94] Pappas M, Buechel FF, DePalma AF (1976) Cylindrical total ankle joint replacement: surgical and biomechanical rationale. Clin Orthop 188: 82–92
[95] Procter P, Paul JP (1982) Ankle joint biomechanics. J Biomech 15: 627–634
[96] Pyevich MT, Saltzman CL, Callaghan JJ, Alvine FG (1998) Total ankle arthroplasty: a unique design. Two to twelve-year follow-up. J Bone Joint Surg Am 80: 1410–1420
[97] Rippstein PF (2003) Clinical experiences with three different designs of ankle prostheses. Foot Ankle Clin 7: 817–831
[98] Rudigier J, Grundei H, Menzinger F (2001) Prosthetic replacement of the ankle in posttraumatic arthrosis. Europ J Trauma 2: 66–74
[99] Saltzman CL (2000) Perspective on total ankle replacement. Foot Ankle Clin 5: 761–775
[100] Saltzman CL, Alvine FG (2002) The AGILITY total ankle replacement. AAOS Instruct. Course Lect., chap 14, pp 129–134
[101] Saltzman CL, Knecht SL, Callaghan JJ, Estin M, Alvine FG (2004) AGILITY total ankle arthroplasty: a 7 to 16 year follow-up study. In: Proc. AAOS Congress, San Francisco, USA
[102] Samuelson KM, Freeman MA, Tuke MA (1982) Development and evolution of the ICLH ankle replacement. Foot Ankle 3: 32–36
[103] Sandberg ST, Kofoed H (1998) Cemented ankle arthroplasty for osteoarthritis and rheumatoid arthritis – long-term results. In: Current status of ankle arthroplasty (Kofoed H, ed), chap 20. Springer, Berlin, pp 94–96
[104] Schernberg F (1998) Current results of ankle arthroplasty: European multi-centre study of cementless ankle arthroplasty. In: Current status of ankle arthroplasty (Kofoed H, ed), Springer, Berlin, pp 41–46
[105] Schill S, Biehl C, Thabe H (1998) Prosthetic replacement of the ankle. Mid-term results with the Thompson-Richards and S.T.A.R. ankles. Orthopäde 27: 183–187
[106] Schill S, Thabe H (1998) Ankle arthroplasty: a clinical follow-up. In: Current status of ankle arthroplasty (Kofoed H, ed), chap 19. Springer, Berlin, pp 90–93
[107] Scholz KC (1976) Total ankle replacement arthroplasty. In: Foot science (Bateman JE, ed). Saunders, Philadelphia, pp 106–135
[108] Scholz KC (1987) Total ankle arthroplasty using biological fixation components compared to ankle arthrodesis. Orthopaedics 10: 125–131
[109] Schreiber A, Dexel M, Zollinger H (1978) A new ankle joint total endoprosthesis. Z Orthop Ihre Grenzgeb 116: 595–596
[110] Stauffer RN (1976) Total ankle joint replacement as an alternative to arthrodesis. Geriatrics 31: 79–85
[111] Stauffer RN (1977) Total ankle joint replacement. Arch Surg 112: 1105–1109
[112] Stauffer RN (1979) Total joint arthroplasty. The ankle. Mayo Clin Proc 54: 570–575
[113] Stauffer RN, Chao EY, Brewster RC (1977) Force and motion analysis of the normal, diseased, and prosthetic ankle joint. Clin Orthop 127: 189–196
[114] Stauffer RN, Segal NM (1981) Total ankle arthroplasty: four years' experience. Clin Orthop 160: 217–221
[115] Swanson SA, Freeman MA, Heath JC (1973) Laboratory tests on total joint replacement prostheses. J Bone Joint Surg Br 55: 759–773
[116] Takakura Y, Tanaka Y, Akiyama S (1996) Results of total ankle arthroplasty. J Foot Surg 11: 9–16
[117] Takakura Y, Yanaka Y, Sugimoto K, Tamai S, Masuhara K (1990) Ankle arthroplasty. A comparative study of cemented metal and uncemented ceramic prostheses. Clin Orthop 252: 209–216
[118] Teigland CJ (1990) Revisional surgery after failure of total replacement prosthesis of the ankle joint in rheumatoid patients. Rheumatology 13: 87–91
[119] Tillmann K, Schaar B (1998) Cemented and uncemented ankle endoprosthesis: clinical and podographic results. In: Current status of ankle arthroplasty (Kofoed H, ed), chap 5. Springer, Berlin, pp 22–28
[120] Tragern D (1981) Follow-up study of 5 St. George ankle prostheses. Unfallheilkunde 84: 390–392
[121] Unger AS, Inglis AE, Mow CS, Figgie HEI (1988) Total ankle arthroplasty in rheumatoid arthritis: a long-term follow-up study. Foot Ankle 8: 173–179
[122] Valderrabano V, Hintermann B, Dick W (2004) Scandinavian total ankle replacement: a 3.7-year average follow-up of 65 patients. Clin Orthop 424: 47–56
[123] Valderrabano V, Hintermann B, Nigg BM, Stefanyshyn D, Stergiou P (2003) Kinematic changes after fusion and total replacement of the ankle, part 1: range of motion. Foot Ankle Int 24: 881–887
[124] Valderrabano V, Hintermann B, Nigg BM, Stefanyshyn D, Stergiou P (2003) Kinematic changes after fusion and total replacement of the ankle, part 2: movement transfer. Foot Ankle Int 24: 888–896
[125] Valderrabano V, Hintermann B, Nigg BM, Stefanyshyn D, Stergiou P (2003) Kinematic changes after fusion and total

References

replacement of the ankle, part 3: talar movement. Foot Ankle Int 24: 897–900
[126] Voegeli AV (1998) Our experience with a spherical ankle replacement. In: Current status of ankle arthroplasty (Kofoed H, ed), chap 23. Springer, Berlin, pp 111–115
[127] Wang Y, Dai K (1995) Long-term results of total ankle replacement. Zhonghua Wai Ke Za Zhi 33: 359–361
[128] Waugh TR, Evanski PM, McMaster WC (1976) Irvine ankle arthroplasty. Prosthetic design and surgical technique. Clin Orthop 114: 180–184
[129] Wiedel JD (1977) Total ankle arthroplasty with Smith prosthesis. Orthop Trans 1: 154–155
[130] Wood PL, Deakin S (2003) Total ankle replacement. The results in 200 ankles. J Bone Joint Surg Br 85: 334–341
[131] Wood PLR (1998) Total ankle replacement (LINK S.T.A.R.) for rheumatoid arthritis. In: Current status of ankle arthroplasty (Kofoed H, ed), chap 7. Springer, Berlin, pp 34–36
[132] Wood PLR (2003) Experience with the STAR ankle arthroplasty at Wrightington Hospital, UK. Foot Ankle Clin 7: 755–765
[133] Wood PLR, Clough TM (2004) Mobile bearing ankle replacement: clinical and radiographic comparison of two designs. In: Proc. AAOS Congress, San Francisco, USA
[134] Wood PLR, Clough TM, Jari S (2000) Clinical comparison of two total ankle replacements. Foot Ankle Int 21: 546–550
[135] Wynn AH, Wilde AH (1992) Long-term follow-up of the CONAXIAL (Beck-Steffee) total ankle arthroplasty. Foot Ankle 13: 303–306

Chapter 6

CURRENT DESIGNS OF TOTAL ANKLE PROSTHESES

Many models of total ankle prosthesis are available on the market today. The designs differ from each other in several ways, including the number and composition of components, biomechanical behavior, and implantation technique. In this chapter, the newest and best-known prostheses have been chosen for discussion. The content, length, and accuracy of the following sections depend on the reports available in the literature about each design at the time of publication.

6.1 AES® Ankle

The AES® (Ankle Evolutive System) was designed in 1998 by a team under the direction of Dr. J. C. Asencio in Nîmes, France, and is manufactured by Biomet Merck, in Dordrecht, The Netherlands.

6.1.1 Background and Design

The modular, three-component AES® ankle (Fig. 6.1) is made of cobalt-chromium material with a hydroxyapatite coating, and is manufactured in three sizes. The prosthetic design is generally similar to the Buechel-Pappas™ ankle, but with some improvements: a thicker tibial component, an improved the tibial stem, and the introduction of a hemiprosthetic situation of the mediolateral malleolar recesses. The tibial component is available in two thickness (5 mm and 10 mm), and the tibial stem is available in two lengths (30 mm and 40 mm). The polyethylene inlay is available in various thicknesses, which helps in the achievement of optimal ligament balancing. The ankle is inserted cementless with hydroxyapatite-enhanced bone ingrowth.

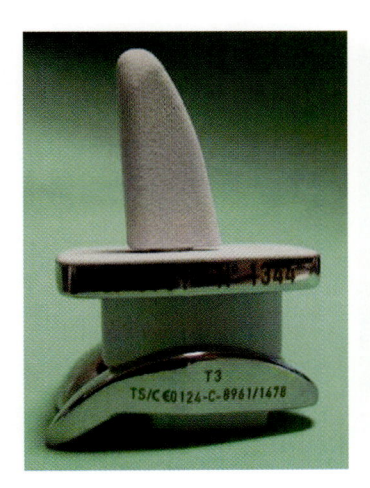

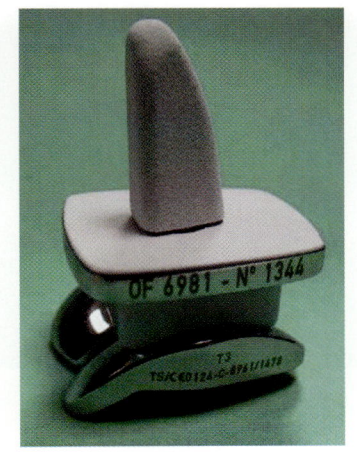

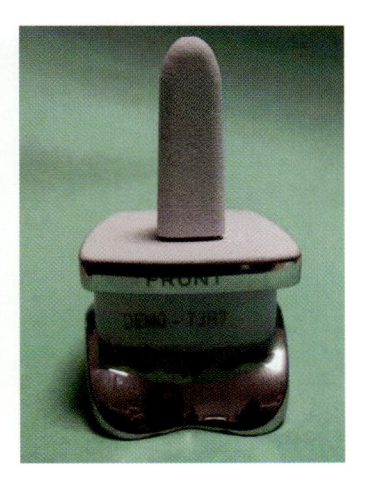

Fig. 6.1. AES® ankle.
The AES® ankle is a three-component total ankle prosthesis (see text). *(Courtesy of Dr. J. Asencio, Nîmes, France)*

6.1.2 Results

Results are not available in the literature. Since 1999, Asencio (Dr. J. Asencio, personal communication 2004) has performed 240 total ankle replacements using the AES® ankle. Sixty-five percent of the cases were complex, necessitating additional surgeries such as osteotomies, fusions, and ligamentoplasties. Using the functional score of the French Association of Foot and Ankle Surgeons (AFCP) with a maximum of 100 points, 204 patients (85%) reached 80 to 95 points at a minimum follow-up of two years, and 24 patients (10%) scored between 70 and 79 points (for example, Fig. 6.2). Twelve ankles (5%) had to be revised to arthrodesis.

6.1.3 Concerns

Because of its similarity to the Buechel-Pappas™ ankle, the AES® prosthesis may eventually show comparable concerns such as weakness of the anterior tibial cortex, loosening around the stem, and mediolateral malleolar impingement pain due to the hemiprosthetic situation.

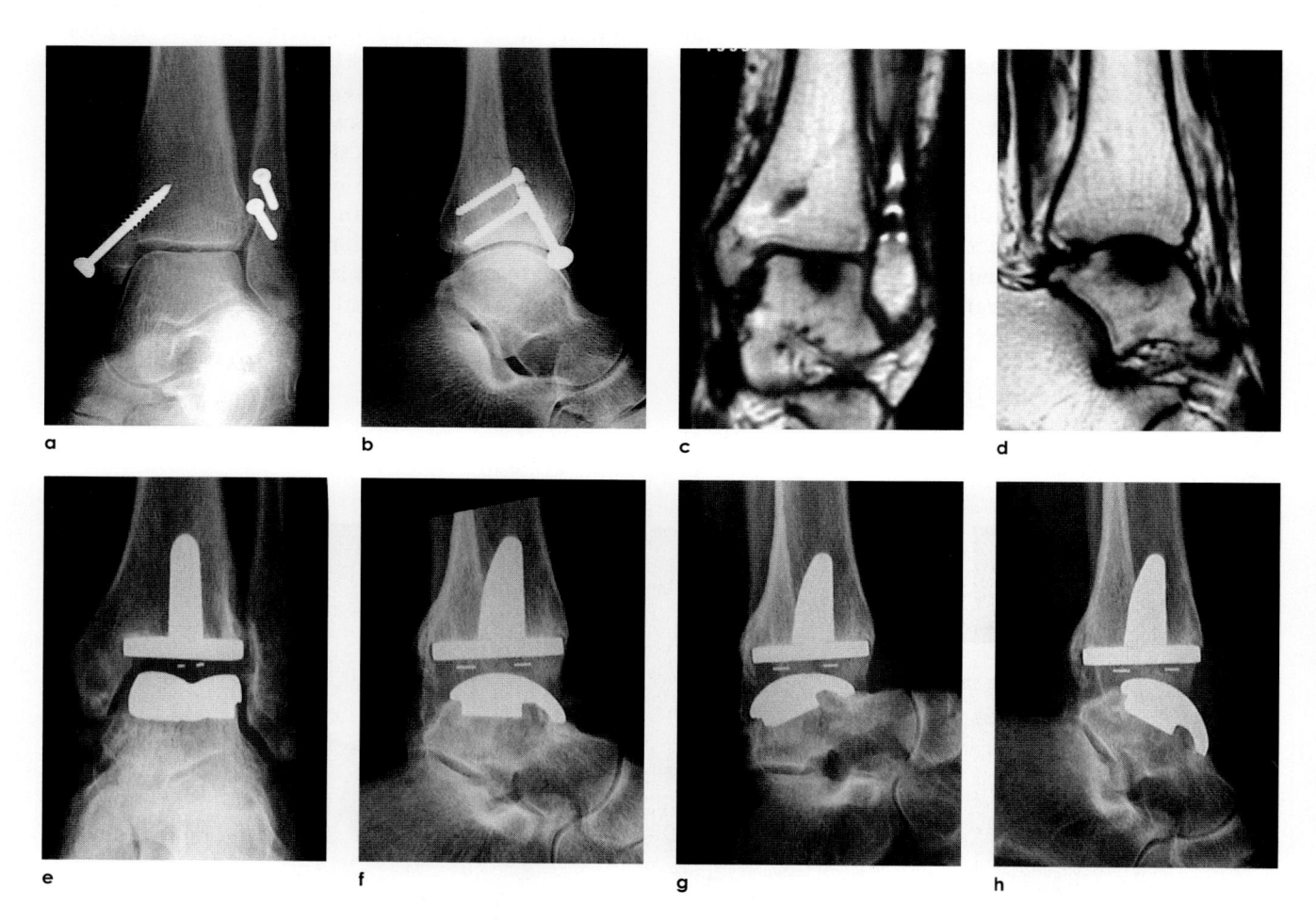

Fig. 6.2. AES® ankle – clinical case.
Three years after ankle fracture (female, 54 years old) (**a, b**), painful post-traumatic osteonecrosis of the central talar body (**c, d**). At three-year follow-up, the ankle is well aligned and stable (**e, f**) with a range of motion of 20° of dorsiflexion (**g**) and 30° of plantar flexion (**h**). The patient is very satisfied and has no pain and no walking limitation. *(Courtesy of Dr. J. Asencio, Nîmes, France)*

6.2 AGILITY™ Ankle

The AGILITY™ Total Ankle System was designed in 1984 by Dr. F. G. Alvine in Sioux Falls, South Dakota, USA, and is manufactured by DePuy Orthopaedics, in Warsaw, Indiana, USA.

6.2.1 Background and Design

Dr. Alvine based the design of the AGILITY™ Total Ankle System on an analysis of one hundred ankle X-rays at DePuy Orthopaedics. The modes of failure of other implants were used in the design process before a prototype was developed in 1983. The first implant of an AGILITY™ ankle occurred in 1984, and although the basic design persists, multiple enhancements have been made since then.

The AGILITY™ Total Ankle System is a two-component, porous-coated, fixed-bearing implant with a partially conforming articulation (Fig. 6.3). The tibial articular surface is wider than that of the talar component, thus allowing some sliding and rotational motion. The modular tibial component is obliquely rectangular and consists of a titanium component and an integrated concave polyethylene insert, available in a variety of thicknesses. The bone-implant interface of the tibial component has a porous coating on its entire superior surface, as well as along the medial and lateral malleoli. Support is achieved by bridging the lateral cortex of the tibia and the medial cortex of the fibula, and also by fusing the tibiofibular syndesmosis, which allows some bearing of weight through the fibula. The convex cobalt-chromium talar component is designed to be semiconstrained in nature and to be wider anteriorly than posteriorly, which provides more stability in the stance phase of gait. It is placed perpendicular to the polyethylene tibial surface, and articulates with the top and sides of the insert, depending on its position in the mortise. This increases the load transfer area and avoids malleolar impingement. The talar component has a porous coating on its inferior surface. A total of 60° of motion is built into the implant. Six different implant sizes and two thicknesses of polyethylene inserts are available.

The unique design of the AGILITY™ ankle theoretically has several advantages over previous designs:

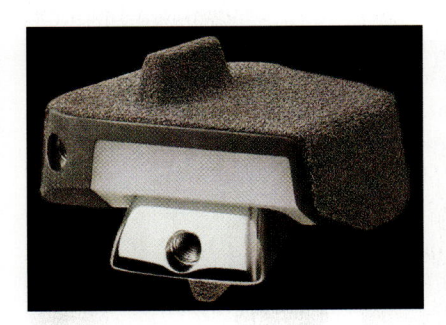

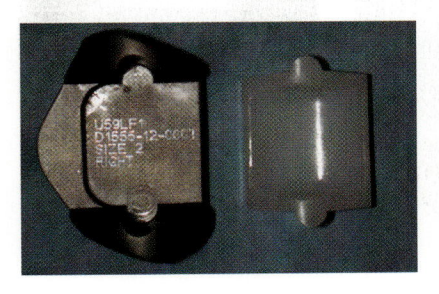

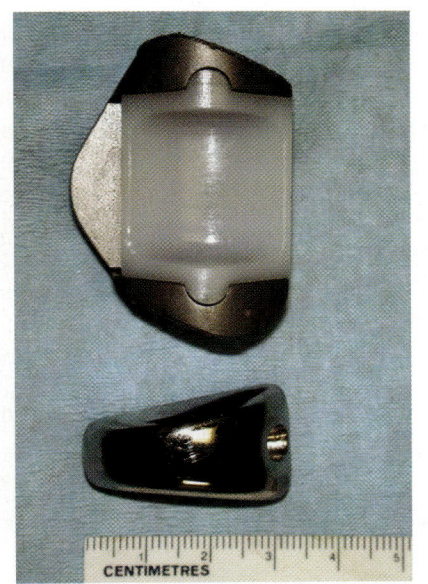

Figure 6.3. The AGILITY™ ankle.
The AGILITY™ Total Ankle System is a two-component semiconstrained total ankle prosthesis (see text). *(From DePuy Orthopaedics, Warsaw, IN, USA, with permission)*

- It allows complete joint replacement, because the two-component design incorporates syndesmotic fusion to permit resurfacing of the entire joint.
- It eliminates fibular motion, thus converting a three-bone joint into a two-bone joint, which should simplify the mechanical problems involving the ankle.
- The syndesmotic fusion provides an increased surface area for tibial component fixation, thus increasing the bone-implant interface to resist subsidence, while also allowing the fibula to share some of the load.
- The tibial articulating surface is placed 23° externally, conforming to the external rotation of the normal ankle joint to simulate normal transmalleolar ankle alignment.
- Slight translation on the coronal plane as well as axial rotation is made possible by the partially conforming design, decreasing load transfer to the bone-implant interface.

Implantation Technique

The implant is put in under distraction using an external ankle distractor, with two skeletal pins in the foot (talus and calcaneus) and two pins in the tibia. This allows the ankle to be brought back to its proper ligamentous tension and the foot to be realigned. The ankle exposure is based on two incisions: one anterior and one lateral. The anterior incision is made between the anterior tibial and extensor hallucis longus tendons. The lateral incision is performed over the distal fibula, allowing the mobilization and bridging of the tibiofibular syndesmosis. After positioning the alignment jig and the correctly sized tibiotalar cutting block, the bone cuts (including a V-shaped tibia cut for the tibial component fin) are carefully made with an oscillating saw blade, in order to avoid fracturing the malleoli. Finally, a V-shaped talar body cut is performed in 20° external rotation to accommodate the talar component fin. Thereafter, the final components are implanted, the ankle distractor is removed, and the syndesmotic fusion is performed by decortication of the tibiofibular syndesmosis and the introduction of two cancellous bone screws.

The AGILITY™ ankle has undergone five different development phases, reflecting the progressive improvement gained through experience:

- Phase 1 (1983–1987): The original design was implanted in the first 22 ankles.
- Phase 2 (1987–1997): A thicker tibial component with a flat back was developed, and the talar component changed from titanium to cobalt-chromium. Implanted in 207 ankles.
- Phase 3 (1997–1998): Posterior augmentation was added to the tibial component. Implanted in 104 ankles.
- Phase 4 (1998–2001): The number of sizes available doubled to six.
- Phase 5 (2001): The talar skirt was widened with a "revision" component.

6.2.2 Results

The first 100 patients who were independently assessed after a mean of 4.8 years (range, 2.8 to 12.3 years) showed overall good function and radiographic stability in most patients (Fig. 6.4) [26]. Of the 82 patients still alive, 54% had no pain, 29% had mild pain, 16% had moderate pain, and none had severe pain. Most patients were satisfied with the results of their surgery, with 79% rating their satisfaction level as extremely satisfied, 13% as satisfied, and 8% as indifferent, disappointed, or unhappy. Of greatest concern was the high association between syndesmotic nonunion or delayed union and migration (19% of ankles), ballooning loosening (37%), and circumferential radiolucency (16%). Five patients had undergone revision, three for component design problems that have since been addressed. Talar loosening occurred in two titanium components, and two tibial components fractured. As a result, the talar component was reformatted to cobalt-chromium, and the tibial component was redesigned to be thicker. One total ankle was converted into an arthrodesis.

More recently, Saltzman and Alvine [30] reviewed the outcomes of 294 ankles (in 280 patients), of which 16 ankles were revisions of initial AGILITY™ ankle failures after a minimum follow-up of one year. Ninety-four percent (262 patients with 275 ankle procedures) stated that they had improved quality of life; 92% (258 patients with 271 ankle procedures) would undergo the procedure again; and 95% (265 patients with 276 ankle procedures) would recommend it to a friend. On a visual analog scale of zero to 10 (with zero being no pain and 10 being the worst imaginable pain), 72% of patients (202 ankle procedures) rated their pain as zero to three, 16% (46 ankle procedures) as four to six, and 9% (26 ankle procedures) as seven to 10. Of 180 ankles that had minimum six-month follow-up radiographs, 33 (18%) had nonunion of the syndesmosis, of which one ankle was revised. Kaplan-Meier survivorship analysis estimated a 14-year survival rate of 61% for Phase 1 ankles, with a revision incidence of 27%, and a nine-year survival rate of 76% for Phase 2 ankles, with a revision incidence of 7%. Survivorship analysis for Phases 3 to 5 ankles has not yet been published, and follow-up data from other current studies are not yet available.

The latest AGILITY™ follow-up showed the results of 132 cases with an average follow-up time of nine years [31]. Of these 132 cases, 36 patients with implants were deceased, 14 implants (11%) had been revised or fused, and one patient underwent an amputation for an unrelated cause. Clinical follow-up of 67 (86%) of the remaining 78 living patients (69 of 81 ankles) was performed. Of these patients, over 90% reported decreased pain, were satisfied with their surgery, and would have it again. Nineteen percent (22 of 117 ankles) had progressive subtalar arthritis, and 15% (17 of 117 ankles) had progressive talonavicular arthritis. Eight percent (nine of 117 ankles) had syndesmotic nonunion. Seventy-six percent (89 of 117 ankles) had some evidence of peri-implant radiolucency, but many of these were stable and had no clinical implications at the time of follow-up.

Most recently, Spirt et al [34], reviewed the complications in 306 consecutive primary total ankle arthroplasties using the AGILITY™ ankle at a mean follow-up of 33 months. Eighty-five patients (85 ankles, 28%) underwent 127 reoperations. The most common reoperations were for debridement of heterotopic bone (34%), correction of axial malalignment (24%), and component replacement (18%). Eight patients (9.4%) underwent below-the-knee amputation, however, seven of these considered below-the-knee amputation prior to total ankle arthroplasty due to severe dysfunction. Five-year survivorship free of reoperation was 54%; survivorship free of failure was 80% for all patients, and 89% in patients greater than 54 years of age. The inability to salvage a prosthesis occurred in nine patients (2.9%) and was most often due to loosening or infection. Age was found to be the only significant predictor of reoperation and failure of total ankle arthroplasty.

6.2.3 Concerns

Delayed union or nonunion of the syndesmotic arthrodesis has been reported to occur in more than one-third of patients, raising concerns about prosthesis stability in these individuals (Fig. 6.5) [26]. Stamatis and Myerson [35] reported on a technique that uses a lateral plate to further compress the fibula against the arthrodesis site and lateral component. They found a decrease not only in the rate of nonunion, but also in the incidence of ballooning loosening.

The syndesmotic arthrodesis is generally performed through a separate lateral incision. This requires considerable soft-tissue dissection and places the anterolateral skin at risk. This concern may be addressed by performing the syndesmotic arthrodesis through a single anterior incision, with a limited lateral approach for the double syndesmotic screw placement.

Another concern is the comparatively wide bone resection that is necessary for resurfacing the medial and lateral recesses. This may make later revision or conversion to arthrodesis more difficult (see Fig. 11.18, Chap. 11: Complications of Total Ankle Replacement), and may also increase the risk of fracture of the malleoli. A further detrimental effect of recess resurfacing is that it narrows the talar component, thus increasing the contact load [32]. The unique design of this implant also requires more bone resection from the talus than other designs, and this, in turn, may result in loss of trabecular bone strength [13] and talar component subsidence, particularly posteriorly where the component is relatively narrow. This problem was addressed in Phase 5 by modifying the talar component to make it wider posteriorly.

Another concern is the use of an external ankle distractor to correct deformity. This method of realignment should not be a substitute for proper ligament balancing and congruent bone resection.

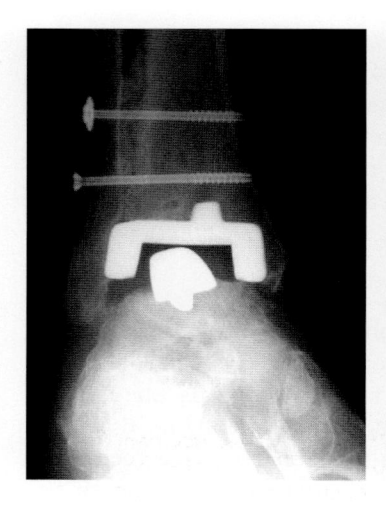

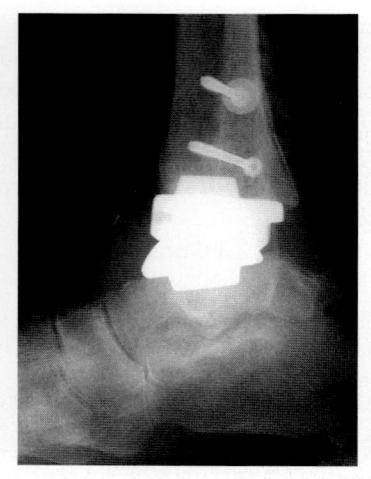

Fig. 6.4. AGILITY™ prosthesis – clinical case 1.
Stable and well-aligned hindfoot two years after total ankle replacement with solid syndesmotic fusion (male, 59 years). Of some concern are the varus tilt of the talar component and potential polyethylene wear resulting from point contact. *(Courtesy of Dr. J. Nunley, Durham, NC, USA)*

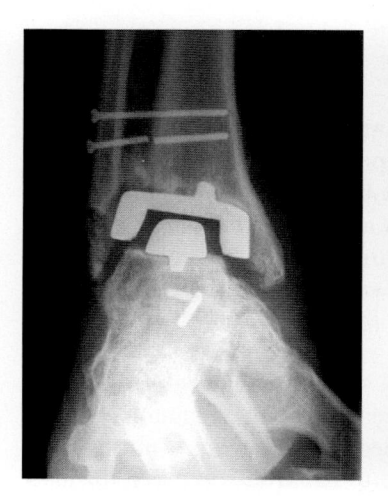

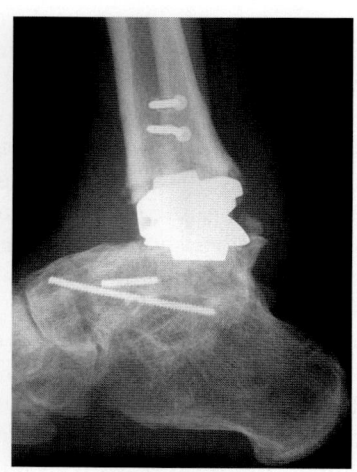

Fig. 6.5. AGILITY™ prosthesis – clinical case 2.
Nonunion of the syndesmotic arthrodesis and implant instability 20 months after total ankle replacement (male, 39 years)

Without proper balancing, the malalignment will persist after the surgery.

Finally, a specific concern related to partially conforming prostheses is the accelerated delamination of the polyethylene at areas of point or edge contact [5]. This wear is exacerbated when the polyethylene is less than 6 mm thick [7]. The standard polyethylene thickness in the AGILITY™ ankle varies from 3.73 mm to 4.7 mm [26], depending on component size. The use of a "plus 2 mm" polyethylene insert may, in part, overcome this problem, but the use of thicker polyethylene requires more bone resection and may raise the shear forces at the bone-implant interface by increasing the lever arms of the acting forces.

6.3 Buechel-Pappas™ Ankle

The Buechel-Pappas™ Total Ankle Replacement was designed in 1989 by Drs. F.F. Buechel and M. J. Pappas, and is manufactured by Endotec Inc., in South Orange, New Jersey, USA.

6.3.1 Background and Design

The Buechel-Pappas™ Total Ankle Replacement is an improved approach to an earlier mobile-bearing prosthesis (the New Jersey LCS [Low Contact Stress] Ankle, Endotec Inc., South Orange, NJ, USA). The current implant was modified to include a deeper talar sulcus to contain the

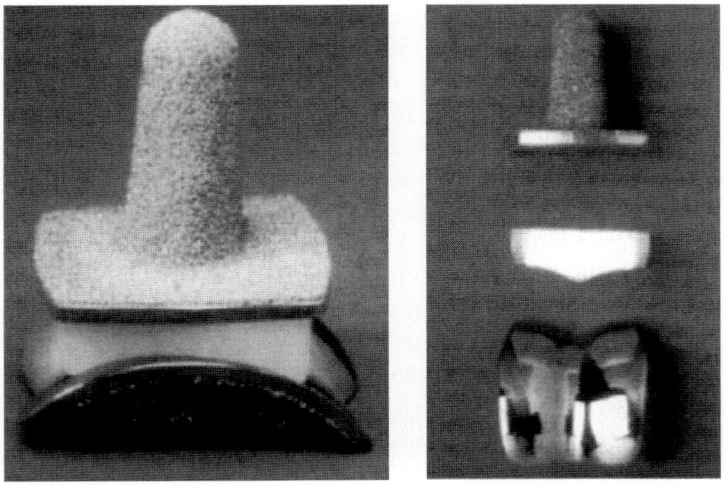

6.3 Buechel-Pappas™ Ankle

Fig. 6.6. Buechel-Pappas™ ankle.
The Buechel-Pappas™ Total Ankle Replacement is a three-component prosthesis. *(From Endotec Inc., in South Orange, NJ, USA, with permission)*

bearing component, an additional talar fixation fin, a thicker tibial component to avoid fracture, and a porous coating covered by titanium nitride thin-film ceramic. The Buechel-Pappas™ ankle is a mobile-bearing, fully conforming, titanium, porous-coated, cementless design (Fig. 6.6). It combines mobility and full conformity in an effort to achieve low wear and low contact forces. The flat, 2-mm thick tibial plateau is supported by a central stem implanted in the tibial metaphysis. The single-radius, concave talar component necessitates the removal of minimal bone and is stabilized by two fins. A congruent ultrahigh molecular weight polyethylene bearing (available in various thicknesses), is inserted between the metallic implants. The upper surface is flat, but the lower surface conforms to the talar dome with a longitudinal sulcus, thereby providing control of medial-lateral translation and preventing dislocation. The sulcus also provides some inversion and eversion without producing edge loading to the polyethylene tray. The design does not resurface the medial and lateral gutters of the ankle. To reduce polyethylene wear, the Buechel-Pappas™ ankle uses a nitride ceramic film on the titanium bearing surfaces that has shown improved wear characteristics with ultrahigh molecular weight polyethylene over cobalt-chromium *in vitro* [25]. The Buechel-Pappas™ ankle is available in six sizes.

6.3.2 Results

A first review of 23 cementless cases in 1988 found that 87% had no pain or mild pain [4]. At a mean follow-up of 10 years (range, 2 to 18 years), the 10-year survivorship was 86.3% and the 18-year survivorship was 74.2% for the 40 New Jersey LCS ankles [3]. Patient satisfaction (good or excellent) was 75%. Lucencies of 2 mm or more persisted around the tibial component between eight and 12 years postoperatively. One tibial component developed a fracture of the loading plate and required revision. Two other tibial components were revised because of excessive wear. No tibial component was clinically loose, and all three revised tibial components were stable at the time of revision. Lucencies of 2 mm or more persisted around three talar components between six and 17 years postoperatively. Only one of these three talar components required revision. Despite the absence of radiolucencies, six other talar components (15%) were noted to have subsidence.

The results with the Buechel-Pappas™ ankle, as reported in the same paper on 50 ankles, were superior (Fig. 6.7). At a mean follow-up of 6.5 years (range, two to 10 years), the 10-year survivorship was 93.5% [3]. Patient satisfaction (good or excellent) was 94%, and subsidence was seen in only 2% of the 40 ankles.

In a series of 30 ankles (20 cases with the New Jersey LCS ankle; 10 cases with the Buechel-Pappas™ ankle), a fracture of the medial malleolus occurred perioperatively in five ankles. One of these five ankles failed because of a painful nonunion and persisting valgus malalignment. Three other ankles, all with the original LCS design, failed due to varus instability. All four failures were successfully revised with arthrodesis. The range of motion obtained at a mean follow-up of six years (range, three to nine years) was 31°, including 6° of dorsiflexion and 25° of plantar flexion.

In a series of 38 independently assessed Buechel-Pappas™ ankles at a mean follow-up of 4.5 years (range, two to eight years), three of the ankles (8%) had undergone revision [20]. Radiographs showed two ankles with eccentric wear and lateral-bearing subluxation. Two of the three patients with a preoperative diagnosis of osteonecrosis sustained lateral talar collapse.

Rippstein [28] reported his first results on 25 cases (20 ankles with post-traumatic osteoathrosis; five ankles with rheumatoid arthritis) after a minimum of one year. In 18 cases (72%), additional surgical procedures were done: gastrocnemius or Achilles tendon lengthening (12 cases), hindfoot fusion (five cases), and Dwyer osteotomy (one case). Severe complications included one oversized talar component, one deep infection, and one tibial nerve entrapment. Overall true ankle motion (as measured radiographically while the foot is bearing full weight), was 22.8° (range, 7° to 20°), including dorsiflexion of 9.2° (range, 2° to 20°) and plantar flexion of 13.6° (range, 7° to 20°). No prosthesis showed any radiographic signs of loosening.

In a comparative prospective randomized clinical study of 100 ankles, Wood and Clough [43] found, at a mean follow-up of 28 months (range, 24 to 37 months), no significant difference between the Buechel-Pappas™ (B-P) and the S.T.A.R. (Scandinavian Total Ankle Replacement, see Sect. 6.8: S.T.A.R. Ankle) ankle prostheses. The mean age of the patients was 64 years (range, 31 to 83). The preoperative diagnosis was inflammatory arthritis in 31 ankles, and osteoarthrosis in 69 ankles. Seven patients died from unrelated causes, but of the 93 remaining ankles, 87 (94%) showed good clinical results. The AOFAS (American Orthopaedic Foot and Ankle Society) score for pain (maximum 40) improved from zero to 34, and the functional score (maximum 60) from 29 to 42. Four replacements required revision (one from early deep infection, one from subluxation, one broken B-P tibial implant, one broken S.T.A.R. insert). Two other ankles (one with aseptic loosening and one with unimproved pain) were unsatisfactory, but did not have further surgery. The radiographs of 10 ankles (five B-P ankles and five S.T.A.R. ankles), including the B-P ankle that was revised for subluxation, showed loss of full contact between the component surfaces. The authors described this phenomenon as "edge loading." It was more likely to occur ($p < 0.01$) when the preoperative varus or valgus deformity was greater than 20° (six of 15 compared with four of 85).

6.3.3 Concerns

Drawbacks with the New Jersey LCS ankle include fracture of the medial malleolus, varus instability, bearing dislocation, fracture of the tibial component, and subsidence of the talar component [3, 6]. Subsequent design changes in the Buechel-Pappas™ ankle included deepening the sulcus to avoid dislocation, however, dislocation remains a concern with any mobile-bearing design, particularly if some frontal plane motion within the prosthesis is allowed, as is the case with the Buechel-Pappas™ ankle. Other design changes included adding a talar fin to avoid subsidence, and thickening the tibial component to avoid fracture. These design modifications, however, may not prevent similar problems from occurring in the long-term.

A major concern is that the tibial component must be implanted through an anterior cortical window (Fig. 6.8), which compromises the cortical integrity proximal to the implant. Despite replacing the fragment during surgery, the anterior cortex of the distal tibia remains weakened, and as a result, load transmission from the implant to the bone may occur mainly through the tibial stem. Another concern with the tibial component is the non-anatomic shape and its small size relative to the tibial bone (that is, it usually has no circumferential cortical bone support, so the tibial loading plate is prone to subsidence in the remaining weak cancellous bone) (Fig. 6.7). This means that the main load transfer has to occur through the tibial stem which,

6.3 Buechel-Pappas™ Ankle

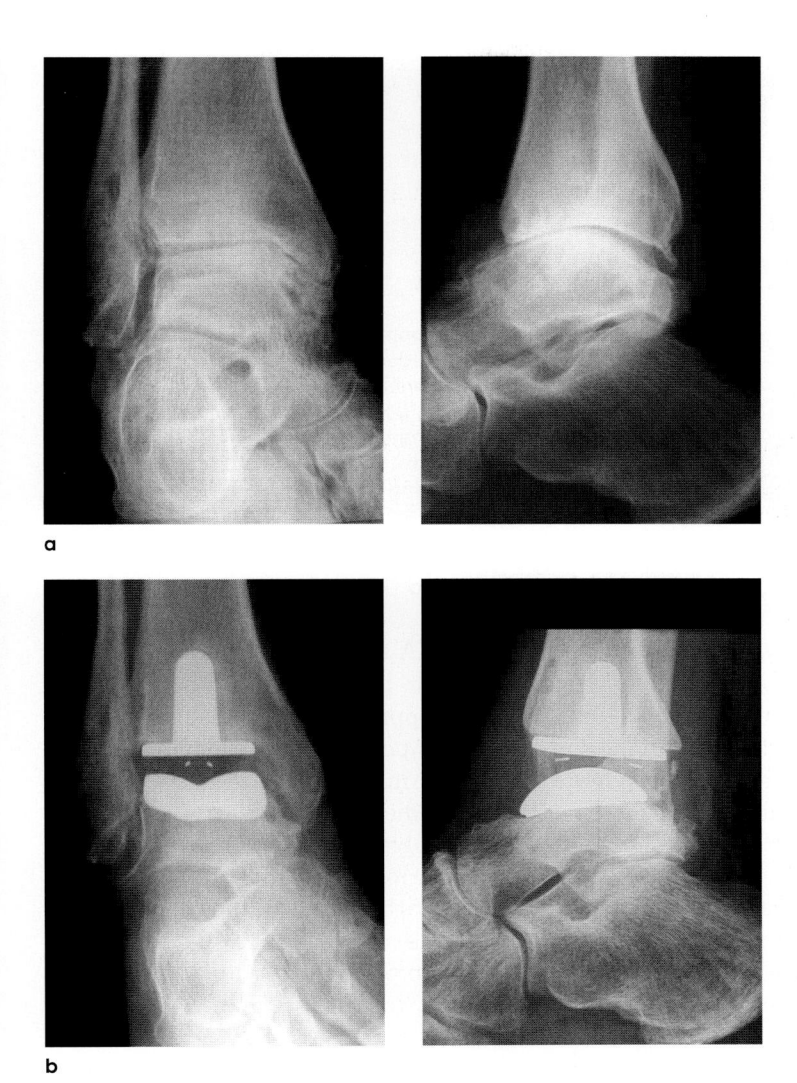

Fig. 6.7. Buechel-Pappas™ ankle – clinical case 1. Post-traumatic osteoarthrosis after ankle fracture with slight varus malalignment (male, 63 years old) (**a**). The window in the anterior cortex is still visible after three months (**b**). Of some concern is that the undersized tibial plateau receives no support from the cortex of the tibial metaphysis. The weakening of the cortical shell of the talar neck (anterior margin of the talar component) is also a concern. *(Courtesy of Dr. T. Perren, Davos, Switzerland)*

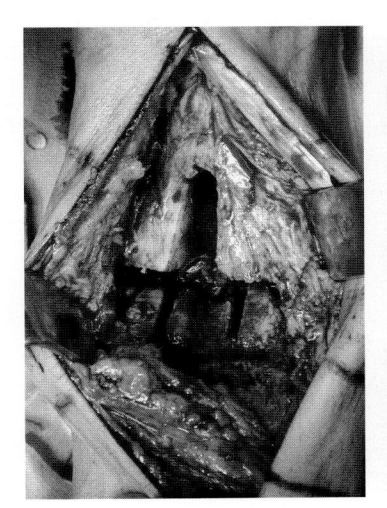

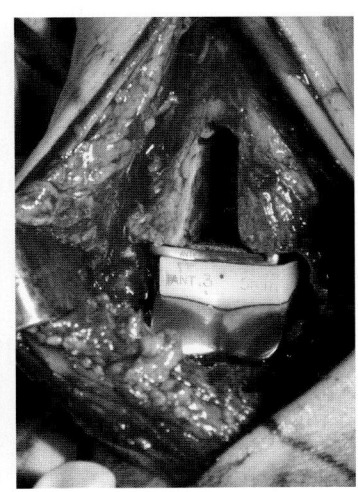

Fig. 6.8. Buechel-Pappas™ ankle – intraoperative *situs*. The anterior cortex of the tibia is disrupted and weakened by the anterior window (same patient as in Fig. 6.7). *(Courtesy of Dr. T. Perren, Davos, Switzerland)*

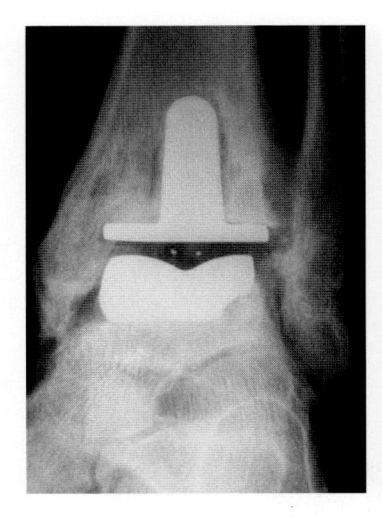

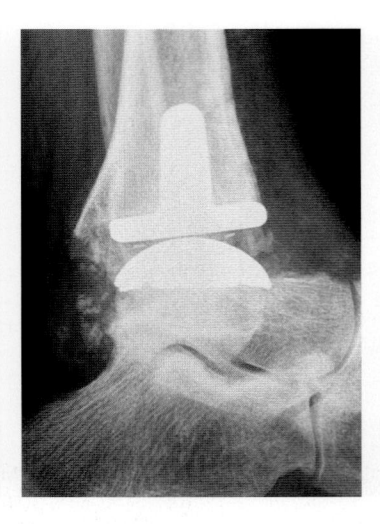

Fig. 6.9. Buechel-Pappas™ ankle – clinical case 2.
Bony overgrowth around the undersized tibial plate and ossification with painful stiffness 14 months after total ankle replacement (female, 52 years old). In addition, there are persisting arthritic changes in the not prosthetically replaced medial and lateral recesses, which may be a source of continuing pain. In addition, the weakening of the cortical shell of the talar neck is of some concern

in turn, may cause stress shielding at the distal bone-tibial loading plate interface.

Of some additional concern is the radiographic observation of tibial bony overgrowth, both anteriorly and posteriorly (Fig. 6.9) [3]. The anterior-posterior dimensions of the tibial loading plate fall short of the true anterior-posterior dimensions of a resected distal tibia, which allows osteogenesis and spur formation to form bony overgrowth that can limit range of motion.

Titanium has intrinsically poor wear characteristics compared with cobalt-chromium [21]. Even though titanium nitride ceramic film shows improved wear *in vitro* against polyethylene, recent studies of similarly treated retrieved femoral heads raise concern about the long-term *in vivo* performance of this technology [10, 27].

A final concern is that the Buechel-Pappas™ ankle does not resurface either the medial or lateral ankle recess. This may be a source of continued pain (Fig. 6.9), especially in a malaligned and severely arthritic ankle. In addition, it may hinder the normalization of ankle mechanics and ankle motion after long-standing deformity and malalignment.

6.4 ESKA Ankle

The ESKA Ankle Prosthesis was designed in 1990 by Dr. J. Rudigier, Offenburg, Germany, and is manufactured by ESKA Implants GmbH & Co, Lübeck, Germany.

6.4.1 Background and Design

The cementless ESKA Ankle Prosthesis is a three-component design for implantation through a lateral (transfibular) approach (Fig. 6.10). Both the tibial and talar components are ridge-shaped to keep bone loss to a minimum and to meet the bone trabeculae as perpendicularly as possible. The fully congruent, mobile polyethylene bearing (or meniscus) articulates superiorly with the flat tibial glide plate and inferiorly with a longitudinally molded talar component. This design feature allows for unconstrained motion of the polyethylene meniscal bearing with respect to internal/external rotation, plus transverse plane rotation at the meniscal-tibial interface, some talar tilt, and dorsiflexion/plantar flexion at the meniscal-talar interface [29]. The current second-generation talar component was changed to a symmetrical shape, because no advantages were seen with the initially asymmetrical shape [29]. A three-dimensional metallic open-pore implant surface (Metal II®) has been selected for optimal osseointegration.

6.4.2 Results

In a study by Rudigier et al [29], pain completely disappeared in 28 of 40 patients (70%) after implantation (Fig. 6.11). Twenty-three patients were able to walk more than 2 km without pain, and 13 patients were able to walk more than 5 km without pain. Three ankles had to be revised to arthrodesis:

6.4 ESKA Ankle

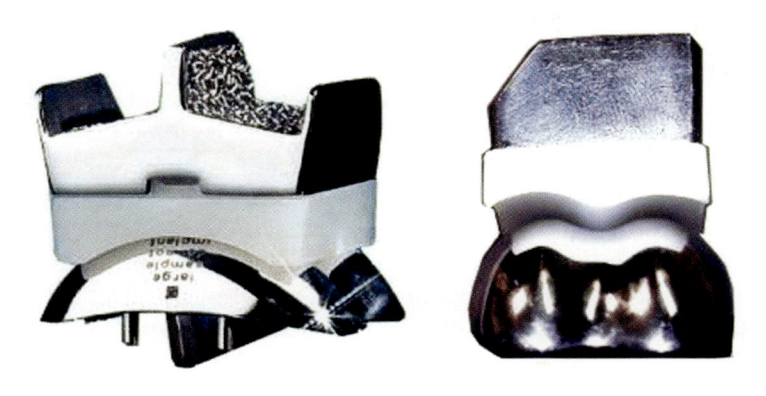

Fig. 6.10. ESKA ankle.
The cementless ESKA Ankle Prosthesis is a three-component design (see text). *(From ESKA Implants GmbH & Co, Lübeck, Germany, with permission)*

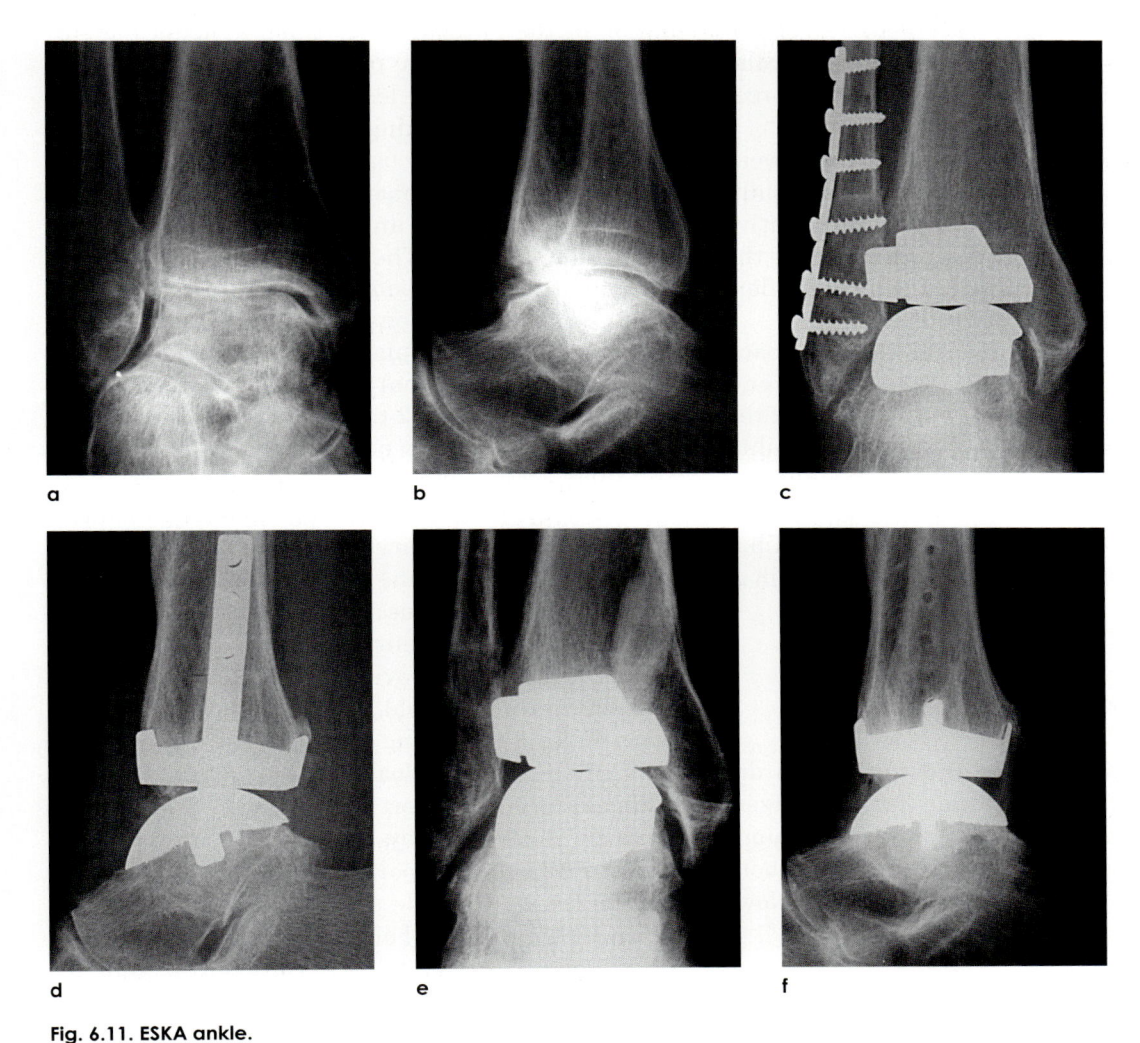

Fig. 6.11. ESKA ankle.
Post-traumatic osteoarthrosis after tibial fracture (female, 57 years old) (**a, b**). Stable implants after eight weeks (**c, d**). At two-year follow-up, the patient exhibits unlimited function, no pain, and a stable ankle. Follow-up X-rays show a well-aligned ankle with good osseointegration (**e, f**). *(Courtesy of Dr. J. Rudigier, Offenbach, Germany)*

two during the first postoperative year because of deep infection, and one after three years because of recurrent ossifications. In another ankle, a fracture of the tibial component occurred nine years after implantation, however, it was successfully revised by changing the tibial component.

6.4.3 Concerns

The non-anatomically shaped tibial component is undersized relative to the tibial bone, so it usually has no posterior cortical bone support, and is therefore prone to subsidence in the remaining weak cancellous bone. Another concern with respect to potential subsidence is the bulky design of the tibial component, which increases the torque and shear forces to the bone-implant interface.

There is a potential risk for polyethylene wear and weakening that results from the implant design. The polyethylene inlay is oversized relative to the tibial component, so it may extend past the surface of the tibial component during dorsiflexion/plantar flexion of the loaded foot.

Another concern is the transfibular approach with the necessary lateral malleolar osteotomy. First, this approach may damage the integrity of the distal tibiofibular ligaments, leading to instability of the ankle mortise. Second, it makes malalignment and instability extremely difficult to address during positioning of the implants. And third, fibular union is needed before full weight-bearing may be allowed.

6.5 HINTEGRA® Ankle

The HINTEGRA® Total Ankle Prosthesis was designed in 2000 by Dr. B. Hintermann (Basel, Switzerland); Dr. G. Dereymaeker (Pellenberg, Belgium); Dr. R. Viladot (Barcelona/Spain); and Dr. P. Diebold (Maxeville, France), and is manufactured by Newdeal® SA in Lyon, France.

6.5.1 Background and Design

The HINTEGRA® Total Ankle Prosthesis is a non-constrained, three-component system that provides inversion/eversion stability (Fig. 6.12). Axial rotation and normal flexion/extension mobility are provided by a mobile bearing element. The HINTEGRA® ankle provides 50° of congruent contact flexion/extension and 50° of congruent contact axial rotation, which provides congruent contact surfaces for normal load-bearing activities, even in the case of a distinct implantation error or pre-existing deformity. Limits of motion are dependent on natural soft-tissue constraints: no mechanical prosthetic motion constraints are imposed for any ankle movement with this device. In the sagittal plane, a 4° posterior tibial inclination angle is used on the tibial component loading plate, approximating the inclination of the natural distal tibial articulating surface. This inclination provides substantial resistance to the posterior load (0.8 times body weight) produced during walking [36], and leaves the loading of the collateral ligaments substantially unaffected after joint replacement.

The HINTEGRA® ankle uses all available bone surface for support. The anatomically shaped, flat tibial and talar components essentially resurface the tibia and talar dome, respectively, and wings hemiprosthetically replace degenerate medial and lateral facets (a potential source of pain and impingement). No more than 2 to 3 mm of bone removal on each side of the joint is necessary to insert the tibial and talar components. On the tibial side, most importantly, the bony architecture remains intact, and in particular, the anterior cortex is preserved. Perfect apposition with the hard subchondral bone is achieved by the flat resection of the bone and the flat surface of the component. Primary stability for coronal plane motion is provided by two screws inserted into the anterior shield, in the upper part of oval holes so that the settling process of the component is not hindered by axial loading. On the talar side, additional anterior support is provided by a shield, and press fit is provided by the slightly curved wings. Two screws, inserted parallel to the main transmission forces, but outside of the main load transmission area between the bone and the implant, provide additional primary stability in the sagittal, and, to a lesser extent, frontal planes.

This fixation concept prevents any stress shielding from occurring, which has been found to be critical with other designs that use stems [9] and bars [39] for fixation. A porous-coated surface covered by porous titanium and hydroxyapatite allows early fixation of the implant through hydroxyapatite bonding and then later secure ingrowth of bone within the beaded interstices.

Contact stress between the articulating surfaces is minimized by an increased contact area as compared with other designs [4, 18, 30]. With regard to the superior secondary articulating surface of the mobile bearing, wear on this surface is expected to be relatively low, because there is relatively little secondary motion (axial rotation, and sagittal and coronal translation) compared with the primary motion (flexion/extension). A longitudinal ridge on both the medial and lateral borders of the component restricts the polyethylene motion on the talus to anterior and posterior translation, preventing rotation.

Unconstrained ankle prostheses rely on restoration of correct soft-tissue tension for stability. Precise adjustment of ligament tension can only be achieved by component surfaces that correspond as closely as possible to the original anatomy of the ankle, as is the case with the HINTEGRA® design. Ligament tension also depends on accurate implantation. Once the device has been fitted, however, there is almost no opportunity to correct the tension. To this end, the HINTEGRA® improved instrumentation has been created to ensure proper alignment of the replaced ankle. For instance, a specialized tibial resection jig makes it possible to adjust the block in the frontal plane, so that the patient's individual tibiotalar angle can be respected.

The HINTEGRA® ankle includes a metal tibial component, an ultrahigh density polyethylene mobile bearing, and a metal talar component, all of which are available in five sizes. The metal components are manufactured of cobalt-chromium alloy with a porous coating that has 20% porosity. The porous coating is covered by titanium fluid and hydroxyapatite. The remaining metallic surfaces are highly polished.

The tibial component employs a flat, 4-mm thick loading plate with pyramidal peaks on the flat surface against the tibia and an anterior shield that allows for fixation by two screws through two oval holes (Fig. 6.13). The anatomically sized flat surface allows for optimal contact with the subchondral bone, as well as optimal support of the cortical bone ring, providing a maximal load-transfer area. It also makes it possible to minimize bony resection to 2 to 3 mm of the subcortical bone. The flat resection makes it possible to preserve the anterior tibial bone intact. In addition to providing a location for screw fixation, the anterior shield prevents the adherence of scar tissue that might restrict motion.

The talar component is conically shaped, with a smaller radius medially than laterally, and an anterior shield for the placement of two screws (Fig. 6.14). It consists of a highly polished articular surface, and a medial and lateral surface. A 2.5-mm high rim on the medial and lateral sides ensure stable position and anterior/posterior translation of the polyethylene on talar surface. The medial and lateral talar surfaces are covered by two wings that are anatomically sized and formed to the original articular, cartilage-covered surfaces. The inner, slightly curved surface of the wings allows for press fit of the component to the bone. The anterior shield increases the bone support on weaker bone at the talar neck, to increase stability in the sagittal plane, to provide a place for screw fixation, and to prevent the adherence of scar tissue that might restrict motion. The current design, as introduced in 2004, includes two pegs to facilitate the insertion of the talar component and to provide additional stability, particularly against anterior-posterior translation.

The high-density polyethylene mobile bearing (ultrahigh molecular weight polyethylene) consists of a flat surface on the tibial side and a concave surface that perfectly matches the talar surface (Fig. 6.15). It has a minimum thickness of 5 mm, but is also available in thicker sizes (7 mm and 9 mm). The size of the bearing is determined by the talar size. Its superior surface is smaller than that of the tibial surface. Thus, it lies entirely within the border of the tibial loading plate during normal activity, even if a talar component one size bigger than the tibial size is chosen. As it fully covers the talar component, it ensures optimal stability against valgus/varus forces and minimal contact stress in both the primary and secondary articulating surfaces. The bearing is restrained by the compressive action of the collateral ligaments and adjacent tissues. Further, compressive muscle forces and gravitational loads across the joint hold the bearing against the metallic articulating surfaces. Thus, when properly positioned, dislocation of the bearing is unlikely.

6.5.2 Results

Hintermann et al [12] reported on a consecutive series of 116 patients (122 ankles) at a mean follow-up of 18.9 months (range, 1 to 3 years). Preoperative diagnosis was post-traumatic osteoarthrosis in 91 cases (75%), primary osteoarthrosis in 16 cases (13%), and systemic arthritis in 15 cases (12%). Eight ankles (6.6%) had to be revised. Four were revised because of loosening of at least one component, one because of dislocation of the meniscus, and three for other reasons. All revisions were successful. Eighty-four percent of patients were satisfied, and the clinical result was rated as good or excellent in 82% of the cases (Figs. 6.16 and 6.17). The AOFAS Hindfoot Score [14] improved from 40 points preoperatively to 85 points at follow-up. Eighty-three ankles (68%) were completely pain free. The average range of motion was clinically 39° (range, 15° to 55°), and under fluoroscopy (that is, true ankle motion) 37° (range, 7° to 62°). Radiographically, the tibial component was stable in all ankles, and no tilting of the component had occurred since the surgery. Migration of the talar component was, however, observed in two ankles.

6.5.3 Concerns

A major concern with the first design was the positioning of the talar component, which tended to slide too posteriorly while press fitting (see Fig. 11.9, Chap. 11: Complications of Total Ankle Arthroplasty). With the addition of two talar pegs, the newer design may resist such translational forces during press fitting.

A potential concern in uncemented resurfacing prostheses is the use of screws that may create stress shielding. The HINTEGRA® ankle, however, uses oval holes on the tibial side so that some settling of the component during osseointegration is possible. On the talar side, the two screws are

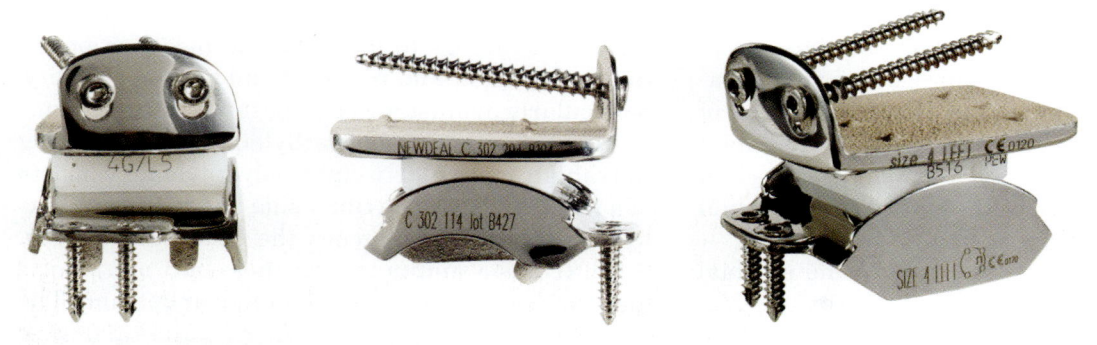

Fig. 6.12. HINTEGRA® ankle.
The HINTEGRA® Total Ankle Prosthesis is a nonconstrained, three-component system. This new version uses pegs (see text). *(From Newdeal® SA in Lyon, France, with permission)*

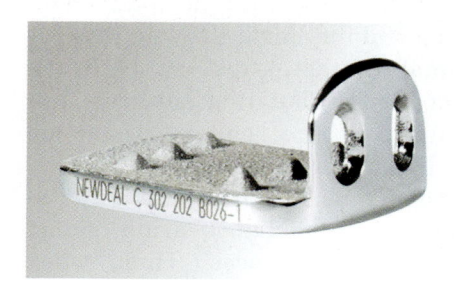

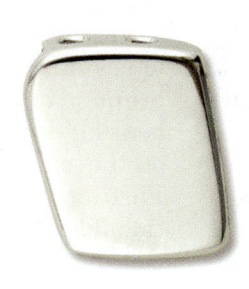

Fig. 6.13. HINTEGRA® ankle – tibial component.
The HINTEGRA® tibial component has a flat, 4-mm thick loading plate with pyramidal peaks on the flat surface against the tibia, and an anterior shield that allows for fixation by two screws through two oval holes (see text). *(From Newdeal® SA in Lyon, France, with permission)*

6.5 HINTEGRA® Ankle

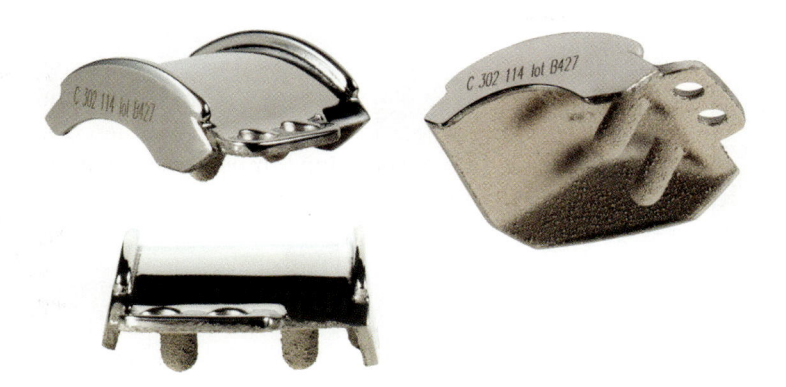

Fig. 6.14. HINTEGRA® ankle – talar component.
The HINTEGRA® talar component is conically shaped, with a smaller radius medially than laterally, and an anterior shield for the placement of two screws (see text).
(From Newdeal® SA in Lyon, France, with permission)

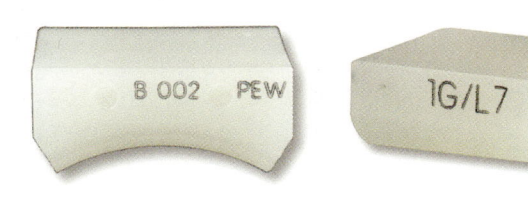

Fig. 6.15. HINTEGRA® ankle – polyethylene mobile bearing.
The HINTEGRA® high-density polyethylene mobile bearing (ultra-high molecular weight polyethylene) consists of a flat surface on the tibial side and a concave surface that perfectly matches the talar surface (see text). *(From Newdeal® SA in Lyon, France, with permission)*

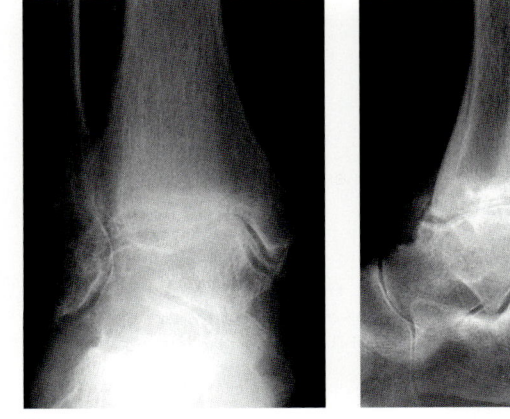

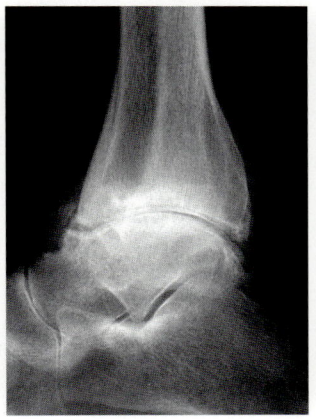

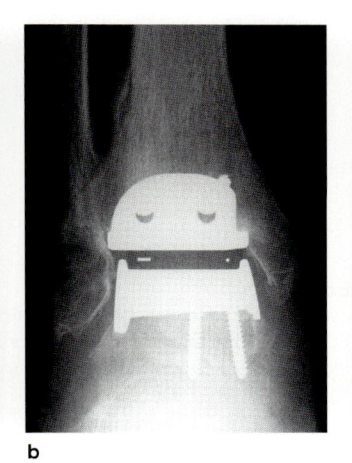

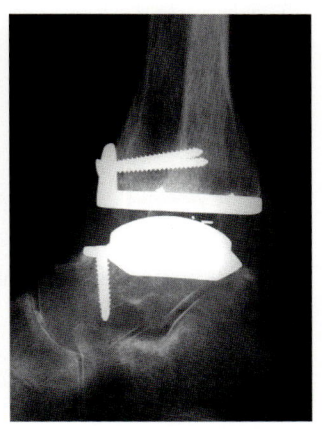

a b

Fig. 6.16. HINTEGRA® ankle – clinical case 1.
The preoperative X-rays show a post-traumatic osteoarthrosis after surgically treated ankle fracture (female, 61 years) (**a**). At 12-month follow-up, the patient exhibits unlimited function, no pain, and a stable ankle. Follow-up X-rays show a well-aligned ankle with good osseointegration (**b**)

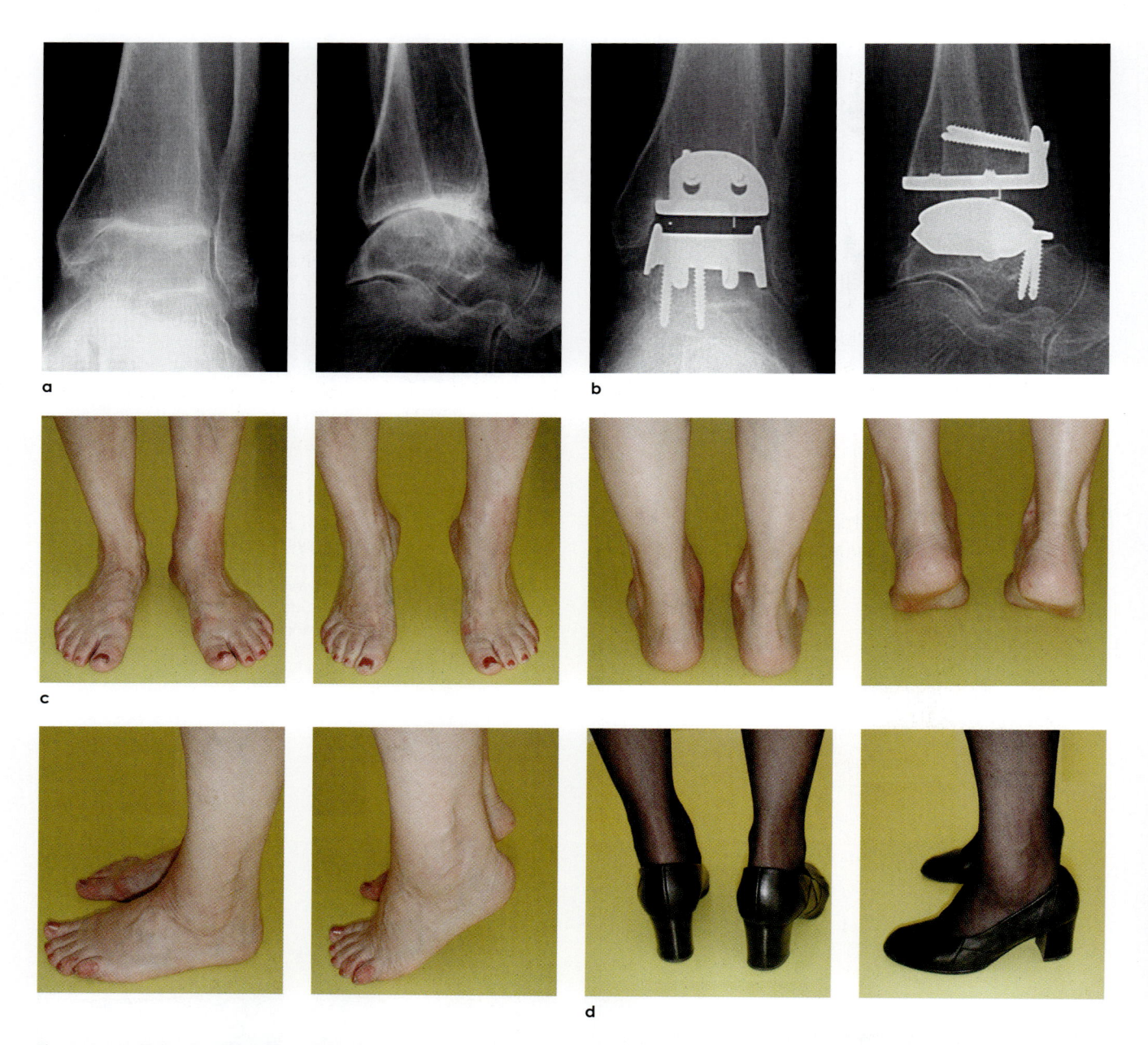

Fig. 6.17. HINTEGRA® ankle – clinical case 2.
Post-traumatic osteoarthrosis 32 years after conservatively treated tibial fracture (female, 70 years) (**a**). Five months after total ankle replacement using the new HINTEGRA® prosthesis with pegged talar component: radiographically well-aligned and stable ankle (**b**), clinically unlimited function (**c**), and no restriction for footwear (**d**). This very active patient went downhill skiing six months after total ankle replacement

positioned perpendicular to the bone surface which again allows settling of the component during the osseointegration process. Finally, screw fixation for both components is located eccentrically to the load transfer area, minimizing the potential for stress shielding.

A final concern is the flat tibial component (which includes only six pyramidal peaks) is potentially not sufficient to resist against translational or rotational forces. Screw fixation was, however, shown to provide sufficient stability until firm osseointegration has occurred (see Fig. 4.16, Chap. 4: Anatomic and Biomechanical Characteristics of the Ankle Joint and Total Ankle Arthroplasty) [12].

6.6 Ramses Ankle

The current Ramses Total Ankle Prosthesis was designed in 1998 by a team under the direction of Dr. G. Mendolia in Boulogne S/Mer, France, and is manufactured by Fournitures Hospitaliers in Mulhouse, France.

6.6.1 Background and Design

The Ramses ankle has a spheroidally shaped talus that allows rotation about multiple axes (Fig. 6.18). The tibial component includes a 2-mm thick loading plate, a rim on both the medial and lateral sides, and two oblique pegs. The lateral rims protect the malleoli and act as guides for the polyethylene bearing that is allowed anterior/posterior translation. The talar component has a spheroidally shaped articulating surface and a flat contact surface to the bone. It also includes one peg to provide stability on the talar body.

Some benefits associated with the use of this design include the preservation of the anterior tibial cortex, the ability to insert the pegged tibial com-

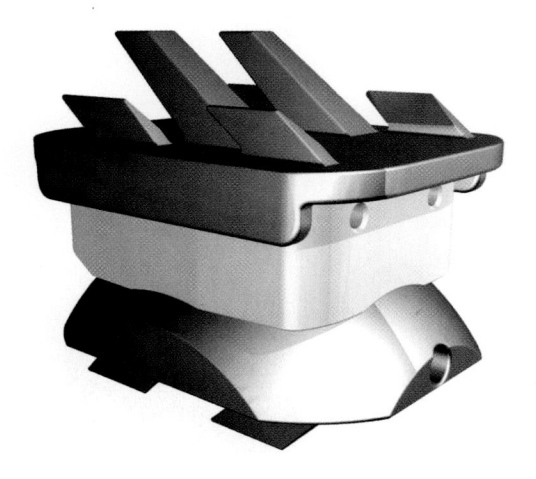

Fig. 6.18. Ramses ankle.
The Ramses ankle has a spheroidally shaped talus that allows rotation about multiple axes (see text). *(Courtesy of Dr. G. Mendolia, Boulogne S/Mer, France)*

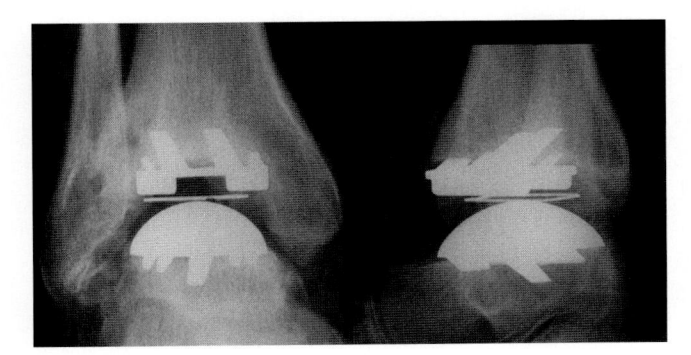

Fig. 6.19. Ramses ankle – clinical case 1.
Benefits of the Ramses ankle are preservation of the anterior tibial cortex, the ability to insert the pegged tibial component from the distal end, and flat resection of the talus. The X-rays show stable and well-aligned implants two years after total ankle replacement. Of some concern are the undersized tibial implant (in relation to the overall tibial resection surface) and the small thickness of the tibial component. *(Courtesy of Dr. G. Mendolia, Boulogne S/Mer, France)*

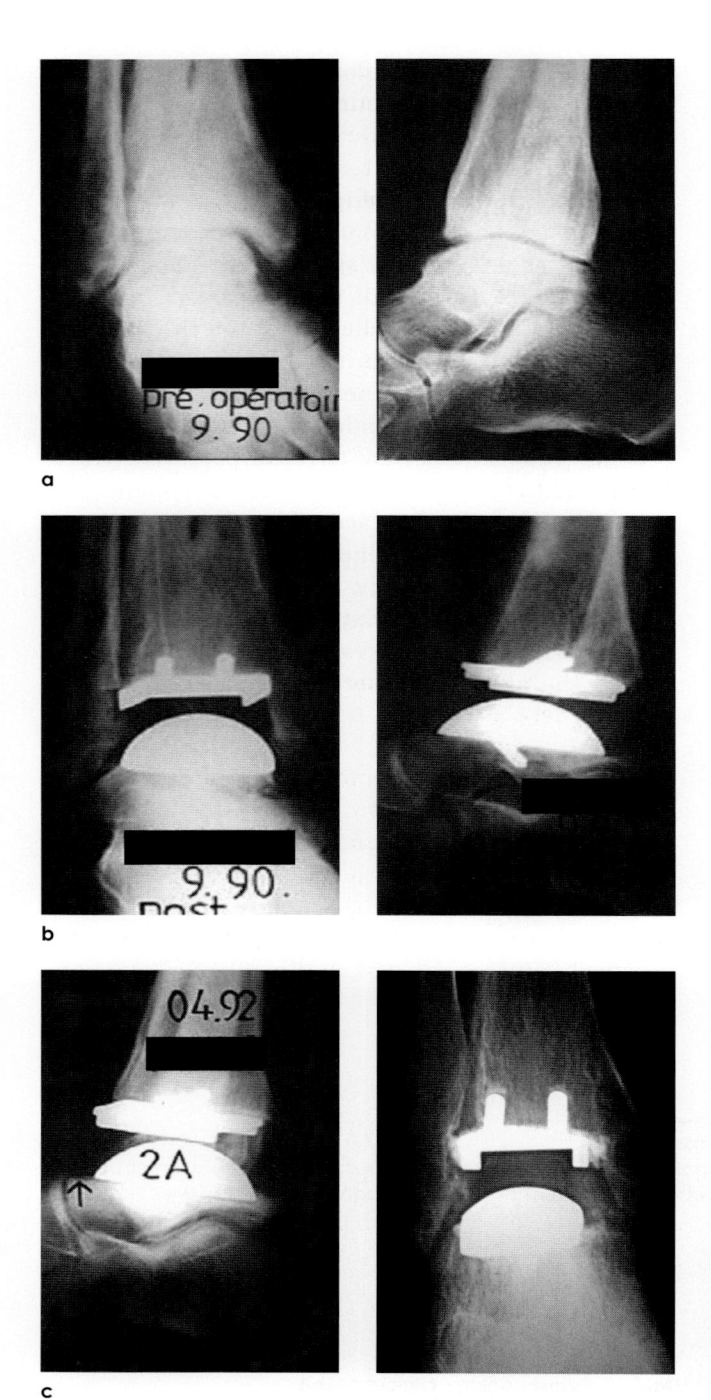

Fig. 6.20. Ramses ankle – clinical case 2.
Post-traumatic osteoarthrosis after tibial pilon fracture (female, 53 years) (**a**). The postoperative X-rays show well-aligned and appropriately sized implants (**b**). Stable implants after two years (**c**) and 10 years (**d**). *(Courtesy of Dr. G. Mendolia, Boulogne S/Mer, France)*

ponent from the distal end, and flat resection of the talus (Fig. 6.19).

6.6.2 Results

Mendolia [23] reported, at a mean follow-up of 4.3 years (range, two to eight years), on a series of 38 patients with 38 uncemented Ramses ankle replacements. The cases were performed by 12 different surgeons. Complications included one malleolar fracture, three varus or valgus malalignments, and two ankle instabilities. There was limited dorsiflexion motion in eight ankles. Five ankles (13%) were revised to arthrodesis because of pain. Five other ankles (13%) had unsatisfactory results because of pain and stiffness.

Most recently, Mendolia (personal communication 2004) reported on a series of 69 ankles. The diagnosis was post-traumatic osteoarthrosis in 32 ankles, avascular necrosis of the talus in seven ankles, rheumatoid arthritis in 12 ankles, and primary osteoarthritis in 11 ankles. An additional heel cord lengthening was performed in 20 ankles (29%), but neglected in eight ankles (12%), which resulted in limited dorsiflexion. Twelve ankles (17%) were revised: six because of loosening of a component (three ankles were revised with a new uncemented component, and three were revised to arthrodesis), and six ankles because of pain (of which four were revised to arthrodesis, and the other two were revised by debridement). The obtained result at a minimum follow-up of 10 years was good or excellent in 53 ankles (77%, of which five were revised to arthrodeses) (Fig. 6.20), fair in 15 ankles (22%, of which one was revised to arthrodesis), and poor in one ankle (1%, revised to arthrodesis). No pain was reported in 35 of the remaining 62 ankles (57%), whereas there was moderate pain in 15 ankles (24%) and severe pain in 12 ankles (19%). While 50 ankles (81%) were stable, 12 ankles (19%) were unstable. A range of motion of more than 30° was found in 39 ankles (63%), but five ankles (8%) were stiff at neutral foot position.

6.6.3 Concerns

With the use of the Ramses ankle, frontal plane stability relies entirely on ligamentous support. This does not correspond to the normal human ankle, where almost 100% frontal plane stability is provided by the articular surfaces [37]. Chronic overstress of the ligaments may cause pain, instability, and submalleolar impingement.

Another concern is the wide talar bone resection, which makes any revision surgery difficult, particularly secondary arthrodesis (Fig. 6.21). A final concern is the thin tibial loading plate that potentially may not resist loading forces in the long term (Fig. 6.19).

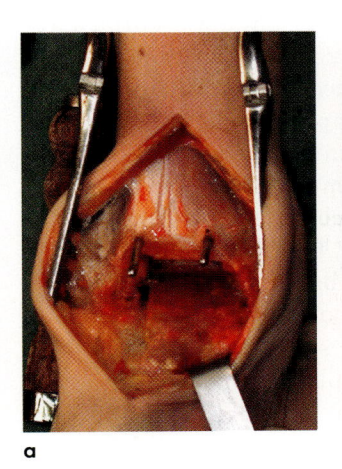

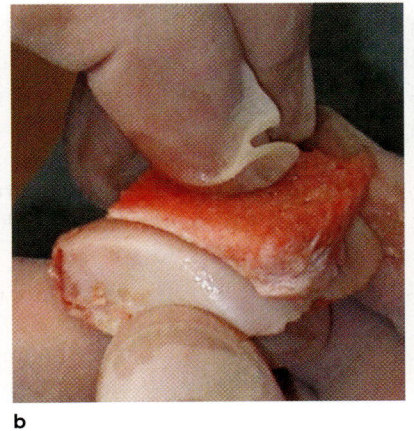

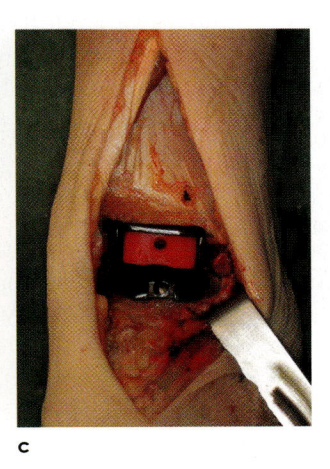

Fig. 6.21. Ramses ankle – intraoperative *situs*.
Wide bone resection (**a**, **b**), particularly on the talar side, is necessary to insert the prosthesis. View (**c**) shows the trial prosthetic components. *(Courtesy of Dr. G. Mendolia, Boulogne S/Mer, France)*

6.7 SALTO® Ankle

The SALTO® Total Ankle Arthroplasty was designed in 1998 by a team under the direction of Dr. Th. Judet, Saint-Ismier, France, and is manufactured by Tornier SA, Saint-Ismier, France.

6.7.1 Background and Design

The cementless SALTO® Total Ankle Arthroplasty is a three-component design that includes an optional polyethylene implant to resurface the fibula (Fig. 6.22). The flat, 2-mm thick tibial plateau is supported by a central keel-like stem with a hollow bar implanted in the tibial metaphysis, and includes a metallic rim on the medial side to protect the medial malleolus. The double-radii (medial radius smaller than the lateral radius), concave talar component necessitates the removal of minimal bone and is stabilized by a cylindrically shaped fin. Two wings hemiprosthetically replace the medial and lateral facets. A congruent, ultrahigh molecular weight polyethylene bearing (available in various thicknesses) is inserted between the metallic implants. The upper surface is flat, but the lower surface conforms to the talar dome with a longitudinal sulcus, thereby providing control of medial/lateral translation and preventing dislocation. The sulcus also provides some inversion and eversion without producing edge loading to the polyethylene tray. The SALTO® ankle also includes a round polyethylene inlay supported by a peg for optional resurfacing of the talofibular facet of the fibula to help prevent bony impingement.

6.7.2 Results

Bonnin et al [2] reported on mid-term results of a first series of 98 consecutive ankle replacements using the SALTO® Total Ankle Arthroplasty (Fig. 6.23). The indications were osteoarthritis (69 ankles) and rheumatoid arthritis (29 ankles). At a follow-up of 35 months (range, 24 to 68 months), two patients (two ankles) were deceased, one patient (one ankle) was lost, and two prostheses were revised to arthrodesis. In the remaining 93 ankles, the AOFAS Hindfoot Score was found to have improved from 32.3 preoperatively to 83.1 at follow-up, and it was slightly (but not significantly) higher in the rheumatoid arthritic ankles (84.2) than in the osteoarthritic ankles (82.5). Seventy-two patients (78%) were pain free, 54 were able to walk unlimited distances, 25 were able to walk more than 1 km, 67 had no limp, but seven needed aid. True ankle motion (as measured radiographically) increased from 15.2° preoperatively to 38.3° at follow-up. At follow-up, two prostheses were removed, two prostheses showed radiographic loosening, and two ankles had required revision surgery (synovectomy and resection of medial calcifications, respectively). Survival rate at follow-up was 98% (best scenario) or 94.9% (worst scenario) with ultimate implant removal, but 93.8% (best scenario) or 91.8% (worst scenario) with ultimate implant removal, X-ray evidenced loosening, or revision.

6.7.3 Concerns

One concern is that a slit and hole must be created in the anterior tibial cortex to insert the tibial component, which compromises the cortical integrity proximal to the implant. Despite replacing the fragment during surgery, the anterior cortex of the distal tibia remains weakened, and as a result, load transmission from the implant to the bone may occur mainly through the tibial keel. Another concern with the tibial component is the non-anatomic shape and its small size relative to the tibial bone (that is, it usually has no circumferential cortical bone support) (Fig. 6.23b), so the tibial loading plate is prone to subsidence in the remaining weak cancellous bone, or to impinging upon or causing lesion the tendons (for example, the flexor hallucis longus) when the tibial component is larger than the tibial bone. If the central cancellous bone of the tibial plateau is too weak, the stability obtained by the keel and the hollow bar against translational and rotation forces may potentially be insufficient. If the tibial bone is very strong, then force transmission between the implant and the bone may occur mainly through the keel and bar, and they may provoke stress shielding to the top of the bar. As a result, bending moments are created within the tibial component, and this may result in rupturing of the implant when it is fully loaded. With this in

6.7 SALTO® Ankle

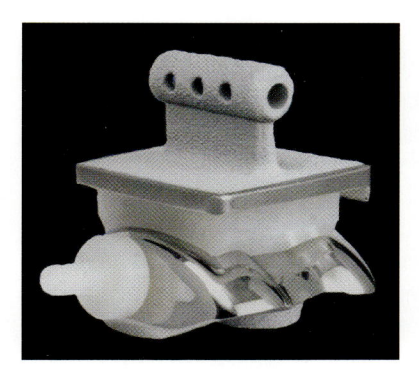

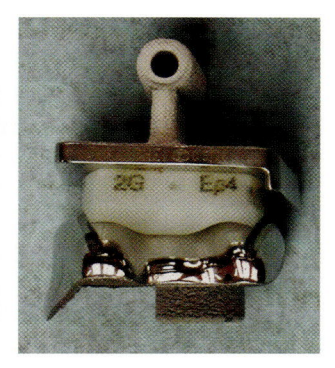

Fig. 6.22. SALTO® ankle.
The cementless SALTO® Total Ankle Arthroplasty is a three-component design that includes an optional polyethylene implant to resurface the fibula (see text)

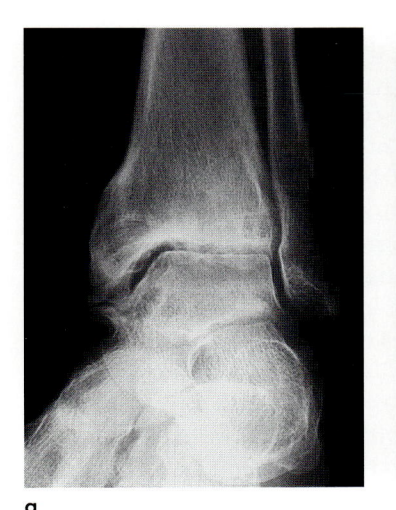

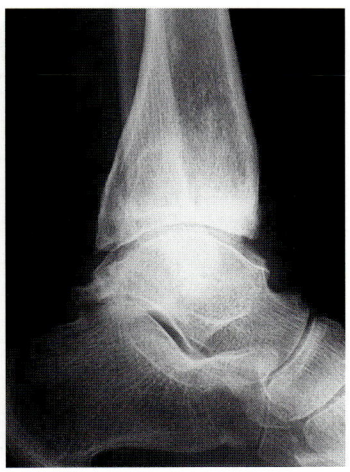

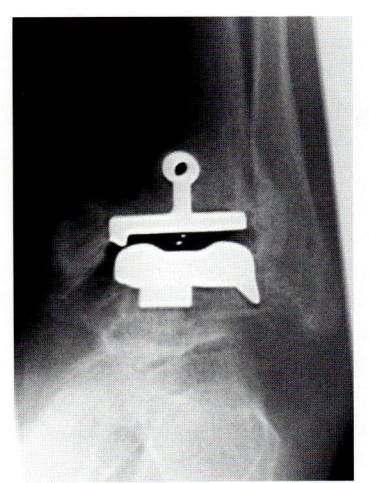

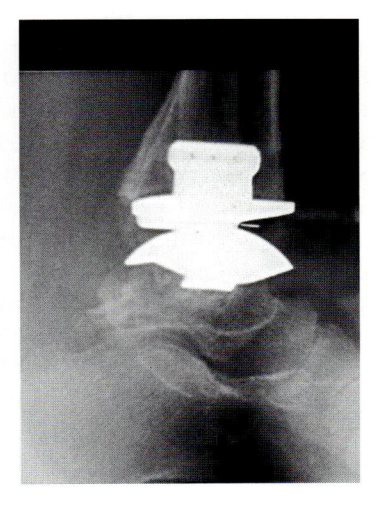

Fig. 6.23. SALTO® ankle – clinical case.
Post-traumatic osteoarthrosis after ankle fracture (female, 27 years) (**a**). Postoperative X-ray after total ankle replacement without resurfacing the talofibular facet with the round polyethylene inlay (**b**). Notice the small size of the implant relative to the tibia, and the lack of circumferential cortical bone support. *(Courtesy of Dr. H. Trouillier, Bielefeld, Germany)*

mind, another concern is the thin, 2.5-mm tibial plateau, which may not be strong enough to resist shear and torque forces.

Of some additional concern is tibial bony overgrowth, both anteriorly and posteriorly. The anterior-posterior dimensions of the tibial loading plate fall short of the true anterior-posterior dimensions of a resected distal tibia, which allows osteogenesis and spur formation to form bony overgrowth that can limit range of motion.

6.8 S.T.A.R. Ankle

The S.T.A.R. (Scandinavian Total Ankle Replacement) ankle was designed in 1981 by Dr. H. Kofoed in Copenhagen, Denmark, and is manufactured by Waldemar Link in Hamburg, Germany.

6.8.1 Background and Design

The first S.T.A.R. (Scandinavian Total Ankle Replacement) ankle was introduced 1981 (refer to Table 5.2, Chap. 5: History of Total Ankle Arthroplasty) as a cemented, two-component implant that included a metallic talar component that covered the medial and lateral facets, and a 33-mm long tibial component made of polyethylene. The current S.T.A.R. implant is a three-component, minimally axially constrained, fully conforming, mobile-bearing prosthesis that is implanted without cement (Fig. 6.24). It includes a flat tibial component with two anchorage bars, an ultrahigh molecular weight polyethylene meniscus, and a convex cylindrical talar component that resurfaces the entire talus (including the mediolateral malleolar recesses). The fully congruent, mobile polyethylene inlay (or meniscus) articulates superiorly with a flat cobalt-chromium tibial glide plate, and inferiorly with a longitudinally ridged convex cobalt-chromium talar component. This design feature allows for unconstrained motion of the polyethylene meniscal bearing with respect to internal/external rotation plus transverse plane rotation at the meniscal-tibial interface, and dorsiflexion/plantar flexion at the meniscal-talar interface, but no talar tilt [15, 16, 19]. The design rationale of this prosthesis is to allow 10° of dorsiflexion, 30° of plantar flexion, and 15° of ankle rotation.

The flat tibial component is only 2 mm thick, and has two cylindrical bars dorsally that insert into parallel, drilled holes in the tibial subchondral bone. When implanted, the bars provide rotational stability to the tibial component. Resection for placement of the tibial component usually requires the removal of 2 to 3 mm of bone. The left and right tibial glide plates are interchangeable. Originally, the tibial component was available in three sizes (small, 30 mm long by 30 mm wide; medium, 35 long by 32.5 mm wide; and large, 40 mm long by 35 mm wide), but recently two other sizes were added.

The cylindrically shaped talar component has wings that replace medial and lateral facets. This allows additional load transfer, and essentially resurfaces the talar dome. The talar cup design creates a large surface area that increases component stability and decreases the risk of subsidence. Preparation of the talus requires approximately 2 to 3 mm of bone resection. The left and right components are separate designs. The 1-cm long by 3-mm wide longitudinal ridge on the talar component restricts the polyethylene motion on the talus to anterior and posterior translation. There are currently five sizes of talar components (up from the original three), varying from extra-small (28 mm by 29 mm) to extra-large (38 mm by 35 mm).

Initially, the coating on the non-articular surface of the talar and tibial implants was a single layer of plasma-sprayed hydroxyapatite (Osprovit), 150 μm in thickness [8], which was applied to the cobalt-chromium. For the American Food and Drug Administration (FDA) Class III version, the coating has been changed to a dual coating, consisting of vacuum plasma-sprayed, commercially pure titanium, approximately 200 μm in thickness and porous, and electrochemically deposited calcium phosphate, approximately 20 μm in thickness.

The mobile polyethylene meniscus is congruent with the articular surfaces of the tibial and talar components, creating a contact area of 600 mm^2 on its tibial surface, and 320 mm^2 on its talar surface. The tibial articulation is flat, whereas the talar articulation is concave, with a central groove that is kept centered on the talar component by a 1-cm long and 3-mm wide ridge on the talus. The meniscus is available in five thicknesses (6 mm, 7 mm, 8 mm, 9 mm, and 10 mm). Similarly, a variety of sizes of meniscal components makes it possible to achieve adequate ligament balancing and soft-tissue stability.

6.8.2 Results

A recent long-term study of 52 cases reported a survival rate at 10 years of 72.7% for osteoarthrosis patients and 75.5% for rheumatoid arthritis patients, with a confidence interval as large as 50% [19]. Six ankles in the osteoarthrosis group and five in the rheumatoid arthritis group required revision or arthrodesis. In this study, however, all ankles were fixed by methyl methacrylate cementation. The intermediate results of the noncemented S.T.A.R. ankle, by contrast, have been much more encouraging. At 3.5 years, only one of 35 ankles required revision for malalignment, and none showed evidence of component loosening or subsidence [18]. At 4.4 years (range, one to 10 years), two of 74 ankles were revised, one for malalignment and one for subsidence [17]. The remaining 72 ankles showed no radiographic loosening or subsidence.

Schernberg [33] reported intermediate results from a European multicenter study of 131 cementless S.T.A.R. ankles. The seven-year survival rate was 87.3%, with all failures occurring in the first two years. This suggests that if the S.T.A.R. ankle is implanted incorrectly, it will fail early.

Schernberg's findings, however, were not supported by other studies that have described a deterioration over time. Hintermann, in a consecutive series of 50 ankles, reported patient satisfaction of 91% at a mean follow-up of 2.2 years [11]. No migration was noted in any case, and all implants were considered to be stable (for example, Fig. 6.25). Seven revisions (all in cases of post-traumatic osteoarthrosis), were necessary: local revision of the fibula for painful lateral impingement (three cases), posteromedial soft-tissue revision for painful restriction of dorsiflexion (two cases) (for example, Fig. 6.26), percutaneous lengthening of the Achilles tendon (one case), and osteotomy and callus distraction for angular correction after stress fracture of the distal tibia (one case).

More recently, Valderrabano et al [39] reviewed results after an average of 3.7 years (range, 2.4 to 6.2 years) on a series of 68 ankles (65 patients: 21 males, 34 females, with a mean age at surgery of 56.1 years [range, 22 to 85 years]), including the 50 ankles reported on by Hintermann in the previous paragraph. Twenty-three ankles (34%; 23 patients) had been revised: nine ankles (13%) because of problems with components (major revisions), and 14 ankles (21%) required secondary revisions (additional operations). The indications were: progressive restriction of range of motion in 11 ankles (48%), ballooning tibial loosening with polyethylene wear in three ankles (13%), valgus malalignment in two ankles (9%), primary tibial loosening in two ankles (9%), fibular impingement in two ankles (9%), overlength of the fibula after talar subsidence in one ankle (4%), overlength of the fibula with lateral subluxation of the inlay in one ankle (4%), and severe subtalar osteoarthrosis in one ankle (4%). All revision surgeries were successful, and no implant had to be removed or converted to an ankle arthrodesis. Twenty-seven ankles (54%) were pain free, while 23 ankles (46%) had mild pain, mostly on the medial side. The patients who had post-traumatic osteoarthritis reported significantly more pain. Patient satisfaction was excellent or good in 63 patients (97%), one patient (1.5%) was indifferent, and one patient (1.5%) was either disappointed or very unhappy with the result. The AOFAS Hindfoot Score [14] improved from 24.7 points (range, three to 44) preoperatively to 84.3 points (range, 44 to 100) at follow-up. Periarticular hypertrophic bone formation (mostly located posteromedially) was noted in 43 ankles (63%; 42 patients), and was associated with a decrease in dorsiflexion/plantar flexion movement. Three ankles (4.4%) showed a ballooning bone lysis on the tibial side.

Anderson et al [1] reported on a series of 51 consecutive ankles replaced with the uncemented, hydroxyapatite-coated S.T.A.R. ankle after a follow-up of 4.5 years (range, three to eight years). Twelve ankles (24%) had to be revised: seven ankles because of loosening of at least one component, two ankles because of fracture of the meniscus, and three ankles for other reasons. A component was exchanged in seven of the 12 revisions, and the ankle was successfully fused in the other five cases.

Another eight ankles showed radiographic signs of loosening of one of the components. Three of these eight cases were scheduled for revision, and the remaining five were considered as pending failures at the time of writing. Thus, 31 ankles (61%) had neither a revision nor radiographic signs of loosening, and patient satisfaction levels with their ankle replacements were: 27 patients (87%) satisfied, two patients (6.5%) somewhat satisfied, and two patients (6.5%) not satisfied. Of the 39 unrevised ankles (including the eight ankles with radiographic signs of loosening), 31 patients (79%) were satisfied with their results after ankle replacement, two patients (5%) were somewhat satisfied, and six patients (16%) were not satisfied. A mean follow-up score of 74 points was recorded for the AOFAS Hindfoot Score [14]. The range of motion in the ankle at the time of follow-up averaged 28° (range, 10° to 55°), which did not differ significantly from the preoperative situation. The preoperative range of motion was, however, highly correlated with the change in the range of motion after the operation. Ankles with a preoperative total range of motion of 15° or less doubled the range postoperatively, and those with 16° to 30° gained an average of 6° of motion, but ankles with a preoperative range of motion of 30° or more lost an average of 10°.

Wood and Deakin [42] reported on a series of 200 ankles replaced with the uncemented S.T.A.R. ankle between 1993 and 2000, with a change from a single hydroxyapatite coating to a dual coating of titanium and calcium phosphate in 1998. At a follow-up of 3.8 years (range, two to nine years), they found a mean improvement in the AOFAS Hindfoot Score [14] from 28 to 70 points, a loosening rate of 12%, and a revision rate of 7%, with a cumulative survival rate at five years of 92.7%. Nine ankles sustained a fracture at the time of surgery and 10 sustained a subsequent fracture. Only one fracture failed to unite by immobilization. Seven patients showed evidence of radiological cavitation behind the tibial implant, and seven ankles showed migration of one component. Ankle replacements in which hydroxyapatite had been applied directly onto cobalt-chromium were 7.5 times more likely to show a line of sclerosis just proximal to the implant and 5.6 times more likely to show a gap between the bone and implant than those with the dual coating of titanium and calcium phosphate. Heterotopic bone formation appeared radiologically in 47% of the ankles, however, there was no association between its presence and the clinical outcome. Edge loading was observed in nine ankles; of these, seven ankles had varus or valgus malalignment preoperatively (as did 32 other ankles in the study), but did not evidence edge loading. Of eleven ankles that were revised to fusion, six united with an acceptable final result, and five did not unite on the first attempt.

6.8.3 Concerns

The non-anatomically shaped tibial component is often undersized relative to the tibial bone, so it lacks fully circumferential cortical bone support, and is prone to subsidence in the remaining weak cancellous bone (see Fig. 11.8, Chap. 11: Complications of Total Ankle Replacement). In cases where the tibial component is oversized relative to the tibial bone, it may impinge upon or cause lesions on the tendons (for example, the flexor hallucis longus). In either case, this is critical because the force vector to the tibial component is often not central, so force is placed "off center" (that is, eccentrically), and this results in a downward force vector on that side. In most instances, the force to the tibial plate is placed anteriorly, because the center of rotation of the talus is located anteriorly to the longitudinal axis of the tibia. This tends to be even more pronounced in osteoarthritic ankles, due to anterolateral talar subluxation out of the mortise. The placement of the two parallel drill holes through the anterior cortex may also potentially weaken cortical support (see Fig. 11.10, Chap. 11: Complications of Total Ankle Replacement). On the tibial side, fixation is obtained by using two small anteroposterior bars. If the central cancellous bone of the tibial plateau is too weak, the stability obtained by the two bars against translational and rotation forces may potentially be insufficient. If the tibial bone is very strong, then force transmission between the implant and the bone may occur through the two bars, and they may provoke stress shielding to the top of the bars (Fig. 6.25). As a result, anterior tibial cavitation with ballooning loosening and trabecular formation to the bars may

6.8 S.T.A.R. Ankle

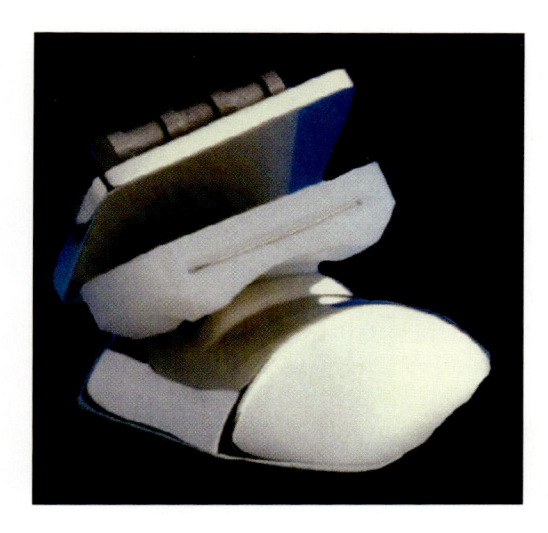

Fig. 6.24. S.T.A.R. ankle.
The cementless S.T.A.R. (Scandinavian Total Ankle Replacement) design is a three-component prosthesis (see text). *(From Waldemar Link in Hamburg, Germany, with permission)*

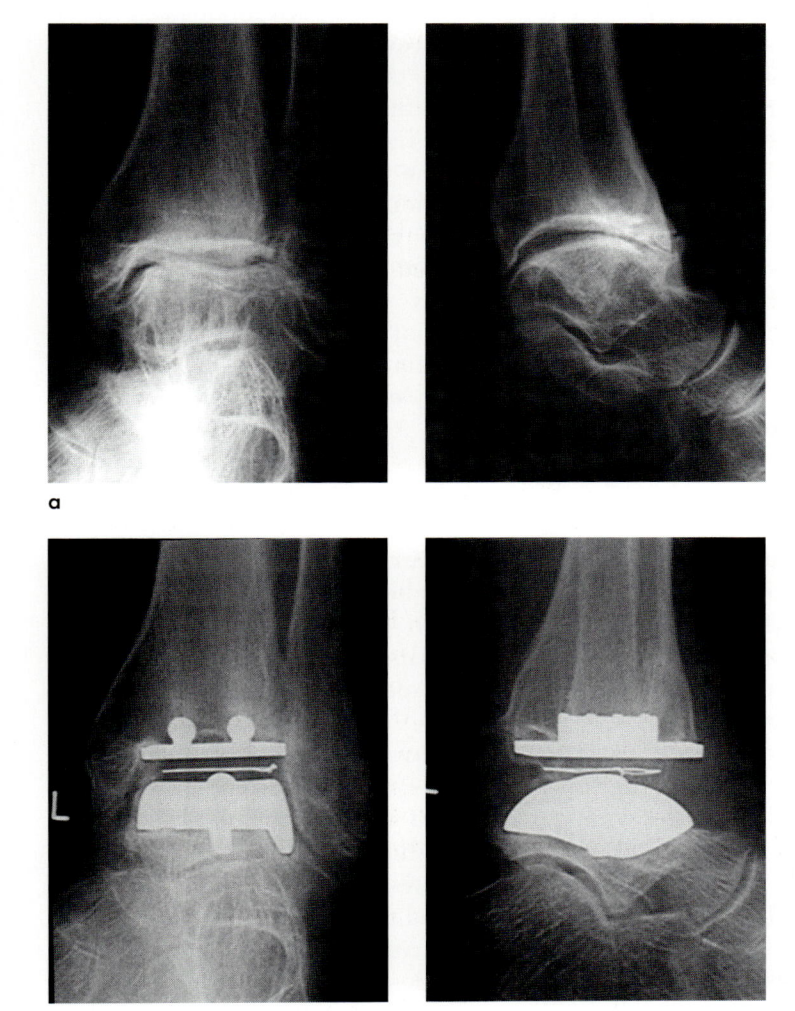

Fig. 6.25. S.T.A.R. ankle – clinical case 1.
Post-traumatic osteoarthrosis after ankle fracture (female, 71 years) (**a**). Unlimited function and extremely satisfied patient after seven years (**b**). Of some concern are the trabeculae running to the fixation bars while there is a cavitation behind the tibial implant

occur. Another concern may be the thin, 2-mm tibial plateau, which may not be strong enough to resist shear and torque forces.

On the talar side, fixation is obtained by press fit and one central fin. Theoretically, a hole in the hard talar body that is either too small or too shallow (for example, in post-traumatic ankles) would hinder the complete settling of the component while squeezing in, or it may lead to fracture of the talus while press fitting the component; whereas, too large a hole would not provide stability to the component.

A specific problem that may result from the non-anatomic, cylindrical design of the talar component is that motion may be restricted and movement transfer may occur about a single axis of rotation relative to the talus [40, 41]. This, in turn, may overstress the medial ankle ligaments and capsule because of the oversized medial radius. This overstress of the medial soft-tissue structures may explain medial ankle pain and posteromedial ossifications that restrict range of motion, as recently reported (Fig. 6.25, see also Fig. 11.14, Chap. 11: Complications of Total Ankle Replacement) [1, 39, 42].

The three-component design has intrinsic congruency between the metal and polyethylene, which is thought to lead to low-peak polyethylene stresses [4, 22, 24]. The contact area of only 320 mm^2 on the talar surface could be critical, particularly because it also incorporates a 10-mm long by 3-mm wide ridge to guide the polyethylene inlay. First, the groove could weaken the meniscal bearing. Second, the short (10-mm long) central ridge of the talar component that moves within this groove could create edge loading to the polyethylene inlay, thus provoking wear along the groove. In three revision cases where significant polyethylene wear occurred, most wear was detected along this capture mechanism [39]. With larger sizes of prosthesis, an additional problem could be size mismatch between the polyethylene inlay and the talar or tibial component mobile bearing, because there is a standard-sized polyethylene inlay.

Inversion and eversion can occur only when the inlay tilts up from one or the other of the two components, a condition that results in edge loading (see Figs. 11.3 and 11.17, Chap. 11: Complications of Total Ankle Replacement). This may cause excessive contact stress on the polyethylene. Theoretically, this effect would be exacerbated by a stiff hindfoot [39].

6.9 TNK Ankle

The TNK (Takakura Nara Kyocera) ankle prosthesis was designed in 1980 by Dr. Y. Takakura, in Nara, Japan, and is manufactured by Kyocera Corporation, Kyoto, Japan, a company that specializes in bioceramic medical products.

6.9.1 Background and Design

The current third-generation TNK ankle has evolved from a variety of previous designs. In its early form, the TNK ankle consisted of metal and polyethylene, and was implanted with the use of cement. Today, it is a fixed-bearing, cementless, ceramic-on-polyethylene prosthesis with a partially conforming articulation (Fig. 6.27a). Bony fixation is achieved through the use of hydroxyapatite-coated beads, cultured stem cells, and a bicortical tibial fixation screw (Fig. 6.27b). The ceramic concave talus articulates with a flat polyethylene tray that includes a flange to resurface the medial recess. The polyethylene tray is secured to the ceramic tibial tray.

6.9.2 Results

In a study by Takakura et al, loosening and subsidence was found to be a major problem with this design (especially in patients with rheumatoid arthritis) [38], involving 100% of ankles implanted with an initial metal-polyethylene design after 9.2 years. Typically the sinking process began to appear about five years postoperatively, especially in the cemented cases, and worsened with time. At 4.1 years, of the 30 uncemented ankles, seven (23%) components showed some degree of subsidence, and six screws (20%) had broken [38]. Six ankles (20%) required revision, five for subsidence or impingement because of subsidence. Despite this, 67% of the ankles were described as good or excellent (Figs. 6.28 and 6.29).

6.9 TNK Ankle

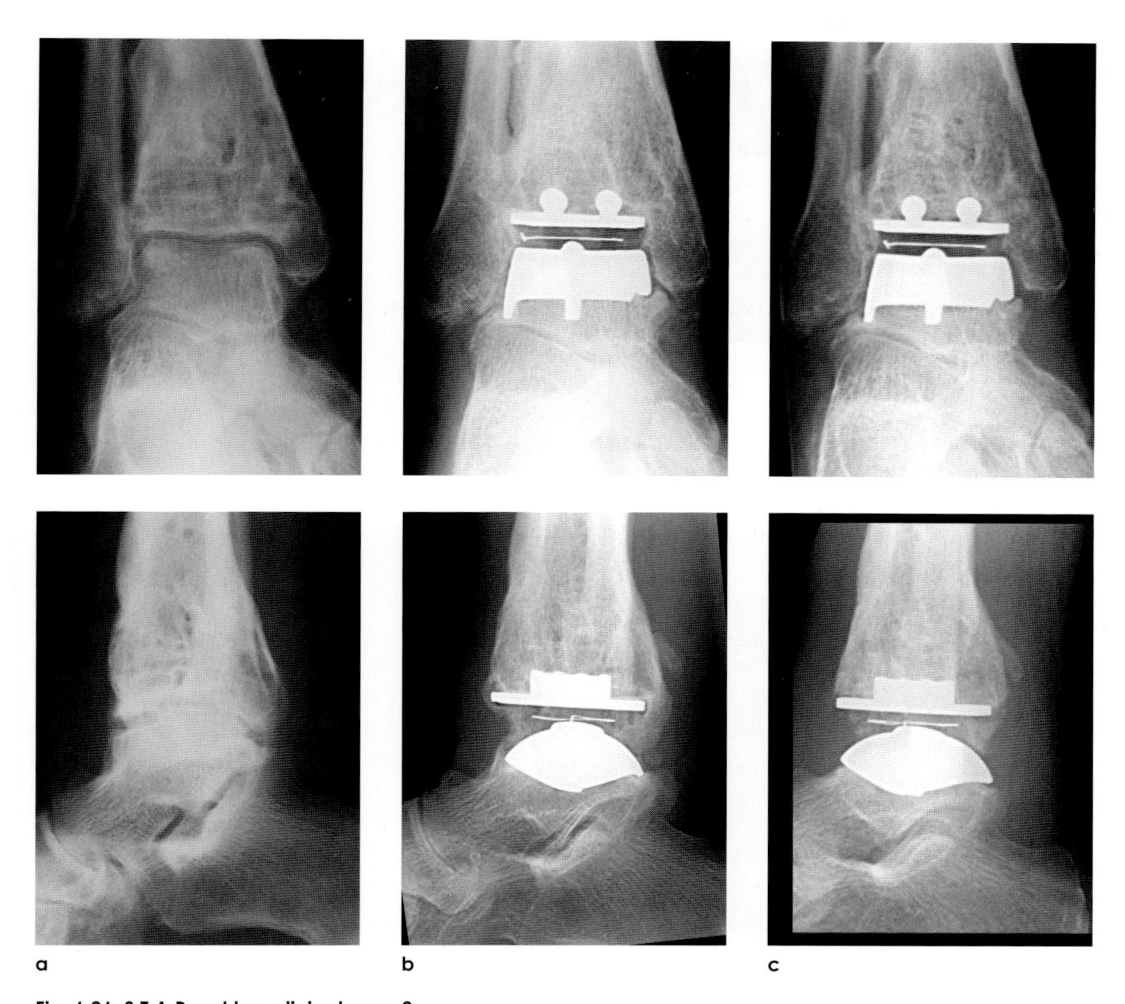

Fig. 6.26. S.T.A.R. ankle – clinical case 2.
Post-traumatic osteoarthrosis six years after tibial pilon fracture (male, 62 years) (**a**). Painful stiffness with peri-articular ossifications 19 months after total ankle replacement (**b**). To rectify the situation, open arthrolysis and resection of the ossifications were done, in combination with prophylactic one-stage irradiation. Since then, the patient has experienced unlimited function without any pain. This X-ray (**c**) shows the ankle 68 months after total ankle replacement

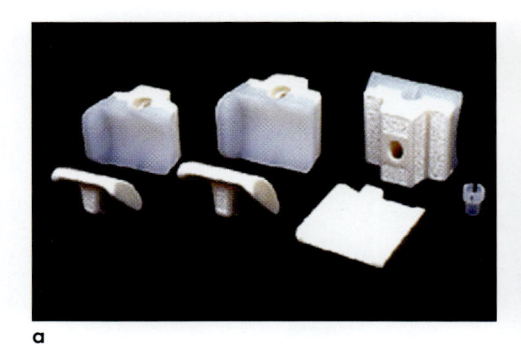

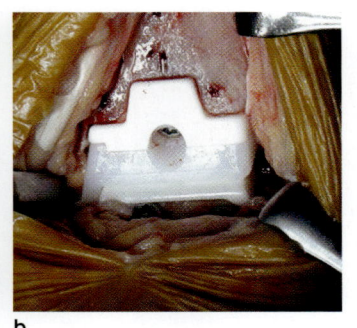

Fig. 6.27. TNK ankle.
The TNK (Takakura Nara Kyocera) ankle prosthesis is a fixed-bearing, cementless, ceramic-on-polyethylene prosthesis with a partially conforming articulation (**a**); third-generation implant with hydroxyapatite coating and used with applied cultured mesenchymal stem cells from patient's bone marrow (**b**). *(Courtesy of Dr. Y. Takakura, Nara, Japan)*

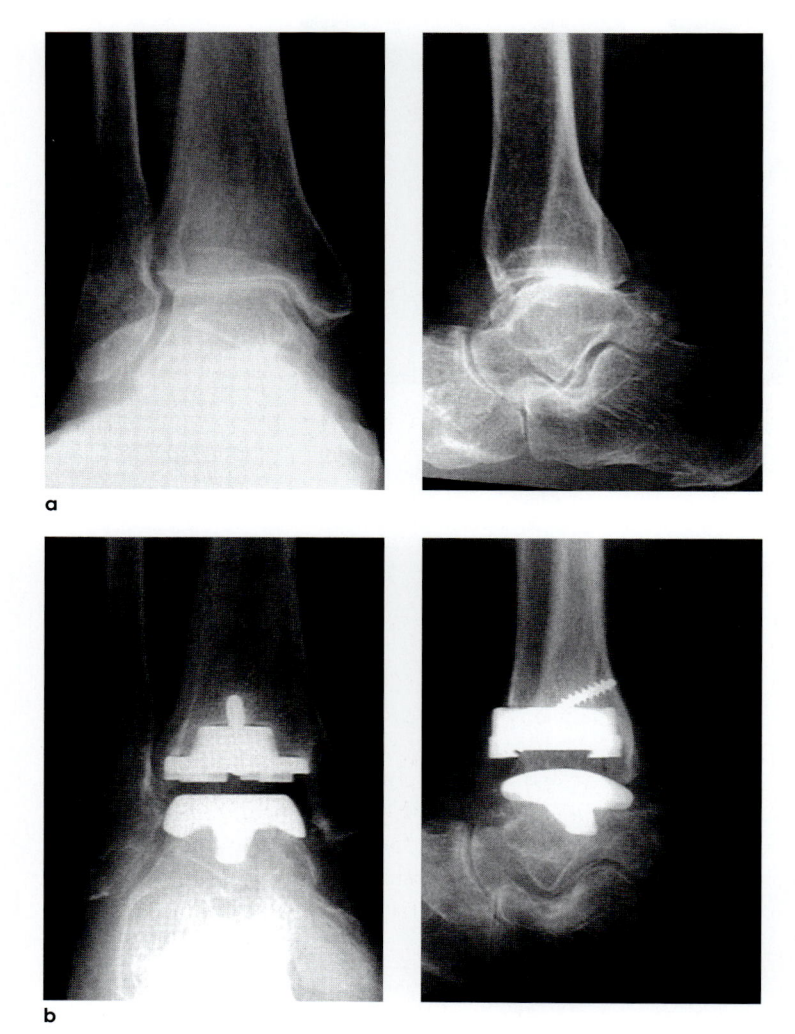

Fig. 6.28. TNK ankle – clinical case 1.
Primary osteoarthritis (female, 64 years) (**a**). Stable and well-aligned implants after one year (**b**). Of some concern is the undersized and bulky tibial component that does not fully cover the posterior aspect of the tibial metaphysis. *(Courtesy of Dr. Y. Takakura, Nara, Japan)*

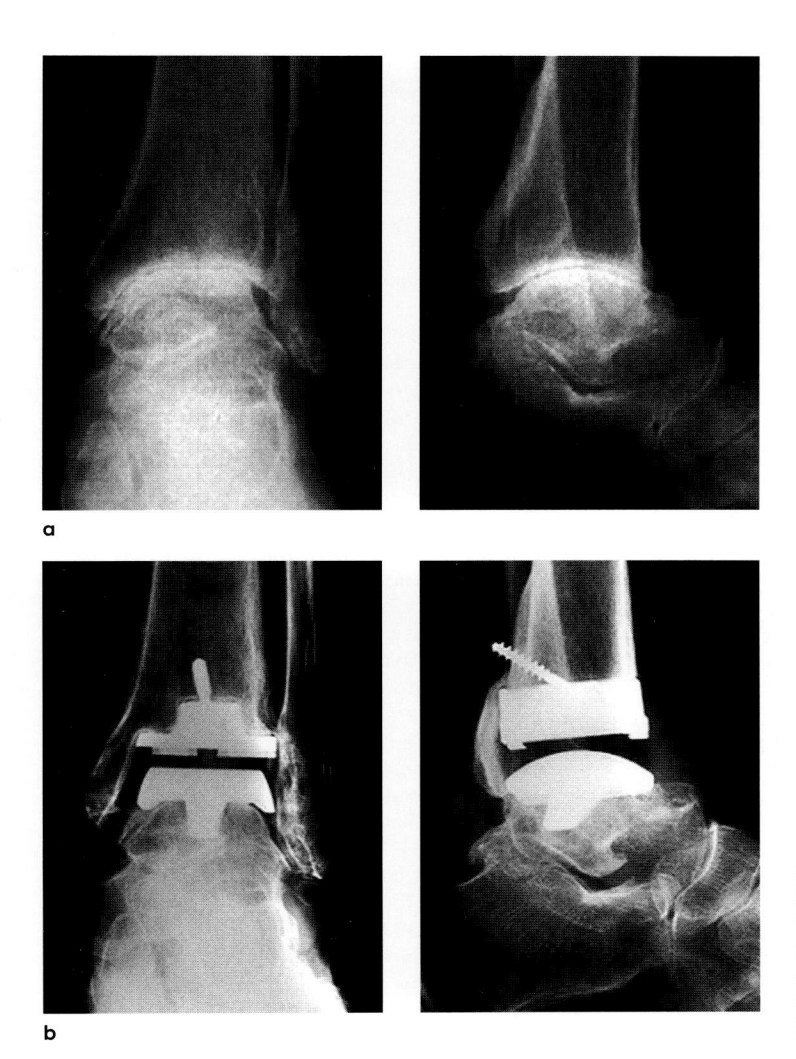

Fig. 6.29. TNK ankle – clinical case 2.
Primary osteoarthritis (female, 65 years) (**a**). Stable and well-aligned implants after 10 years (**b**). Patient has unlimited function and is extremely satisfied. Of some concern are the lucency lines along the tibial component and the extensive posterior ossification. *(Courtesy of Dr. Y. Takakura, Nara, Japan)*

6.9.3 Concerns

The TNK ankle has the same articulation as earlier two-component prostheses, which may transfer excessive shear and torque to the prosthesis-bone interface. These forces may be additionally increased by the bulky design, especially on tibial side. The TNK ankle requires removal of more bone stock than other designs (particularly the mobile-bearing designs), which results in fixation into mechanically inferior bone.

The TNK differs from previous two-component designs only in fixation method. The performance of hydroxyapatite-coated ceramic in osseointegration is, however, unknown. The long-term outcome of a partially conforming ceramic-polyethylene implant is also unknown.

6.10 Conclusions

With the exception of the TNK and AGILITY™ ankles, the current prostheses are three-component designs that include a mobile insert system. All but one (the titanium Buechel-Pappas™) prosthesis are composed of cobalt-chromium and rely on cementless fixation by bony ingrowth. The first-to-intermediate results have been superior to those of the first-generation prostheses. For long-term success, however, further efforts may be necessary to properly address alignment and ligament balancing, which can be better achieved the more closely the normal anatomy and biomechanics of the ankle are mimicked.

References

[1] Anderson T, Montgomery F, Carlsson A (2003) Uncemented S.T.A.R. total ankle prosthesis. Three to eight-year follow-up of fifty-one consecutive ankles. J Bone Joint Surg Am 85: 1321–1329

[2] Bonnin M, Judet T, Colombier J, Piriou P, Gravaleau N, Buscayret F (2004) Mid-term results of the SALTO total ankle prosthesis. Clin Orthop 424: 6–18

[3] Buechel FF, Buechel FF, Pappas MJ (2002) Eighteen-year evaluation of cementless meniscal bearing total ankle replacements. AAOS Instruct. Course Lect., chap 16, pp 143–151

[4] Buechel FF, Pappas MJ, Iorio LJ (1988) New Jersey low contact stress total ankle replacement: biomechanical rationale and review of 23 cementless cases. Foot Ankle 8: 279–290

[5] Collier JP, Mayor MB, McNamara JL, Surprenant VA, Jensen RE (1991) Analysis of the failure of 122 polyethylene inserts from uncemented tibial knee components. Clin Orthop 273: 232–242

[6] Doets HC (1998) The low contact stress Buechel-Pappas total ankle prosthesis. In: Current status of ankle arthroplasty (Kofoed H, ed), chap 6. Springer, Berlin, pp 29–33

[7] Engh GA, Dwyer KA, Hanes CK (1992) Polyethylene wear of metal-backed tibial components in total and unicompartmental knee prostheses. J Bone Joint Surg Br 74: 9–17

[8] Furlong RJ, Osborn JF (1991) Fixation of hip prostheses by hydroxyapatite ceramic coatings. J Bone Joint Surg Br 73: 741–745

[9] Gill LH (2002) Principles of joint arthroplasty as applied to the ankle. AAOS Instruct. Course Lect., chap 13, pp 117–128

[10] Hartman MK, Banks SA, Hodge WA (1997) Wear analysis of a retrieved hip implant with titanium nitride coating. J Arthroplasty 12: 938–945

[11] Hintermann B (1999) The S.T.A.R. ankle. Short- to midterm experience. Orthopäde 28: 792–803

[12] Hintermann B, Valderrabano V, Dereymaeker G, Dick W (2004) The HINTEGRA ankle: rationale and short-term results of 122 consecutive ankles. Clin Orthop 424: 57–68

[13] Hvid I, Rasmussen O, Jensen NC, Nielsen S (1985) Trabecular bone strength profiles at the ankle joint. Clin Orthop 199: 306–312

[14] Kitaoka HB, Alexander IJ, Adalaar RS, Nunley JA, Myerson MS, Sanders M (1994) Clinical rating systems for the ankle-hindfoot, midfoot, hallux, and lesser toes. Foot-Ankle Int 15: 349–353

[15] Kofoed H (1986) A new total ankle joint prosthesis. In: Material sciences and implant orthopaedic surgery (Kossowsky R, Kossowsky N, eds). Martinus-Nijhoff, Dordrecht, pp 75–84

[16] Kofoed H (1995) Cylindrical cemented ankle arthroplasty: a prospective series with long-term follow-up. Foot Ankle Int 16: 474–479

[17] Kofoed H (1998) Medium-term results of cementless Scandinavian total ankle replacement prosthesis (LINK S.T.A.R.) for osteoarthrosis. In: Current status of ankle arthroplasty (Kofoed H, ed), chap 24. Springer, Berlin, pp 116–120

[18] Kofoed H, Danborg L (1995) Biological fixation of ankle arthroplasty. Foot 5: 27–31

[19] Kofoed H, Sorensen TS (1998) Ankle arthroplasty for rheumatoid arthritis and osteoarthritis: prospective long-term study of cemented replacements. J Bone Joint Surg Br 80: 328–332

[20] Lin S, Drzala M (1998) Independent evaluation of Buechel-Pappas 2nd generation cementless total ankle arthroplasty; intermediate-term results. In: Proc. American Orthopaedic Foot and Ankle Society Specialty Day Meeting, New Orleans, USA

[21] Long M, Rack HJ (1998) Titanium alloys in total joint replacement: a materials science perspective. Biomaterials 19: 1621–1639

[22] McIff TE (2002) Design factors affecting the contact stress patterns in a contemporary mobile bearing total ankle replacement. In: Proc. of the 4th Biomechanics World Congress, 4th–9th August, Calgary, Canada

[23] Mendolia G (1998) Ankle arthroplasty – the Ramses prosthesis. In: Current status of ankle arthroplasty (Kofoed H, ed), chap 21. Springer, Berlin, pp 99–105

[24] Pappas A, Buechel FF (2002) Principles of condylar joint replacement – design and design evaluation. In: Proc Sir John Charnley International Arthroplasty Symposium, Total Ankle Arthroplasty, June 28th, Wrightington Hospital, UK

[25] Pappas MJ, Makris G, Buechel FF (1995) Titanium nitride ceramic film against polyethylene. A 48 million cycle wear test. Clin Orthop 317: 64–70

[26] Pyevich MT, Saltzman CL, Callaghan JJ, Alvine FG (1998) Total ankle arthroplasty: a unique design. Two to twelve-year follow-up. J Bone Joint Surg Am 80: 1410–1420

[27] Raimondi MT, Pietrabissa R (2000) The *in vivo* wear performance of prosthetic femoral heads with titanium bitride coating. Biomaterials 21: 907–913

[28] Rippstein PF (2003) Clinical experiences with three different designs of ankle prostheses. Foot Ankle Clin 7: 817–831

[29] Rudigier J, Grundei H, Menzinger F (2001) Prosthetic replacement of the ankle in posttraumatic arthrosis. Europ J Trauma 2: 66–74

[30] Saltzman CL, Alvine FG (2002) The AGILITY total ankle replacement. AAOS Instruct. Course Lect., chap 14, pp 129–134

[31] Saltzman CL, Knecht SL, Callaghan JJ, Estin M, Alvine FG (2004) AGILITY total ankle arthroplasty: a 7 to 16 year follow-up study. In: Proc. AAOS Congress, San Francisco, USA

[32] Saltzman CL, McIff TE, Buckwalter JA, Brown TD (2000) Total ankle replacement revisited. J Orthop Sports Phys Ther 30: 56–67

[33] Schernberg F (1998) Current results of ankle arthroplasty: European multi-centre study of cementless ankle arthroplasty. In: Current status of ankle arthroplasty (Kofoed H, ed). Springer, Berlin, pp 41–46

References

[34] Spirt AA, Assal M, Hansen ST Jr (2004) Complications and failures after total ankle arthroplasty. In: J Bone Joint Surg Am 86: 1172–1178

[35] Stamatis ED, Myerson MS (2002) How to avoid specific complications of total ankle replacement. Foot Ankle Clin 7: 765–789

[36] Stauffer RN (1979) Total joint arthroplasty. The ankle. Mayo Clin Proc 54: 570–575

[37] Stormont DM, Morrey BF, An KN, Cass JR (1985) Stability of the loaded ankle. Am J Sports Med 13: 295–300

[38] Takakura Y, Yanaka Y, Sugimoto K, Tamai S, Masuhara K (1990) Ankle arthroplasty. A comparative study of cemented metal and uncemented ceramic prostheses. Clin Orthop 252: 209–216

[39] Valderrabano V, Hintermann B, Dick W (2004) Scandinavian total ankle replacement: a 3.7-year average follow-up of 65 patients. Clin Orthop 424: 47–56

[40] Valderrabano V, Hintermann B, Nigg BM, Stefanyshyn D, Stergiou P (2003) Kinematic changes after fusion and total replacement of the ankle, part 1: range of motion. Foot Ankle Int 24: 881–887

[41] Valderrabano V, Hintermann B, Nigg BM, Stefanyshyn D, Stergiou P (2003) Kinematic changes after fusion and total replacement of the ankle, part 2: movement transfer. Foot Ankle Int 24: 888–896

[42] Wood PL, Deakin S (2003) Total ankle replacement. The results in 200 ankles. J Bone Joint Surg Br 85: 334–341

[43] Wood PLR, Clough TM (2004) Mobile bearing ankle replacement: clinical and radiographic comparison of two designs. In: Proc. AAOS Congress, San Francisco, USA

Chapter 7

PREOPERATIVE CONSIDERATIONS FOR TOTAL ANKLE ARTHROPLASTY

No consensus exists regarding the indications and contraindications for total ankle arthroplasty. The indications for first-generation total ankle arthroplasty were initially broad and included patients of all ages and diagnoses. These indications narrowed rapidly when poor intermediate-term results and high complication rates became apparent, as described in Chap. 5: History of Total Ankle Arthroplasty [5, 30, 34, 44, 46, 52]. As more experience is gained using modern second-generation arthroplasty techniques, surgical confidence in the outcome of ankle joint replacement is rising, and ankle replacement is being more frequently performed [10, 24, 41]. Perhaps the most critical aspect of promoting a successful outcome (aside from intraoperative factors) is proper patient selection.

The ideal patient for a total ankle arthroplasty is an elderly person with low physical demands, who is of normal weight, and who has good bone stock, normal vascular status, no immunosuppression, intact soft tissues, excellent hindfoot-ankle alignment, and a stable ankle that still has some motion left [24, 40, 41, 46]. By contrast, the use of total ankle arthroplasty in middle-age patients, manual laborers, and those with high physical demands, should be considered only when there is no other reasonable alternative [18, 41, 46].

7.1 Indications

In general, total ankle arthroplasty is indicated for severe, end-stage primary osteoarthrosis, inflammatory arthritis, and post-traumatic osteoarthrosis of the tibiotalar joint that is refractory to conservative measures (Table 7.1). A patient with bilateral ankle arthritis or ipsilateral hindfoot arthritis who has or will require a subtalar (fusion of the talocalcaneal joint) or triple arthrodesis (fusion of the talocalcaneal, talonavicular, and calcaneocuboid joints) is a particularly appropriate candidate for total ankle arthroplasty, because bilateral ankle and pantalar (ankle and triple) arthrodeses drastically reduce the physiology of the hindfoot [24, 41]. Another consideration is that the patient should be a mature individual, probably over the age of 50 years [18]. Some surgeons also consider using total ankle arthroplasty in

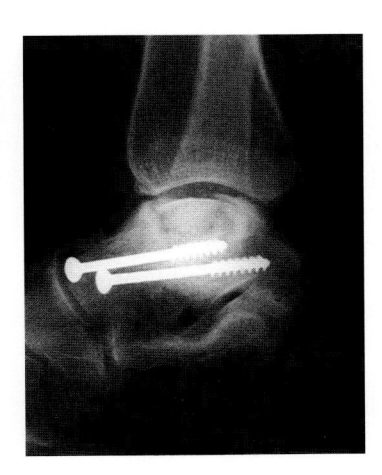

Fig. 7.1. Post-traumatic osteoarthrosis of the ankle after talus fracture.
Extensive osteonecrosis of the talar body with painful secondary osteoarthritis 6.5 years after talus fracture (male, 49 years old)

Table 7.1. Indications and contraindications of total ankle replacement

Indications:
- Primary osteoarthrosis
- Secondary/systemic osteoarthritis (that is, inflammatory arthritis)
  - rheumatoid arthritis
  - hemochromatosis (that is, hemophiliac arthritis)
  - mixed connective tissue disorders (that is, scleroderma, lupus erythematosus)
  - synovial inflammatory conditions
  - psoriatic arthritis
  - septic arthritis (if there is no current or active infection)
- Post-traumatic osteoarthrosis
  - after ankle fracture
  - after tibial pilon fracture
  - after talus fracture (if there is no severe dislocation)
  - after ankle sprains (chronic ankle instability)
  - avascular osteonecrosis (AVN) (if limited to less than 25% of the talar body)

If there is:
- Good bone stock
- Normal vascular status
- No immunosuppression
- Correct hindfoot-ankle alignment
- Well-preserved ankle joint motion
- Sufficient medial and lateral ankle stability
- Low physical demand sports activities (for example, biking, swimming, walking, golfing)

Relative contraindications:
- Previous severe trauma
  - open fracture of the ankle
  - fracture with dislocation of the talar body
  - with segmental bone loss (talus or tibia)
- Avascular necrosis (AVN) of the talus (of 25% to 50% of the talar body)
- Severe osteopenia or osteoporosis
- Long-term use of steroids (systemic, local)
- Insulin-dependent diabetes mellitus
- Demanding sports activities (for example, tennis, jogging, alpine skiing)

Absolute contraindications:
- Neuroarthropathic degenerative disease (Charcot's ankle)
- Active or recent infection
- Avascular necrosis (AVN) of the talus (of more than 50% of the talar body)
- Severe benign joint hypermobility syndrome
- Non-reconstructable malalignment (of 20° or greater varus or valgus)
- Severe soft-tissue problems around the ankle
- Sensory or motor dysfunction of the foot or leg
- High physical demand sports activities (for example, contact sports)

younger patients with post-traumatic osteoarthrosis [18, 24, 32] or rheumatoid arthritis [4, 24, 33, 49], despite the fact that these patients normally have higher physical demands. To some extent, partial avascular necrosis of the talar dome is also an indication for total ankle arthroplasty. This may be particularly true for osteochondral defects after failed alternative treatments. In the case of osteonecrosis secondary to a talus fracture, however, arthroplasty is not indicated (Fig. 7.1).

The final determination of the clinical indications for total ankle arthroplasty, however, should be influenced by intermediate and long-term results, comparison of results with those of other treatment options (for example, arthrodesis), and the feasibility of salvage after failure.

7.2 Contraindications

The contraindications for total ankle arthroplasty are better defined than the indications. Most current contraindications, derived from patient factors in previous studies that were associated with unacceptably high rates of complications and early failure, can be divided into absolute and relative contraindications [35].

Absolute contraindications (Table 7.1) include neuroarthropathic degenerative joint disease (Charcot's ankle), active or recent infection, significant avascular necrosis of the talus (more than 50% of the talar body; especially for cementless talar fixation), a compromised soft-tissue envelope around the ankle, neurological dysfunction of the foot or leg, severe non-reconstructable malalignment (20° or greater varus or valgus deformity), or ligamentous instability (for example, chronic ankle instability) of the ankle or hindfoot [10, 18, 24, 41, 40, 46].

Relative contraindications (Table 7.1) include young age, high physical demands, previous and successfully treated osteomyelitis of the ankle, previous severe open fracture of the ankle, previous dislocation fracture of the talus, segmental bone loss, long-term steroid use (for example, in cases of rheumatoid arthritis, ulcerative colitis, Crohn's disease, etc.), insulin-dependent diabetes mellitus, and severe osteoporosis [10, 18, 24, 35, 37, 44].

7.3 Considerations Specific to Total Ankle Replacement Surgery

The successful outcome of a total ankle replacement is closely related to the evaluation and correct management of potential pre- or intraoperative risk factors.

7.3.1 Rheumatoid Arthritis and Inflammatory Arthropathy

In patients with rheumatoid arthritis and other inflammatory arthropathies, first-generation cemented and constrained implants have been associated with an increased risk of prosthetic subsidence caused by poor bone quality. There was also an increased risk of perioperative complications such as postoperative wound infection, and late aseptic loosening owing to chronic synovitis in the subtalar joint [10, 12]. Several reports on patients with rheumatoid arthritis who underwent total ankle arthroplasty with first-generation implants concluded that the implants were prone to early failure and that clinical results deteriorated with time, resulting in an unacceptably high revision rate [8, 9, 22, 28, 27, 29, 30, 31, 47, 52]. Conversely, Kofoed and Sorensen [33], using a second-generation implant with cement fixation, reported no difference in implant survival or clinical outcome between patients with rheumatoid arthritis and those with osteoarthrosis. Overall implant survival was 75% at an average follow-up of nine years. Similar favorable results for patients with rheumatoid arthritis were reported for second- and third-generation semi- and nonconstrained, uncemented implants [4, 23, 25, 48, 49, 50, 51]. These newer implants require less bony resection for implantation, thus preserving the underlying subchondral bone that is so critical for long-term stability [3, 7, 16, 17, 24, 25, 45].

Because patients with rheumatoid or inflammatory arthritis often have progressive, symmetric involvement in the surrounding joints of the hindfoot and transverse tarsal joints over time [1], ankle arthrodesis potentially accelerates the degeneration of these adjacent joints [35]. These patients will, therefore, be subjected to further arthrodesis. Given the generally poor functional results after pantalar arthrodesis [41], an alternative treatment (such as total ankle arthroplasty) that preserves some ankle joint motion is particularly favorable for these rheumatoid patients, who have generally low physical demands.

There is still, however, need for careful patient selection. Total ankle arthroplasty should be avoided in patients with significant vasculitis because of increased wound infection [1, 12], and used cautiously in patients who are taking immunosuppressive agents (for example, methotrexate or prednisone) in an active phase of the disease [10, 41]. To a small extent, total ankle replacement is also contraindicated in rheumatoid arthritis patients who have ligament insufficiency (deltoid, spring, or lateral ligament complex), significant ankle deformity (Fig. 7.2), or significant bony erosion (severe cystic deformation) in the ankle joint [10, 35, 36]. Rheumatoid arthritis patients with preserved or restored (that is, with subtalar or triple arthrodesis) alignment and ligamentous integrity, however, may be particularly well suited for total ankle arthroplasty.

> **The Author's Approach**
> In rheumatoid patients, if there is deformity, realignment of the ankle and foot must be achieved before total ankle replacement. In most instances, stable correction can only be obtained by arthrodesis of the hindfoot (either subtalar or triple arthrodesis), particularly in cases with associated ligamentous insufficiency. Such additional procedures can usually be performed in conjunction with total ankle replacement.

7.3.2 Infection

There is consensus that active or recent infection is a contraindication for total ankle arthroplasty or arthroplasty in general. There has been little discussion, however, in the orthopedic literature about ankle replacement in patients with previous infection of the ankle joint or the surrounding soft tissues (Fig. 7.3). Theoretically, there may be an increased risk of reinfection or reactivation of a subclinical infection after total ankle arthroplasty in these patients. In patients after total joint replacements (hip or knee), postoperative infection rates that are two to three times higher than in rheuma-

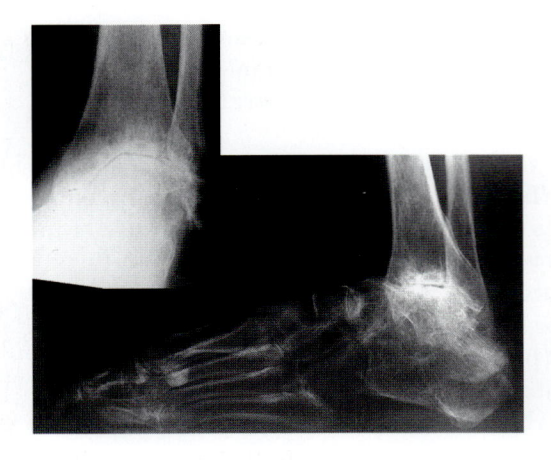

Fig. 7.2. Rheumatoid osteoarthritis of the ankle with severe malalignment.
In this rheumatoid arthritis patient (female, 54 years old), severe arthritis of the ankle with lateral ligament insufficiency resulted in an ankylotic varus and supinatus deformity

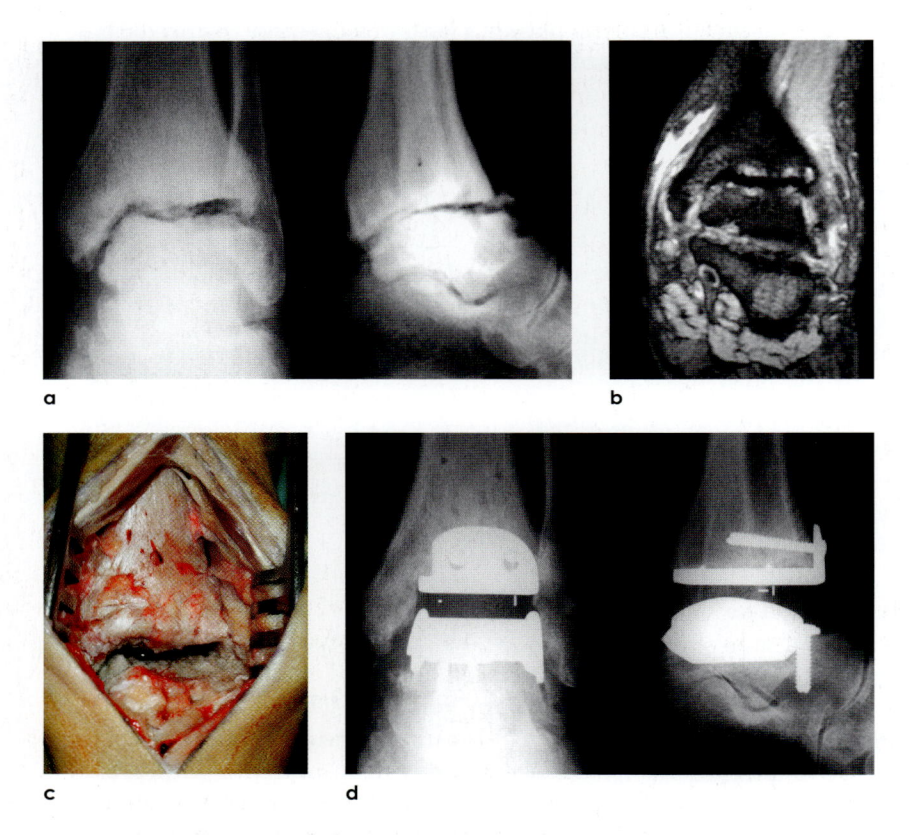

Fig. 7.3. Secondary ankle arthritis after septic arthritis.
Severe destruction of the ankle joint after septic arthritis (staphylococcus areus) following an intra-articular corticosteroid injection nine months prior (male, 55 years old). The X-rays (**a**) and MRI (**b**) reveal an extensive subchondral delamination and edema with cyst formation, and surgical exposure (**c**) shows the destruction process. View (**d**) shows the implants well integrated into the bone 12 months after replacement, with no evidence of recurrent infection

toid arthritis patients have been reported [21]. Diabetes mellitus, obesity, malnutrition, and oral corticosteroid use also have been associated with an increased risk of infection [21].

It is, therefore, necessary to perform a careful evaluation of patients with previous infection or predisposing factors, including a thorough history, physical examination, and assessment of the overlying skin and soft tissue. Laboratory analysis may include an evaluation of the differential leukocyte count, and C-reactive protein level. Additional work-up may include a technetium-99 bone scan or, for a higher specificity and sensitivity for active infection, an indium-111 leukocyte scan [10]. Magnetic resonance imaging (MRI) may further help to identify osteomyelitic processes in the subchondral bone.

> **The Author's Approach**
> Once an active infection and/or osteomyelitis process have been excluded or appropriately treated, total ankle replacement is undertaken without any additional modalities. During surgery, however, bone biopsies are harvested for bacteriologic analysis, which allows (if necessary) specific long-term antibiotic therapy. To date, late infection has not been observed in any case after total ankle arthroplasty in a previously infected ankle (see Fig. 7.3).

7.3.3 Osteopenia and Osteoporosis

The primary concern with total ankle replacement in patients with osteopenia or osteoporosis is inadequate bony fixation and early subsidence of the components, particularly in the tibial component (Fig. 7.4). Previous studies by Hvid et al [26] have emphasized that the tibial bone is up to 40% weaker than the corresponding talar bone, and that, after removing only 5 mm of bone, there is a tremendous loss of trabecular strength in the distal tibia. Theoretically, this problem can be solved by using a larger implant with a larger corresponding surface area of contact, as is the case with the AGILITY™ ankle [3]. This prosthesis, however, also requires tibiofibular fusion and the removal of more bone, including the subchondral plate. The HINTEGRA® ankle, by contrast, offers three significant advantages:

- it requires minimal bone resection, thus preserving the subchondral plate,
- it has an anatomically shaped large implant, which allows bony support of the prosthesis on cortical bone,
- it has a flat design, and so does not weaken the cortical architecture of the distal tibia.

In a consecutive series of 122 HINTEGRA® ankles, no subsidence was observed in any patient, even though they were allowed to weight-bear immediately postoperatively [25].

Nevertheless, severe osteopenia or osteoporosis should generally be considered a relative contraindication to total ankle arthroplasty [10, 13, 40].

> **The Author's Approach**
> In cases with severe osteopenia or osteoporosis, special care is taken not to damage the bone surface after resection. For instance, no lamina spreader is inserted into the joint for distraction; instead, an externally fixed spreader with two K-wires (Hintermann™ Distractor, Newdeal®, Lyon, France) is used. In addition, the implant should be slightly larger than the resected bone surface to achieve fully circumferential cortical bone support, particularly on tibial side (Fig. 7.5).

7.3.4 Weight Restrictions

The specific configuration of the ankle joint with its considerable surface area of contact can tolerate joint reactive forces of four to six times body weight during gait [14, 35, 38, 43]. Patients with arthritic changes at the ankle joint tend to alter their gait to compensate for the decreased range of motion, thereby decreasing forces across the ankle to three times body weight, which has been shown to remain constant up to one year after total ankle arthroplasty [43]. Because stiffness usually increases with arthritic changes of the ankle and hindfoot joints, rotational and shear forces are suggested to be higher in patients with foot and ankle arthritis. Theoretically, the greater the body weight of the individual, the greater the forces that are transmitted to the implants after ankle replacement. However, the ratio of body mass index to im-

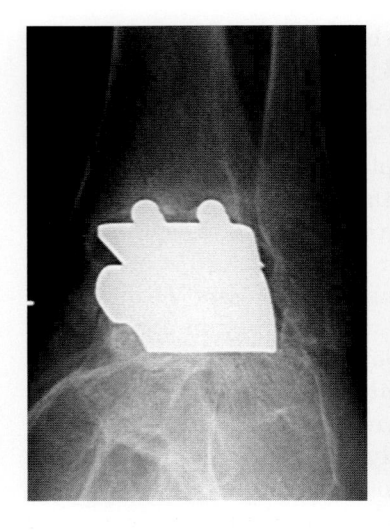

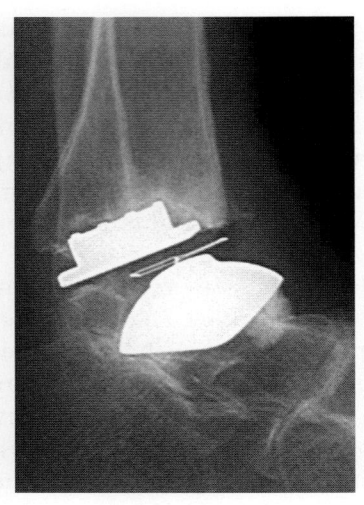

Fig. 7.4. Scleroderma-caused secondary osteoarthritis.
Breakdown of the implants immediately after implantation (first radiological control at six weeks) in severe osteopenia following chronic cortisone medication and immunosuppression because of aggressive scleroderma disease (female, 37 years old). The implants were left in place and did not show further subsidence. The patient has no pain in her prosthetic left ankle, can walk without aids, and is still happy with the result after 6.8 years

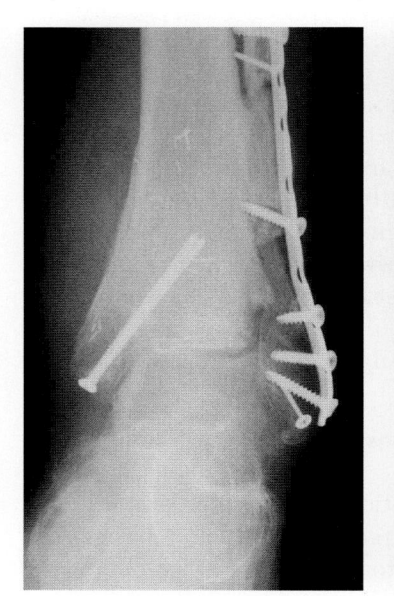

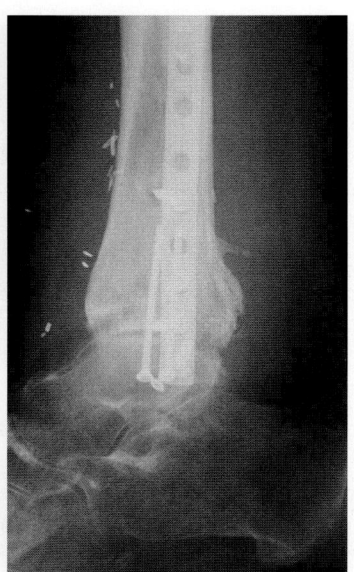

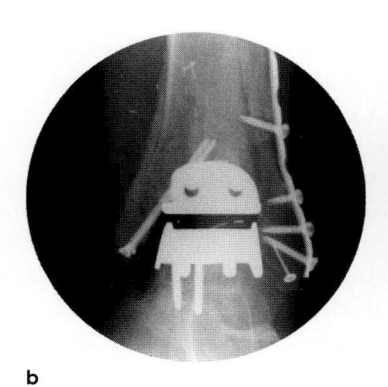

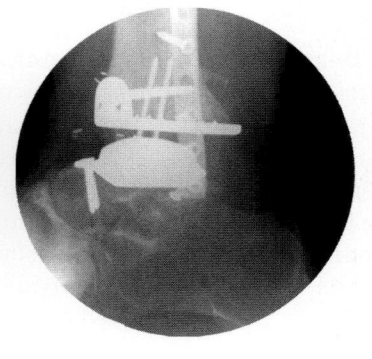

Fig. 7.5. Post-traumatic osteoarthrosis after open tibial pilon fracture.
Forty-two-year-old male patient with severe post-traumatic ankle arthritis 3.2 years after an open fracture of the tibial pilon that necessitated soft-tissue reconstruction by a vascularized flap. In order to cover the complete pericortical rim, relatively oversized TAR implants were used and the former osteosynthesis implants left in place. Preoperative X-rays (**a**); X-rays after total ankle replacement (**b**)

plant size is probably even more important than weight alone, especially with respect to potential subsidence of the talar component [12]. On the other hand, the few studies that have included patient weight in evaluating the outcome after total ankle arthroplasty have failed to show a correlation between patient weight and implant failure or pain [39].

> **The Author's Approach**
> Large or heavy patients require basically the same precautions as patients with severe osteopenia or osteoporosis. A thicker polyethylene inlay should also be considered, however, because of potential increased wear. A minimum thickness of 7 mm may be recommended.

7.3.5 Adjacent Joint Arthritis

The management of adjacent joint arthritis (subtalar and transverse tarsal joints) in the presence of an arthritic ankle is still a matter of considerable debate. The surgeon must first determine the severity of involvement of the adjacent joints, and must identify any deformity that may be present throughout these joints. Some surgeons propose to proceed with total ankle arthroplasty before subtalar or triple arthrodesis, particularly if there is no evidence of structural or rigid deformity [18]. On occasion, the affected joints (especially the subtalar and midfoot joints) will realign themselves while the prosthesis is being implanted because of the tension in the ankle and lengthening of the medial column that result from the procedure. Sometimes, especially in the post-traumatic population, even though significant radiographic changes are present and patients may have loss of motion, once the ankle is replaced, the adjacent joints no longer seem to be symptomatic, apparently due to the stress reduction that results from restoring normal motion at the ankle (Fig. 7.6). Conversely, some surgeons propose to proceed with subtalar or triple arthrodesis before total ankle arthroplasty in order to obtain a rigid plantigrade foot, particularly in the presence of fixed deformity, or in rheumatoid patients [12, 13, 18].

> **The Author's Approach**
> In post-traumatic patients, if there is no fixed deformity, total ankle arthroplasty may be done first. If this does not result in a properly aligned foot, additional fusion is considered at the same stage. If the foot is well aligned and stable after the total ankle arthroplasty, additional surgery

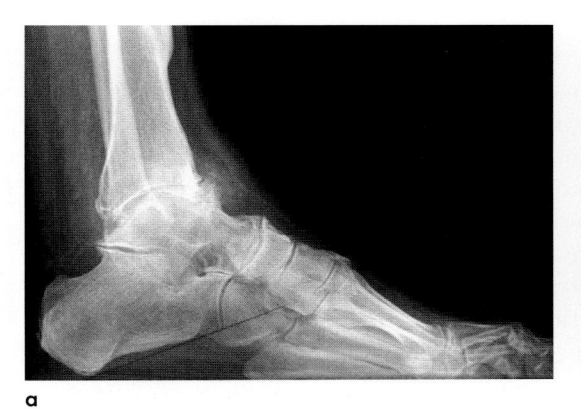

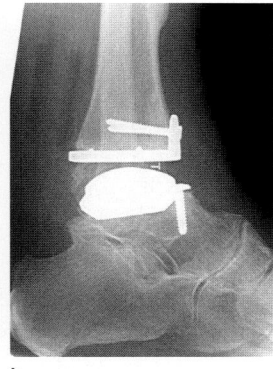

Fig. 7.6. Post-traumatic osteoarthrosis with pes equinus malalignment.
Painful post-traumatic osteoarthrosis 22 years after ankle fracture with fixed equinus position and significant degenerative changes in the adjacent joints, particularly the subtalar and talonavicular joints (male, 63 years old) (**a**). Preoperative examination revealed pain exclusively at the ankle joint, whereas the left pronation/supination movement (about 50% of the contralateral side) was pain free. Twelve months after total ankle replacement, the patient had no pain, was able to walk more than three hours at a stretch, and was extremely satisfied with the result (**b**)

> may be considered later, if necessary. In fact, such potential secondary surgery is very seldom necessary (estimated to be less than 5%). In rheumatoid patients, and particularly if there is a fixed deformity, a subtalar or triple arthrodesis is done first. If there are no special compromises, especially with regard to the soft-tissue envelope, total ankle arthroplasty is done later during the same surgery.

7.3.6 Lower Limb, Ankle, or Hindfoot Malalignment

Relevant deformity above the ankle can be either at the level of the knee joint or the tibial bone itself [20]. Unilateral compartment osteoarthrosis of the knee joint often results in secondary varus or valgus deformity, respectively. Post-traumatic malunion of a tibial shaft fracture leads predictably to ankle osteoarthrosis over the long-term. Such deformities or malalignments of the lower leg significantly affect the morphology of the ankle joint and should therefore be considered prior to implantation of a total ankle replacement.

In the case of deformity at the level of the knee joint, usually from degenerative wear of one femorotibial compartment (medial or lateral) of the joint, correction of the deformity should occur prior to total ankle arthroplasty. After the exclusion of multi-compartmental knee osteoarthrosis, high tibial valgisation osteotomy (when there is varus deformity) or supracondylar varisation femoral osteotomy (when there is valgus deformity) can realign the limb proximally in preparation for total ankle arthroplasty. When the knee joint is symptomatic, however, the patient should undergo a total knee replacement prior to total ankle arthroplasty.

Malalignment in the supramalleolar or distal tibial region that is greater than 10° in any plane (as is typically the case with post-traumatic malunion) requires corrective osteotomy at the level of the deformity before ankle arthroplasty (Fig. 7.7) [10, 12, 13, 19, 41]. Based on the author's preference, valgus deformity may be corrected by medial closed-wedge osteotomy, and varus deformity by medial open-wedge osteotomy. Additional fibular correction osteotomy or even multiplanar lower leg osteotomy may be necessary in certain cases.

Deformity also can occur at the level of the ankle joint itself. In most instances, this occurs in patients with post-traumatic osteoarthrosis (Fig. 2.2, Chap. 2: Characteristics of the Diseased Ankle). A patient with a severe lower leg fracture or pilon injury can end up with a varus tilt of the mortise if the fibula heals out to length but the tibia shortens. Similarly, valgus deformity may be seen when the fibula is shortened. Minor amounts of deformity can be corrected with bone cuts during replacement surgery.

Deformities in the foot may be the most common source of malalignment in patients with ankle osteoarthrosis. A varus ankle is commonly seen after recurrent ankle sprains (that is, chronic ankle instability). Frequently, the hindfoot and forefoot are in varus as well (Fig. 2.3, Chap. 2: Characteristics of the Diseased Ankle). A valgus ankle is the end result of severe acquired flatfoot, in which medial column support has been lost (Fig. 7.8). In either case, placing an ankle prosthesis onto a foot with persisting deformity leads to recurrent tilting of the talus, inlay subluxation, and early failure. Correcting the foot deformity before or simultaneously with total ankle arthroplasty is essential for optimal long-term results.

> **The Author's Approach**
> In the case of malalignment of the lower leg, the supramalleolar region should be corrected first, and total ankle replacement considered when the osteotomy has healed. By contrast, malalignment at the level of the ankle and foot is, in most instances, corrected at the time of total ankle replacement. As stated above, sometimes the insertion of a prosthesis into a collapsed ankle sufficiently realigns the foot and ankle by ligament tensioning, and no additional bony procedure is necessary.

7.3.7 Hindfoot-Ankle Instability

Ligamentous instability in the ankle can be managed either simultaneously or in a staged fashion through soft-tissue reconstruction. Valgus defor-

7.3 Considerations Specific to Total Ankle Replacement Surgery

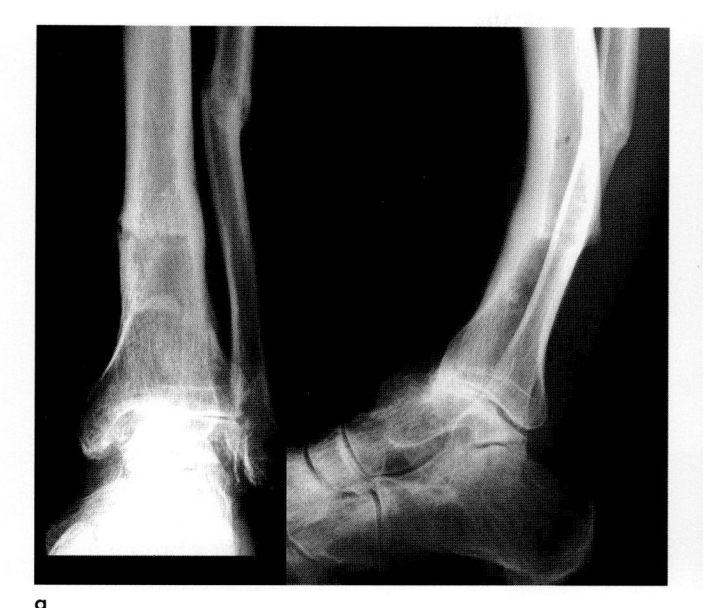

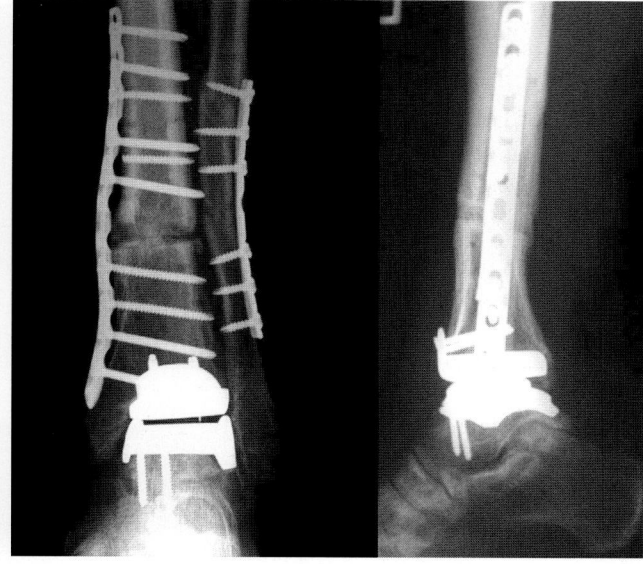

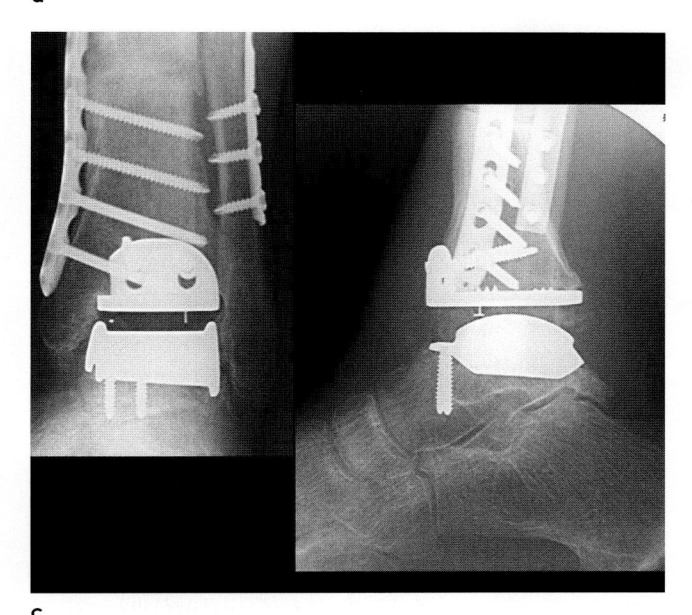

Fig. 7.7. Post-traumatic ankle osteoarthrosis and severe lower leg malunion.
Secondary osteoarthrosis of the left ankle 34 years after a midshaft fracture of the tibia and fibula (skiing accident) that healed in a recurvatum malunion of 35° (male, 68 years old, former downhill ski racer, still very active and skiing) (**a**). A one-stage correction of the malalignment and total ankle replacement was chosen for insurance reasons; although the author did not encounter any postoperative problems, he would definitively not recommend the one-stage approach because of the increased risk of soft-tissue problems. The patient was allowed free mobilization and full weight-bearing after four months, and he reported at the 12-month follow-up (**b**, **c**) that he had started downhill skiing 10 months after surgery

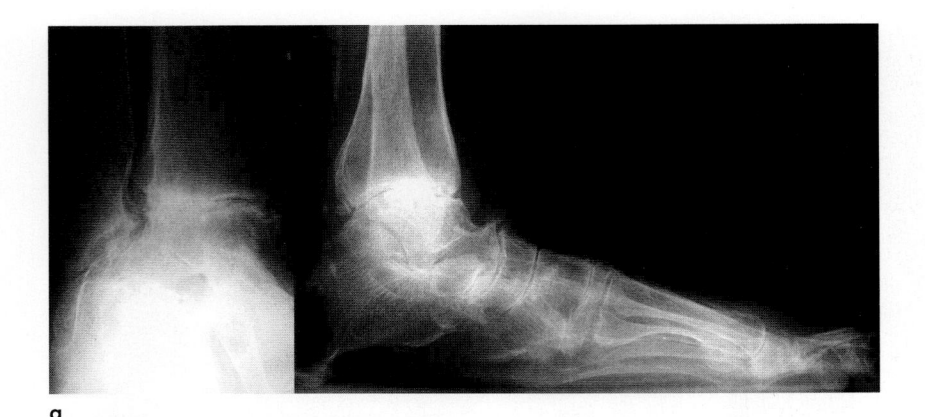

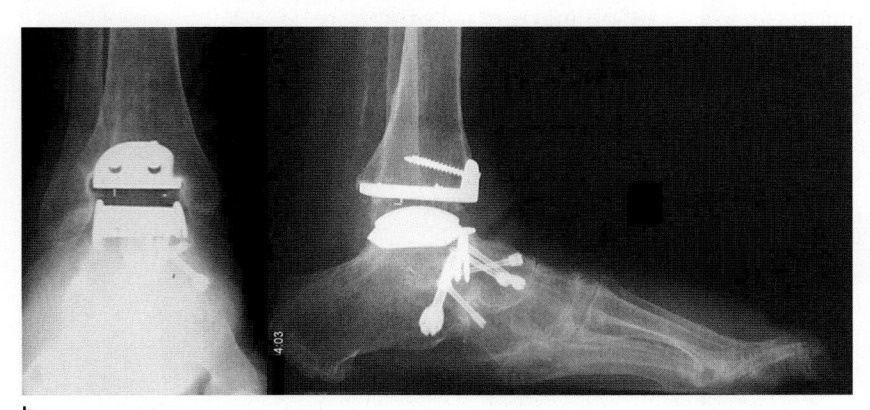

Fig. 7.8. Post-traumatic osteoarthrosis with hindfoot valgus.
Acquired valgus and flatfoot deformity seven years after ankle fracture, syndesmotic insufficiency and progressive posterior tibial tendon dysfunction with severe and painful lateral ankle/subfibular impingement (male, 69 years old) (**a**). The hindfoot and ankle are well aligned and stable two years after one-stage triple arthrodesis and total ankle replacement (**b**). At last follow-up the patient reported a high level of satisfaction, complete pain relief, and unlimited walking ability

mity associated with an incompetent deltoid-spring ligament complex is generally considered to be far more technically difficult than a varus deformity, and may be a contraindication to ankle arthroplasty [35]. Varus deformity that is associated with lateral ligamentous instability can be managed with direct anatomic lateral reconstruction, with or without medial release of the deltoid ligament, particularly for long-standing instability [19]. Results after total ankle arthroplasty in patients with ligamentous instability have been somewhat unpredictable, and those who have a clinically deficient deltoid ligament are at higher risk for subsequent failure of the arthroplasty [10].

The Author's Approach
In the case of mild but relevant pathology of the anterior talofibular ligament (for example, elongation or partial tear), this ligament may be reconstructed anatomically with local structures, if possible (that is, the Broström technique). In the case of anterior subluxation of the talus (for example, with total loss of anterior talofibular ligament function), plasty of the anterior talofibular ligament is necessary. The short peroneal tendon is split (in a modification of the Evans procedure) and then routed from posterior to anterior through a drill hole in the lateral mal-

leolus, to be attached under tension to the lateral talar neck. Although the author never performs such a non-anatomic ligament reconstruction in a normal foot, it seems to work well for this application.

In the case of varus ankle (for example, with loss of calcaneofibular ligament function), it is imperative to identify the location of any bony deformity prior to ligament reconstruction. A plantar-flexed first ray is common, and dorsiflexion osteotomy of the first metatarsal should be performed through a second small incision. If the heel remains in varus after ligament reconstruction (using anatomic locative or tendon plastic techniques), a lateral Z-shaped calcaneal osteotomy is performed, which allows the calcaneal tuber to be slid laterally and tilted into a physiological valgus. In most instances, muscular imbalance may be also present. If abnormal tightness of the long peroneal tendon is observed, it is tenodesed through a small incision over the cuboid to the base of the fifth metatarsal.

In the case of a valgus ankle, the resulting flatfoot is carefully examined to identify the collapsed joints and the incompetence pattern of the medial ligaments. First, the medial column is restored and the deltoid-spring ligament complex tensioned. If the hindfoot remains in valgus after the ankle and forefoot are realigned, then a medial sliding osteotomy of the calcaneus is performed through a lateral incision just posterior to the peroneal tendons, and the tuber is slid medially at least 1 cm. Advanced cases of flatfoot deformity and valgus ankle may require a triple arthrodesis in addition to medial column stabilization to achieve proper alignment.

7.3.8 Heel Cord Contracture

The question of whether a heel cord contracture or pes equinus deformity should be addressed by lengthening of the Achilles tendon is still a matter to debate [10, 19, 20]. Heel cord contracture can typically be managed at the time of total ankle arthroplasty. Technical options include superficial release of the gastrocnemius at the musculotendinous junction, open (Z-type) lengthening of the Achilles tendon, and percutaneous lengthening methods. One must take extreme care to avoid overlengthening the tendon distally, as this decreases plantar flexion, push-off power, and significantly affects gait. Conversely, a gastrocnemius release seems to offer the theoretic advantage of improving dorsiflexion without significantly affecting plantar flexion power [19]. Nevertheless, it must be emphasized that aponeurotomy always leads to substantial postoperative loss of muscle power [6].

The Author's Approach
Adequate decompression of the dorsal joint with meticulous removal of the entire dorsal capsule (and sometimes additional release of the dorsal aspect of the deep deltoid ligament) is usually sufficient to obtain about 5° to 10° of dorsiflexion, even in an ankle that has been in equinus for many years. The body then has the ability to stretch out the Achilles tendon over time and slowly regain the lost elasticity. If, however, a minimal dorsiflexion of 5° cannot be achieved through total ankle replacement, gastrocnemius release may be considered. This situation is encountered in nearly 3% of patients.

7.3.9 Soft-Tissue Considerations

Either contract skin scars or unstable chronic wound problems may be encountered in post-traumatic cases, or those with previous surgeries. Early referral to a plastic surgeon and competent examination of the cutaneous soft tissues may be of prophylactic importance, and may prevent unexpected postoperative exacerbations. In such cases, evaluation of macro- and microcirculation, sensitivity, neurological functions, and soft-tissue elasticity, clinically and by imaging techniques (for example, MRI, MR angiography, ultrasound), represents the golden standard.

7.3.10 Age Considerations

The ideal patient for total ankle arthroplasty is an elderly person with low physical demands. Because of the post-traumatic origin of up to 80% of ankle arthritis, however, patients with a painful end-stage arthritis are typically younger than those with severe hip or knee arthritis [12, 15].

Previous studies have suggested an increased risk of implant failure in younger patients with post-traumatic osteoarthrosis. Kitaoka and Patzer [30] reported, at an average follow-up of nine years after total ankle arthroplasty, a failure rate of 43% in patients younger than 57 years of age and of 26% in patients over 57 years of age. Stauffer and Segal [44], based on their outcome analyses, proposed that total ankle arthroplasty should not be considered in patients under 60 years of age with post-traumatic osteoarthrosis, and Alvine [2] recommended the procedure only for patients over 55 years of age. Spirt et al [42], in a five-year survivorship analysis on a series of 306 consecutive total ankle replacements using the AGILITY™ prosthesis, found age to be the only significant predictor of reoperation and failure of total ankle replacement.

On the other hand, Kofoed and Lundberg-Jensen [32] reported at a follow-up of six years, an implant survival rate of 75% in patients younger than 50 years of age (n=30; median age, 46 years [range, 22 to 49 years]) and of 81% in patients older than 50 years of age (n=70; median age, 63 years [range, 51 to 83 years]). This difference in implant survival was not significant. The authors did not find a statistical difference in the clinical outcome, the frequency of revision procedures, and/or conversion to ankle arthrodesis between the two groups of patients. Similar results have been reported by others [4, 48, 49].

Although a "recommended" range of age for candidates for total ankle arthroplasty has not been established, the longevity of an implant is clearly related to the amount of loading placed on the implants [41]. Younger, more active patients typically want to resume more vigorous activities after total ankle arthroplasty than do older, more sedentary patients [10, 46]. Therefore, younger patients must be counseled appropriately about activity restrictions after total ankle arthroplasty. The problem remains, however, that the only alternative to total ankle arthroplasty is ankle arthrodesis. When counseling a younger patient with regard to the potential long-term effects of ankle arthrodesis, then, it should be explained that if the patient lives long enough, he or she can expect to develop symptomatic secondary osteoarthrosis in the adjacent joints of the hind- and midfoot.

The Author's Approach
When discussing arthrodesis versus total ankle arthroplasty with a younger patient who suffers from painful end-stage ankle arthritis, one may clearly explain that that total ankle arthroplasty may be a viable option for an initial period of time. If the implant fails over time, and revision arthroplasty is not feasible at that time, then conversion to ankle arthrodesis can be performed. This "two-stage approach" to ankle arthrodesis may effectively preserve the adjacent joints from overuse and secondary osteoarthrosis. Therefore, one should use only total ankle implants that require minimal bone resection, thereby saving bone for further revisions or later isolated ankle joint fusion. Implants that (because of the extensive bone resection) require tibiocalcaneal fusion once they have failed should not be considered for younger patients.

7.3.11 Activity Limitations

Implant longevity is clearly related to the loading history placed on an ankle prosthesis. Vigorous, repetitive, impact-type loading will likely result in early mechanical failure of an implant. Shear forces in the sagittal and coronal planes have been estimated to reach levels of up to two times body weight during gait, and even higher with more strenuous activities [35, 38, 43]. With some ankle designs, the vertical loads applied to the trabecular bone at the bone-implant interface during normal daily activities may exceed the inherent strength of the bone. Although bone remodeling may occur over time, thereby increasing the inherent trabecular strength, it must increase to at least three times the applied load to prevent collapse of the components [26].

There is general consensus in the literature that total ankle arthroplasty is designed to support the stresses associated with activities of daily living, and is not intended to allow resumption of high-impact, strenuous exercise [10]. Patients should, therefore, be generally restricted from any high-impact or stop-

and-go exercises, including jogging, competitive sports, and heavy lower-body weightlifting. Low-impact or sedentary activities such as walking, swimming, golfing, and biking, however, are allowed.

> **The Author's Approach**
> In addition to the above-mentioned low-impact activities, the author also generally permits patients to participate in downhill and cross-country skiing (classical technique only), having not observed any related problems thus far.

7.3.12 Smoking

Although little is reported in the literature regarding the success rates for total ankle arthroplasty in smokers as compared with non-smokers, it is generally thought that smoking may indirectly influence outcomes, because smoking increases the immediate perioperative risks. The systemic vasoconstrictive effects of nicotine are known to inhibit wound healing, and delayed wound healing and wound necrosis are common complications of ankle replacement surgery (up to 40% in some series) [2, 5, 44]. The continued presence of nicotine can also adversely affect bony ingrowth into uncemented components. Finally, nicotine significantly increases the risk of nonunion of arthrodeses in smokers as compared with non-smokers [11]. This is of utmost importance when considering the use of total ankle prostheses that rely on syndesmotic fusion (for example, the AGILITY™ ankle) or need additional complex hindfoot reconstruction including osteotomies and arthrodeses.

7.4 Conclusions

Adequate evaluation of potential pre- or intraoperative risk factors may be the most critical aspect of promoting a successful outcome. Knowledge of the indications, as well as both relative and absolute contraindications, is of great importance (see Table 7.1). The ideal patient for a total ankle arthroplasty is an elderly person with low physical demands, who is of normal weight, and who has good bone stock, normal vascular status, no immunosuppression, intact soft tissues, excellent hindfoot-ankle alignment, and a stable ankle that still has some motion left.

References

[1] Abdo RV, Iorio LJ (1994) Rheumatoid arthritis of the foot and ankle. Am J Orthop Surg 2: 326–332
[2] Alvine FG (2000) Total ankle arthroplasty. In: Foot and ankle disorders (Myerson MS, ed), chap 45. Saunders, Philadelphia, pp 1085–1102
[3] Alvine FG (2002) The AGILITY ankle replacement: the good and the bad. Foot Ankle Clin 7: 737–754
[4] Anderson T, Montgomery F, Carlsson A (2003) Uncemented STAR total ankle prosthesis. Three to eight-year follow-up of 51 consecutive ankles. J Bone Joint Surg Am 85: 1321–1329
[5] Bolton-Maggs BG, Sudlow RA, Freeman MA (1985) Total ankle arthroplasty. A long-term review of the London Hospital experience. J Bone Joint Surg Br 67: 785–790
[6] Brunner R, Jaspers RT, Pel JJ, Huijing PA (2000) Acute and long-term effects on muscle force after intramuscular aponeurotic lengthening. Clin Orthop 378: 264–273
[7] Buechel FF, Pappas MJ, Iorio LJ (1988) New Jersey low contact stress total ankle replacement: biomechanical rationale and review of 23 cementless cases. Foot Ankle 8: 279–290
[8] Carlsson AS, Henricson AS, Linder L (1994) A survival analysis of 52 Bath-Wessex ankle replacements. Foot 4: 34–40
[9] Carlsson AS, Henricson AS, Linder L, Nilsson JA, Redlund-Johnell I (2001) A 10-year survival analysis of 69 Bath-Wessex ankle replacements. Foot Ankle S 7: 39–44
[10] Clare MP, Sanders RW (2002) Preoperative considerations in ankle replacement surgery. Foot Ankle Clin 7: 703–708
[11] Cobb TK, Gabrielsen TA, Campbell DC, Wallrichs SL, Ilstrup DM (1994) Cigarette smoking and nonunion after ankle arthrodesis. Foot Ankle Int 15: 64–67
[12] Conti SF, Wong YS (2001) Complications of total ankle replacement. Clin Orthop 391: 105–114
[13] Conti SF, Wong YS (2001) New developments in total ankle arthroplasty. Orthopedic Special Edition 7: 9–11
[14] Deland JT, Morris GD, Sung IH (2000) Biomechanics of the ankle joint. A perspective on total ankle replacement. Foot Ankle Clin 5: 747–759
[15] Demetriades L, Strauss E, Gallina J (1998) Osteoarthritis of the ankle. Clin Orthop 349: 28–42
[16] Easley ME, Vertullo CJ, Urban WC, Nunley JA (2002) Total ankle arthroplasty. J Am Acad Orthop Surg 10: 157–167
[17] Gill LH (2002) Principles of joint arthroplasty as applied to the ankle. AAOS Instruct. Course Lect., chap 13, pp 117–128
[18] Gould JS, Alvine FG, Mann RA, Sanders RW, Walling AK (2000) Total ankle replacement: a surgical discussion. Part I. Replacement systems, indications, and contraindications. Am J Orthop 29: 604–609

[19] Gould JS, Alvine FG, Mann RA, Sanders RW, Walling AK (2000) Total ankle replacement: a surgical discussion. Part II. The clinical and surgical experience. Am J Orthop 29: 675–682

[20] Greisberg J, Hansen ST, Jr. (2002) Ankle replacement: management of associated deformities. Foot Ankle Clin 7: 721–736

[21] Hanssen AD, Rand JA (1998) Evaluation and treatment of infection at the site of total hip or knee arthroplasty. J Bone Joint Surg Am 80: 910–922

[22] Helm R, Stevens J (1986) Long-term results of total ankle replacement. J Arthroplasty 1: 271–277

[23] Hintermann B (1999) The S.T.A.R. ankle. Short- and mid-term experience. Orthopäde 28: 792–803

[24] Hintermann B, Valderrabano V (2003) Total ankle replacement. Foot Ankle Clin 8: 375–405

[25] Hintermann B, Valderrabano V, Dereymaeker G, Dick W (2004) The HINTEGRA ankle: rationale and short-term results of 122 consecutive ankles. Clin Orthop 424: 57–68

[26] Hvid I, Rasmussen O, Jensen NC, Nielsen S (1985) Trabecular bone strength profiles at the ankle joint. Clin Orthop 199: 306–312

[27] Jensen NC, Kroner K (1992) Total joint replacement: A clinical follow-up. Orthopaedics 15: 236–239

[28] Kaukonen JP, Raunio P (1983) Total ankle replacement in rheumatoid arthritis: a preliminary review of 28 arthroplasties in 24 patients. Ann Chir Gyn 72: 196–199

[29] Kirkup J (1985) Richard Smith ankle arthroplasty. J R Soc Med 78: 301–304

[30] Kitaoka HB, Patzer GL (1996) Clinical results of the Mayo total ankle arthroplasty. J Bone Joint Surg Am 78: 1658–1664

[31] Kitaoka HB, Patzer GL, Strup DMI, Wallrichs SI (1994) Survivorship analysis of the Mayo total ankle arthroplasty. J Bone Joint Surg Am 76: 974–979

[32] Kofoed H, Lundberg-Jensen A (1999) Ankle arthroplasty in patients younger and older than 50 years: a prospective series with long-term follow-up. Foot Ankle Int 20: 501–506

[33] Kofoed H, Sorensen TS (1998) Ankle arthroplasty for rheumatoid arthritis and osteoarthritis: prospective long-term study of cemented replacements. J Bone Joint Surg Br 80: 328–332

[34] McGuire MR, Kyle RF, Gustilo RB, Premer RF (1988) Comparative analysis of ankle arthroplasty versus ankle arthrodesis. Clin Orthop 226: 174–181

[35] Neufeld SK, Lee TH (2000) Total ankle arthroplasty: indications, results, and biomechanical rationale. Am J Orthop 29: 593–602

[36] Newton SE, III (1982) Total ankle arthroplasty. In: Disorders of the foot and ankle (Jahss MH, ed). Saunders, Philadelphia, pp 816–825

[37] Newton SE, III (1982) Total ankle arthroplasty. Clinical study of 50 cases. J Bone Joint Surg Am 64: 104–111

[38] Nigg BM, Hintermann B (1996): Biomechanics of the ankle joint complex and the shoe. In: Musculoskeletal disorders in the workplace – principles and practice (Nordin M, Andersson GBJ, Pope MH, eds), chap 45. Mosby, St. Louis, pp 558–569

[39] Pyevich MT, Saltzman CL, Callaghan JJ, Alvine FG (1998) Total ankle arthroplasty: a unique design. Two to 12-year follow-up. J Bone Joint Surg Am 80: 1410–1420

[40] Saltzman CL (1999) Total ankle arthroplasty: state of the art. Instr Course Lect 48: 263–268

[41] Saltzman CL (2000) Perspective on total ankle replacement. Foot Ankle Clin 5: 761–775

[42] Stauffer RN, Chao EY, Brewster RC (1977) Force and motion analysis of the normal, diseased, and prosthetic ankle joint. Clin Orthop 127: 189–196

[43] Spirt AA, Assal M, Hansen ST Jr (2004) Complications and failures after total ankle arthroplasty. J Bone Joint Surg Am 86: 1172–1178

[44] Stauffer RN, Segal NM (1981) Total ankle arthroplasty: four years' experience. Clin Orthop 160: 217–221

[45] Takakura Y, Yanaka Y, Sugimoto K, Tamai S, Masuhara K (1990) Ankle arthroplasty. A comparative study of cemented metal and uncemented ceramic prostheses. Clin Orthop 252: 209–216

[46] Thomas RL, Daniels TR (2003) Current concepts review: Ankle arthritis. J Bone Joint Surg Am 85: 923–936

[47] Unger AS, Inglis AE, Mow CS, Figgie HEI (1988) Total ankle arthroplasty in rheumatoid arthritis: a long-term follow-up study. Foot Ankle 8: 173–179

[48] Valderrabano V, Hintermann B, Dick W (2004) Scandinavian total ankle replacement: a 3.7-year average follow-up of 65 patients. Clin Orthop 424: 47–56

[49] Wood PL, Deakin S (2003) Total ankle replacement. The results in 200 ankles. J Bone Joint Surg 85-B: 334–341

[50] Wood PLR (1998) Total ankle replacement (LINK S.T.A.R.) for rheumatoid arthritis. In: Current status of ankle arthroplasty (Kofoed H, ed), chap 7. Springer, Berlin, pp 34–36

[51] Wood PLR, Clough TM, Jari S (2000) Clinical comparison of two total ankle replacements. Foot Ankle Int 21: 546–550

[52] Wynn AH, Wilde AH (1992) Long-term follow-up of the Conaxial (Beck-Steffee) total ankle arthroplasty. Foot Ankle 13: 303–306

Chapter 8

SURGICAL TECHNIQUES

Although many surgical approaches have been described in the literature, most current total ankle prostheses are implanted using the standard anterior ankle approach. Because of the fragility of the soft tissues around the ankle, however, and scars from previous injuries or surgeries, the approach sometimes demands a modified technique in order to prevent wound healing problems. Various techniques are used to implant current ankle prostheses. In most cases, however, a jig is used to align a tibial resection block with respect to the longitudinal axis of the tibia. Talar resection is made, to some extent, as a free-hand surgery. In some cases (with the AGILITY™ ankle, for example), an external fixator/distractor is used to realign the ankle and tension the ligaments.

8.1 Preoperative Planning

Recognizing critical preoperative risk factors and doing careful preoperative planning are important factors for limiting complications and obtaining satisfactory results. Meticulous clinical and radiological assessment is required. Clinically, the surgeon should examine and document the soft-tissue conditions, hindfoot alignment, ankle stability, foot deformities, foot vascularization, and sensibility. Lateral and anteroposterior weight-bearing radiographs of the foot and ankle are mandatory, and may help to identify possible osteoarthritis in adjacent joints, as well as varus and valgus deformities of the hindfoot and longitudinal arch. The use of MRI may also help to determine the condition of the subchondral bone, particularly with respect to potential osteonecrosis.

8.2 Surgical Approach to the Ankle

Most of the current total ankle prostheses (the Buechel-Pappas™ ankle [15], the HINTEGRA® ankle [8], the TNK ankle [19], the Ramses ankle [16], the SALTO® ankle [2], and the S.T.A.R. ankle [14]) are implanted using the standard anterior ankle approach, which uses a single incision between the anterior tibial and extensor hallucis longus tendons. The AGILITY™ ankle uses the same anterior incision, as well as a lateral incision over the distal fibula to mobilize and bridge the tibiofibular syndesmosis [17]. The ESKA ankle, by contrast, is implanted using a single lateral (transfibular) approach [18].

8.2.1 Anterior Approach to the Ankle

The patient is positioned supine, with the heel of the foot on the edge of the table. A support beneath the ipsilateral hip, and/or tilting the table serves to get the foot in an upright position so that the ankle is seen from the front side of the leg (Fig. 8.1). A longitudinal skin incision is made over the center of the ankle (Fig. 8.2), taking care to identify and retract the medial branch of the superficial peroneal nerve (Fig. 8.3). The approach is made longitudinally between the extensor hallucis longus and anterior tibial tendons, through the tendon sheet of the extensor hallucis longus [5, 21] or of the anterior tibial tendon [8, 10]. Once the distal tibia is exposed just beneath the anterior tibial tendon ("safety area"), the soft tissues are pushed sideways using a raspatory subperiosteally. Then, the neurovascular bundle is retracted laterally, and two Hohmann retractors are inserted (Fig. 8.4). The ankle capsule is incised vertically over the midpoint of the ankle. Note that it may be necessary to excise the central part of this capsule to gain good exposure. A self-retaining retractor is inserted, and the Hohmann retractors are removed (Fig. 8.5). The anterior osteophytes of the tibia are removed to expose the extent of the depression in the tibial plafond and to clearly expose the anterior aspect of the medial malleolus at the level of the tibial plafond ("anteromedial corner") (Fig. 8.6). Similarly, the anterior osteophytes of the talus are removed (Fig. 8.7), and the medial and lateral sides of the talus are cleared of any fibrosis and osteophytes. To achieve an optimal ankle exposure, a distractor is usually positioned on the medial side. When there is severe valgus deformity, a distractor is sometimes positioned on the lateral side.

Once this has been done and any distractor has been removed, it is possible to assess whether soft-tissue procedures are needed to realign the foot. Varus deformity requires a medial release of the deltoid ligament to restore the joint height, which may be sufficient to correct the alignment and restore normal tension to the lateral ligament. If it does not do so, then lateral ligament reconstruction is required (see Chap. 8, Sect. 8.6.1: Lateral Ligament Reconstruction). Valgus deformity, by contrast, can be corrected without ligamentous release. Correction of malalignment requires experience, however, and the author strongly advises that surgeons initially limit their surgery to ankles with minimal varus or valgus deformity. In view of potential surgical difficulties, severe deformity (that is, varus or valgus malalignment of the talus of more than 20° within the ankle mortise) should generally be regarded as a contraindication for total ankle replacement.

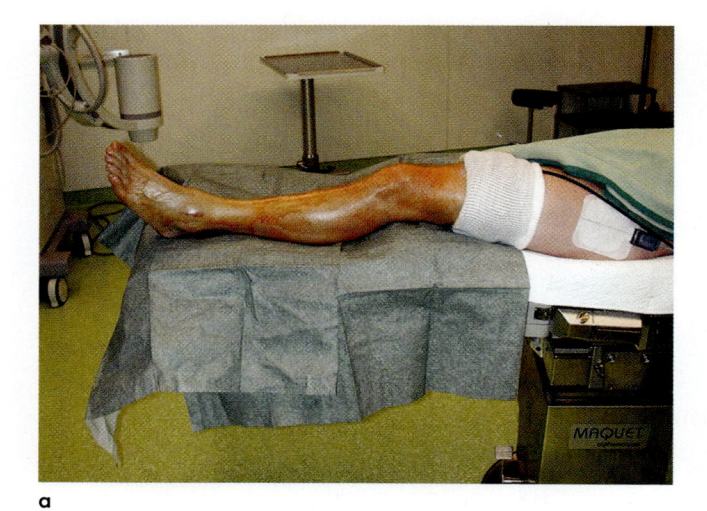

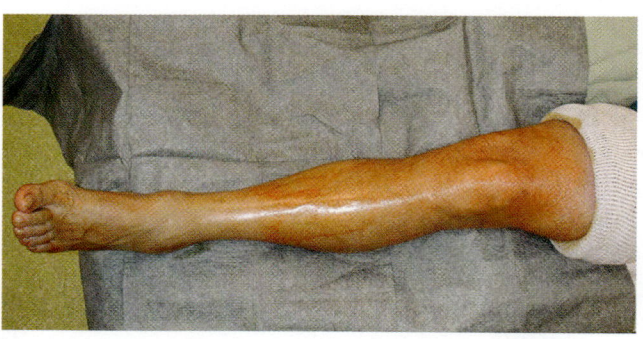

Fig. 8.1. Positioning of the patient.
The patient is positioned supine with the heel of the foot on the edge of the table (**a**), and a support beneath the ipsilateral hip to get the foot in an upright position (**b**)

8.2 Surgical Approach to the Ankle

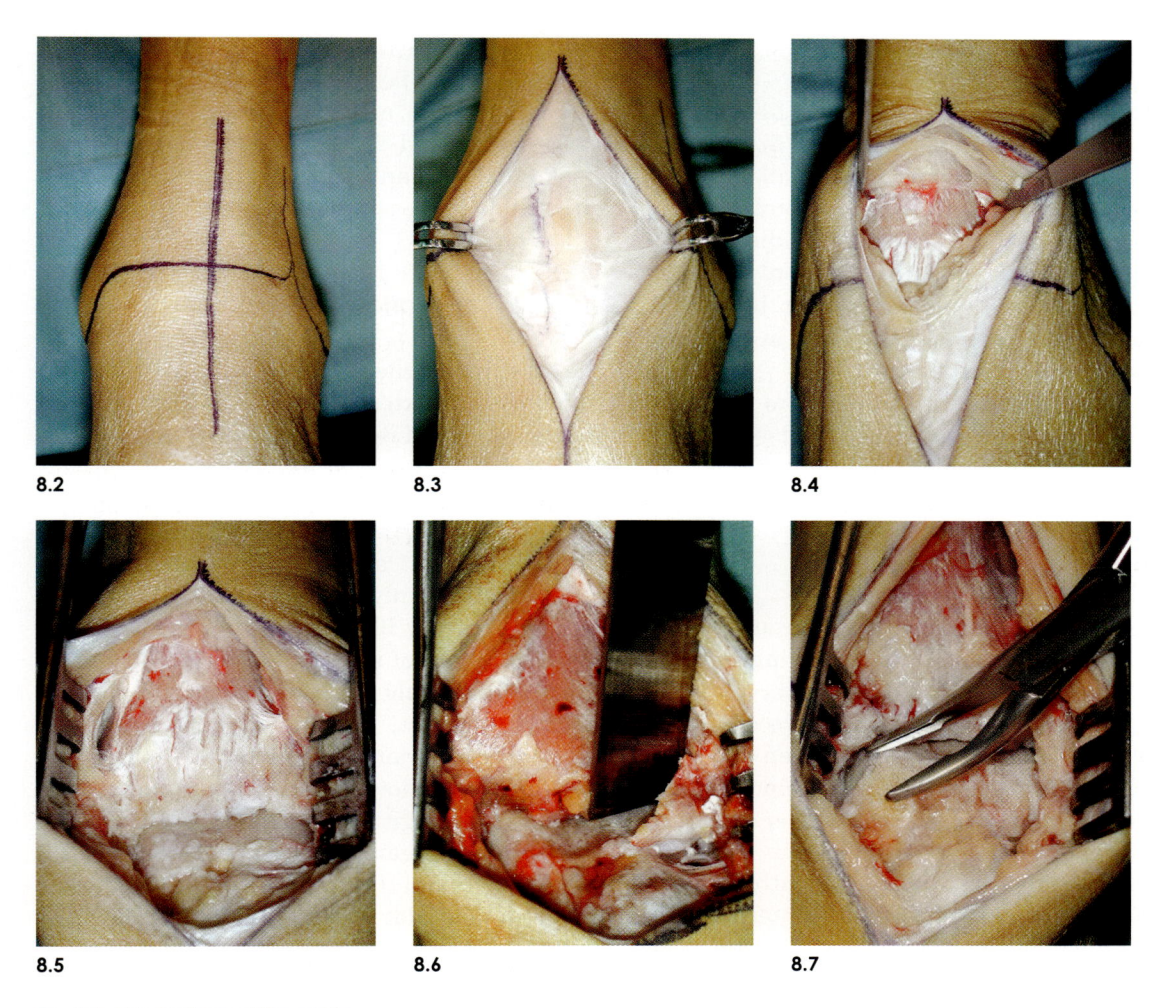

Fig. 8.2. Skin incision of the ankle.
A longitudinal incision 10 to 12 cm long is made

Fig. 8.3. Subcutaneous preparation.
The extensor retinaculum is exposed by paying attention to the superficial peroneal nerve (see text)

Fig. 8.4. Exposure of the distal tibia.
The distal tibia is exposed through an incision between the extensor hallucis longus and the anterior tibial tendon (see text)

Fig. 8.5. Arthrotomy of the ankle joint and insertion of a self-retaining retractor.
After arthrotomy and partial resection of the anterior capsule, a self-retaining retractor is inserted (see text)

Fig. 8.6. Removal of tibial osteophytes.
Osteophytes on the tibial side are removed first to clearly expose the medial malleolus and the tibiotalar joint line (see text)

Fig. 8.7. Removal of talar osteophytes.
Osteophytes on the talar side are removed as well (see text)

8.2.2 Lateral Approach to the Ankle

A lateral skin incision is made along the distal fibula and is continued from the distal tip of the fibula more distally. Lateral osteotomy of the fibula allows anterior to posterior exposure of the ankle joint as the distal fibula is folded back in the plantar direction (meaning that the fibula remains fixed only to the posterior fibulotalar and calcaneofibular ligaments). The anterior syndesmosis is included in the anterior soft-tissue flap.

By comparison to the anterior approach to the ankle, a lateral approach to the ankle limits the ability to assess varus and valgus malalignment and/or instability.

8.2.3 Complications

Incisional complications include releasing the anterior tibial tendon from its sheath, and scarring or transecting the superficial or deep peroneal nerves. Most descriptions of an anterior approach recommend deeper dissection in the interval between the anterior tibial and extensor hallucis longus tendons. Some surgeons even prefer to perform the deeper dissection more laterally, and purposely take the extensor hallucis longus tendon out of its sheath, in an attempt to preserve the restraints of the anterior tibial tendon [6]. Immediately below this lies the deep peroneal nerve, which must be identified and retracted during incision of the capsule. In the author's experience, however, problems with the anterior tibial tendon are uncommon, even though in most instances its sheath is opened or disrupted during surgery. Thus, he recommends using a more medial approach to prevent injuries to the neurovascular bundle.

Wound healing problems are a major complication of total ankle arthroplasty [6, 8]. Throughout the procedure, particular care needs to be exercised with skin retraction to avoid pressure necrosis of the skin and delayed wound healing. Plantar flexion of the foot draws the skin together, and if a self-retaining retractor has been inserted when the foot is 90° to the leg, the force will dramatically increase when the foot is plantar flexed, as is often necessary to gain adequate access. Self-retaining retractors should thus be inserted while the foot is in plantar flexion, or they should be released and reapplied with the foot in a new position to ensure that damage does not occur, or else they should not be used at all. In the author's experience, however, a self-retaining retractor is, when properly applied, far less dangerous to the skin than hooks or Hohmann retractors because it does not exercise direct pressure on the skin (Fig. 8.8).

8.3 Surgical Preparation of the Ankle

With the exception of the AGILITY™ Total Ankle System (which uses an external fixator/distractor to first tension ligaments and realign the ankle), the surgical preparation for all current three-component designs (as well as for the two-component TNK design) is similar. Because of the author's extensive experience with the HINTEGRA® ankle, however, the following description refers mainly to the use of this ankle.

The tibial cutting block is positioned, using the anteromedial corner of the ankle as the distal reference and the tibial tuberosity as the proximal reference (Fig. 8.9). First, the rod is strictly aligned parallel to the anterior border of the tibia, which means that the resection block and the connected rod are aligned in the sagittal plane (Fig. 8.10). Second, to obtain balanced ligaments, the resection block is aligned in the coronal (frontal) plane with respect to the individual tibiotalar line. This is best achieved by pulling the talus in a distal direction (using, for instance, a raspatory) to tension the medial and lateral collateral ligaments. Then the resection block is aligned parallel to the superior talar border (Fig. 8.11). Based on Knupp's finding [12] that there is no intra-individual difference between the tibiotalar angles of the lower limbs, the tibiotalar angle as calculated from an X-ray of the contralateral ankle can also be used to determine the frontal plane adjustment for the tibial resection block. Inman, in his *in vitro* study of 107 specimens [11], demonstrated that the empirical axis of the ankle is obliquely oriented to the long axis of the leg, and when projected on a coronal plane, is directed laterally and downward at a mean angle of 82° (Fig. 8.12). Therefore, there is theoretical reason to insert the components at 82° to the longitudinal axis of the leg, which may be particularly necessary when the talar implant has a cylindrical configuration. In a standing position, however, one would expect it to be best to have the components oriented to the individual line of the tibial plafond. As described above, the author's recommendation is to insert the tibial component so that its orientation is parallel to the upper surface of the talus, while pulling the talus out of the mortise and tensioning the collateral ligaments.

Once this has been done, the tibial resection block is fixed to the tibia by two to four pins, and moved proximally to the desired position. The tibial cut will usually skim the top of the depression in the tibial plafond (Fig. 8.13), but for ankles with extensive subchondral sclerosis or some avascular osteonecrosis, a resection of an additional 2 to 3 mm may be needed to locate suitable bone quality within the resected surface. Some surgeons also advise this for particularly stiff ankles with minimal deformity to gain more postoperative mobility [13, 21]. Extensive bone resection of the distal tibia (that is, resection of the whole subchondral bone plate) may, however, result in loss of bony support for the inserted implant. For this reason, the author strongly advises the resecting of as little bone as possible on the tibial metaphysis. Care should also be taken to avoid fracturing the medial and lateral malleoli (Fig. 8.14).

Some controversies exist about the angle of resection in the sagittal plane with respect to the posterior slope of the inserted tibial component [3, 13, 21]. Although Buechel and Pappas [3] found that any angle between 80° and 90° gave good results, they advise that the tibial component should be inserted with an angle of 83°. Angles less than 80° seem to be associated with poorer range of motion [21], or cause chronic tendonitis of the posterior tibial tendon because of chronic overuse [20]. Statistical proof of this, however, is not forthcoming. Given by the resection block, the Buechel-Pappas ankle uses a posterior slope of 7°, the S.T.A.R. ankle of 6°, and the HINTEGRA® ankle of 4°.

After the tibial cut is done, the distal tibia is removed, including the scarred posterior capsule. This allows the insertion of the HINTEGRA® talar cutting block which is mounted on the tibial block. With the foot held strictly in neutral position, the talar block is fixed to the talus by two pins, and the talar cut is done (Fig. 8.15). The objective is to remove the minimum amount of bone necessary to create a flat surface that is about 1 cm from front to back, and is parallel to and centrally placed under the cut surface of the tibia (Fig. 8.16). A spacer that is the thickness of the implants is inserted into the created joint space to check hindfoot alignment and ligamentous stability of the ankle (Fig. 8.17). While maintaining the correct orientation to the long axis of the foot (that is, the longitudinal axis of the second metatarsal), further talar cuts are made with a second talar jig (Fig. 8.18). The appropriate size of talar component is determined, and the selected resection block is fixed to the talus by two pins, using the anterior border of the tibia as the reference for positioning the talar component. The medial and lateral, and then the posterior cuts are done and the bones are removed (Fig. 8.19). Special attention is paid to the anterior-posterior position of the talar component. A bone resection of 2 to 3 mm from the posterior talus is required to achieve the correct position (Fig. 8.20). Finally, after complete removal of the dorsal capsule (Fig. 8.20) the length of the tibial resection surface is measured to determine the correct size of tibial component (Fig. 8.21).

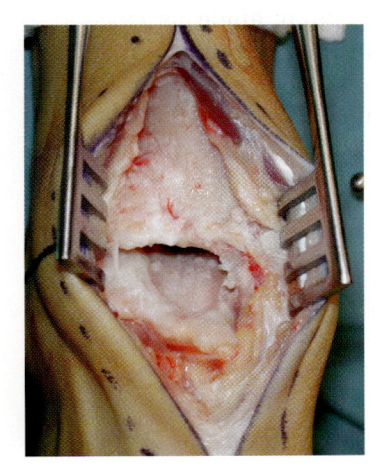

Fig. 8.8. Self-retaining retractor.
A self-retaining retractor exposes the anterior ankle joint without applying traction forces to the skin (as happens when using hooks or Hohmann retractors) (see text)

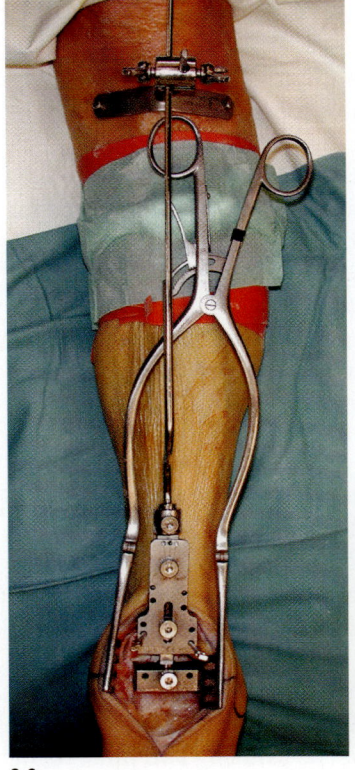

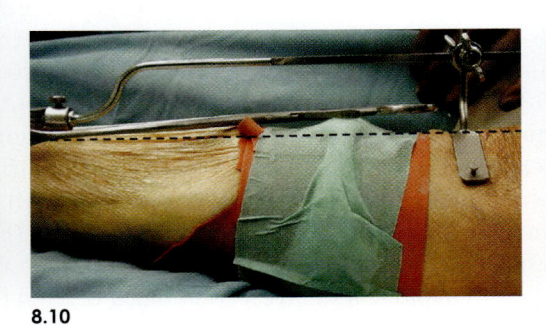

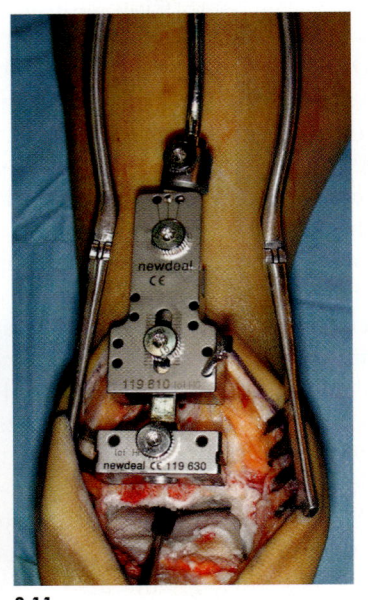

8.9

8.10

8.11

Fig. 8.9. Tibial resection block.
The tibial resection block is positioned with the anteromedial corner of the ankle as the distal reference, and the tibial tuberosity as the proximal reference (see text)

Fig. 8.10. Sagittal alignment of the rod.
The rod is aligned with regard to the tibia in the sagittal plane (see text)

Fig. 8.11. Coronal plane adjustment of the tibial resection block.
The tibial resection block can best be aligned in the coronal plane while pulling the talus in a distal direction, tensioning the medial and lateral ligaments. The upper surface of the talus serves as the reference (see text)

8.12

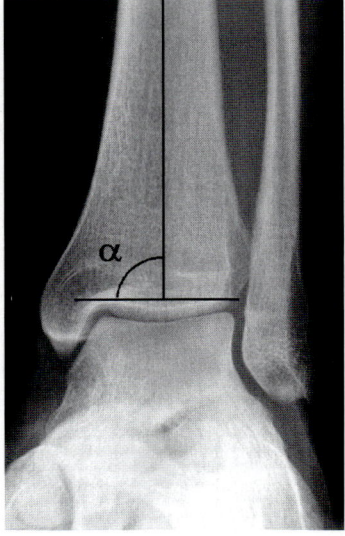

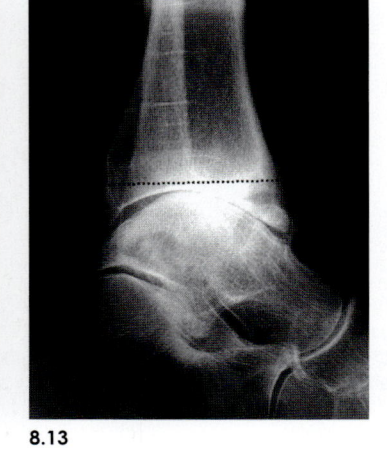

8.13

Fig. 8.12. Tibiotalar angle.
The tibiotalar angle varies significantly between individuals, but not between the two ankles of the same person (see text)

Fig. 8.13. Tibial cut.
The tibial cut is planned to skim the top of the depression in the tibial plafond so that no more than 1 to 2 mm of bone are removed (see text)

8.3 Surgical Preparation of the Ankle

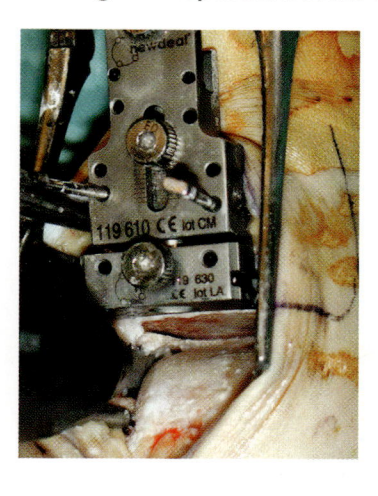

Fig. 8.14. Protection of the malleoli.
To avoid fractures of the medial and lateral malleoli, the saw blade is inserted strictly frontwards, and then the edges are prepared using a reciprocating saw, as shown for the medial side. The author never uses a chisel to complete the cuts (see text)

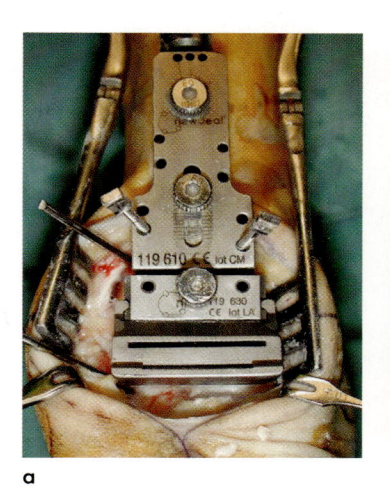

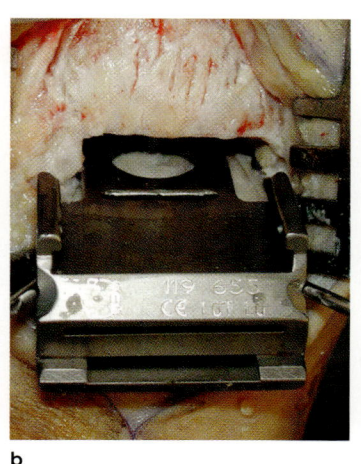

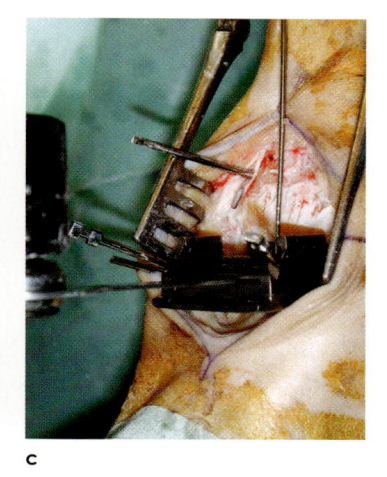

a b c

Fig. 8.15. Talar cut.
With the foot held strictly in neutral position, the talar cutting block is inserted and fixed with two pins to the talus (**a**). Once the tibial resection block is removed, the position of the talar block can be checked, particularly whether it has an appropriate fit to the talus (**b**). The upper slot provides an access point to insert the saw blade for performing the talar cut, while the lower slot provides an access point to prepare the anterior edge of the talar component (**c**) (see text)

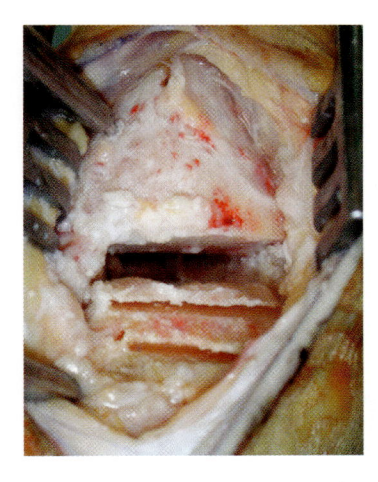

Fig. 8.16. Talar bone cuts.
This figure shows the bone cuts after removal of the talar resection block (see text)

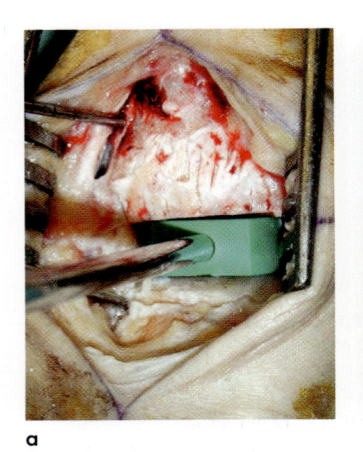

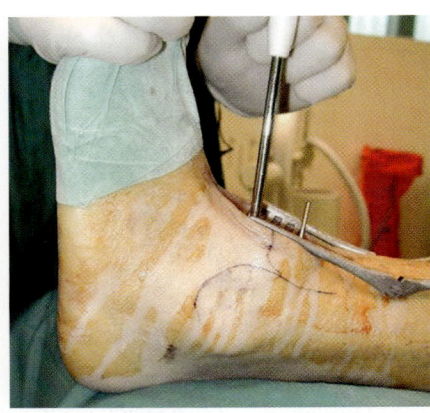

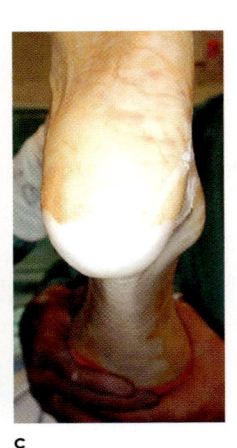

Fig. 8.17. Alignment and stability check
A spacer of 12 mm thickness (corresponding to the thickness of the smallest implant) is inserted (**a**). This makes it possible to check the stability of the ankle (**b**) and alignment of the hindfoot (**c**) while the ligaments are under tension

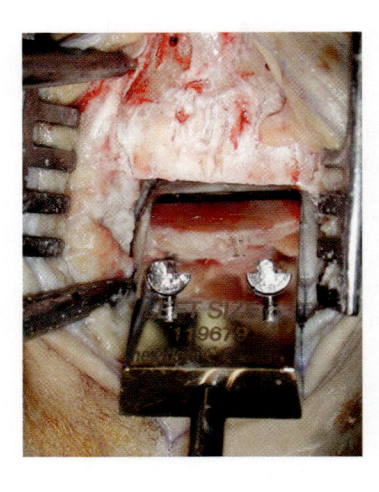

Fig. 8.18. Positioning of the talar resection block.
The appropriate size of talar resection block is selected so that 2 mm of bone will be resected on both the medial and lateral sides. It is also important to perform a bone resection of at least 2 mm on the posterior side to ensure that the talar component will not be situated too posteriorly. The resection block is fixed by two pins (see text)

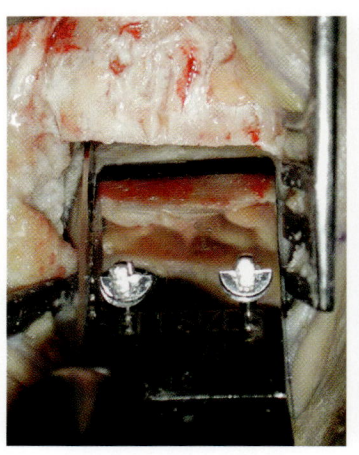

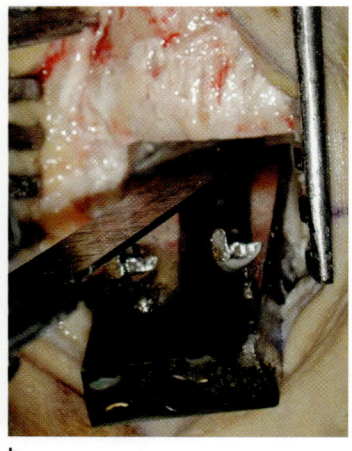

Fig. 8.19. Medial, lateral, and posterior cut of the talus.
The medial and lateral cuts are done using the reciprocating saw (**a**), and the posterior cut using the oscillating saw (**b**) (see text)

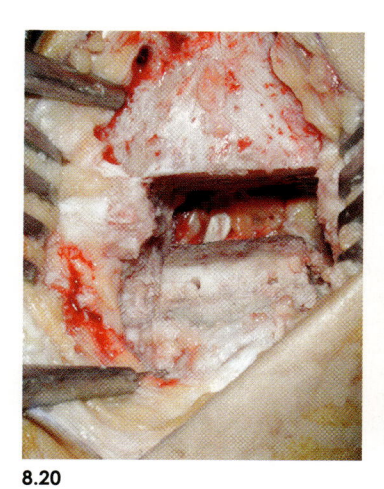

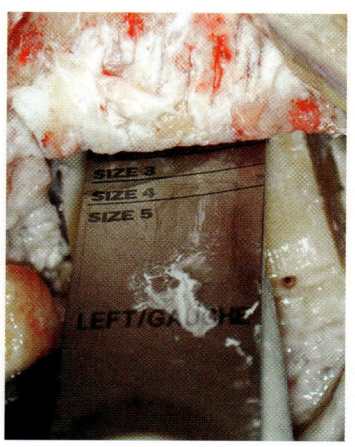

Fig. 8.20. Removal of the dorsal capsule.
The dorsal capsule is completely removed until fat tissue and the flexor hallucis longus tendon are seen (see text)

Fig. 8.21. Measurement of the tibial length.
The length of the tibial resection surface is measured (see text)

8.4 Insertion of the Implants

Note that in cases exhibiting malalignment, ligamentous instability, and concomitant osteoarthrosis of hindfoot joints, additional surgeries are considered prior to prosthetic implantation.

First the trial talus is inserted, and it is positioned to get a proper press fit on talar bone. Then, the trial tibia and bearing are inserted (Fig. 8.22). The achieved alignment, stability, and joint motion are checked clinically, and the component position is checked by image intensification (Fig. 8.23). With the foot held in neutral position, the tip of the talar component indicates the central area of contact with the tibial component, which should be anterior to the imaginary longitudinal axis of the tibia (that is, anterior to the middle of the tibial component as given by the anatomy of the normal ankle) (Fig. 8.24). If the trial talar component is situated too posteriorly, then the next smaller talar resection block is fixed to the talus using the same holes for the pins. Then, a further bone cut is done only posteriorly, removing about 1.2 mm more bone (Fig. 8.25).

Once the trial implants are properly positioned, the anterior resection of the talus is finished using a luer or a saw (Fig. 8.26). The implants are then removed, and the second trial talar component is inserted. The window on the top makes it possible to check the appropriate position and fit to the resected bone surfaces (Fig. 8.27). Two holes are drilled (Fig. 8.28) to receive the two pegs of the talar component. This ensures that the talar component will be positioned in exactly the desired position (Fig. 8.29), as determined before impaction (Fig. 8.30). The tibial component is

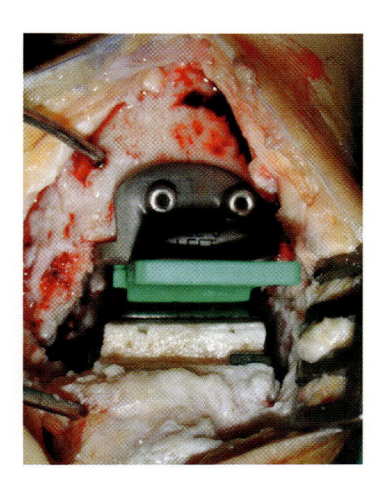

Fig. 8.22. Insertion of the trials.
The trial talus is inserted first, then the trial tibia is inserted, and finally the trial inlay is inserted (see text)

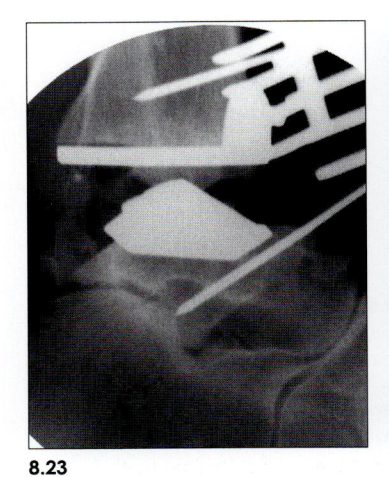

Fig. 8.23. Intraoperative radiological check.
The position of the trial components is checked by image intensifier (fluoroscan) (see text)

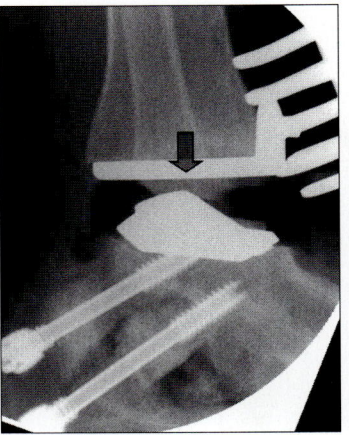

Fig. 8.24. Anterior-posterior positioning of the talus.
While the foot is held in neutral position, the center of the talar component should be in contact with the tibial component on its anterior part. The desired contact point is usually between 40% and 45% of the tibial component, with 0% taken to be the anterior margin, and 100% the posterior margin. In this case, the contact point is between 50% and 55%, thus the talar component should be positioned more anteriorly (see text)

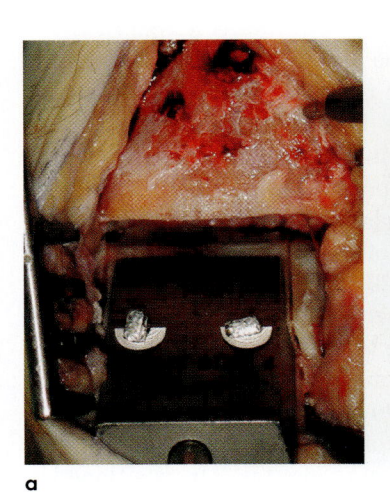

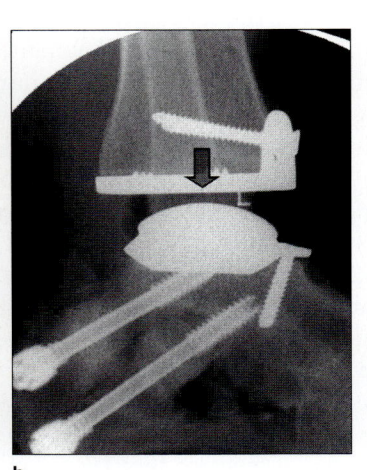

Fig. 8.25. Additional cut on posterior talus.
The next smaller talar resection block is fixed to the talus and the posterior cut is repeated, removing 1 to 1.5 mm more bone from the posterior aspect of the talus (**a**). The final implant now shows a point of contact with the tibial component at 45% (**b**, same patient as Fig. 8.24)

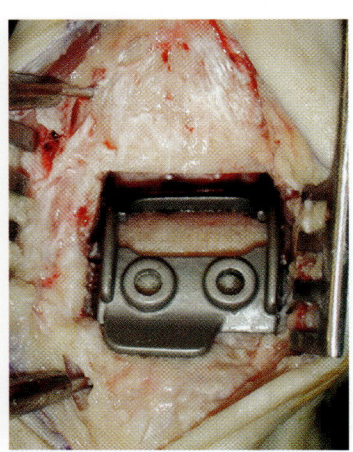

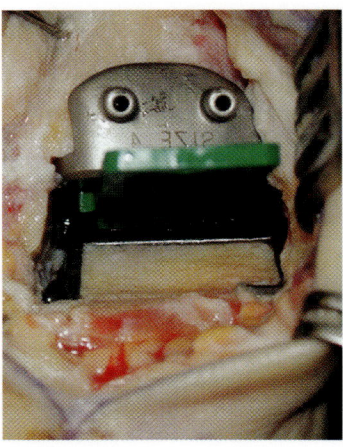

Fig. 8.26. Anterior cut on talus.
Once the anterior-posterior position of the talus is considered to be perfect, the anterior surface of the talus is resected (see text)

Fig. 8.27. Second talar trial component.
The second talar trial component is inserted to check the resected surfaces and the contact between the implant and the bone (see text)

8.4 Insertion of the Implants

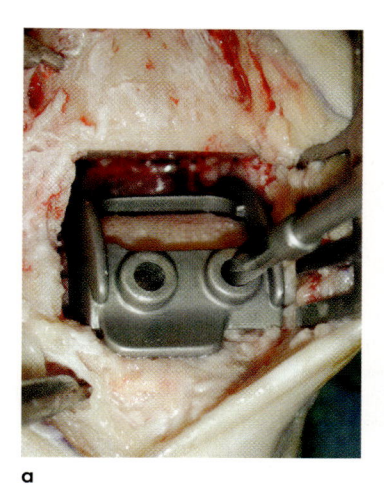

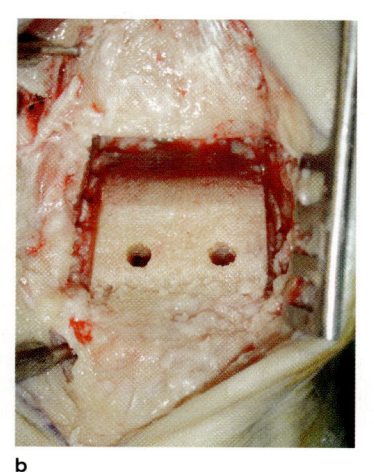

a b

Fig. 8.28. Peg holes for the talar component
Once the position of the talar component is perfect, two holes are drilled to receive the pegs of the talar component (**a**), and the trial is removed (**b**) (see text)

8.29 8.30 8.31

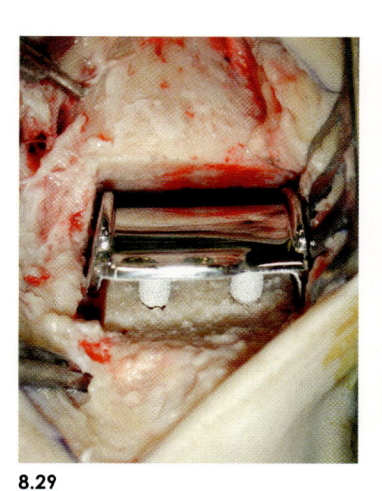

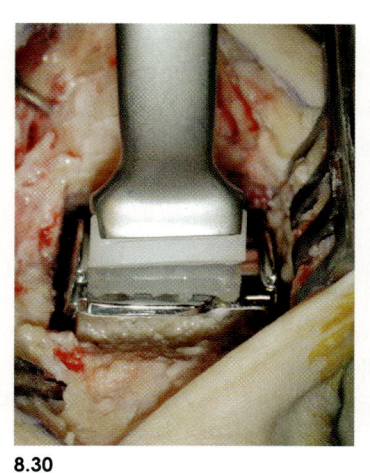

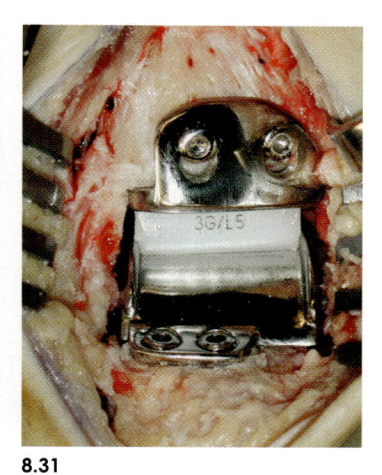

Fig. 8.29. Insertion of the talar component.
The talar component is inserted using the two pegs as a guide (see text)

Fig. 8.30. Impaction of the talar component.
The talar component is impacted using an impactor and a heavy 750 g hammer to achieve a proper press fit of the implant (see text)

Fig. 8.31. Insertion of the polyethylene inlay and the screws.
The polyethylene inlay is inserted, and after checking the mobility and stability of the ankle, screws to the tibia and optionally to the talus are inserted (see text)

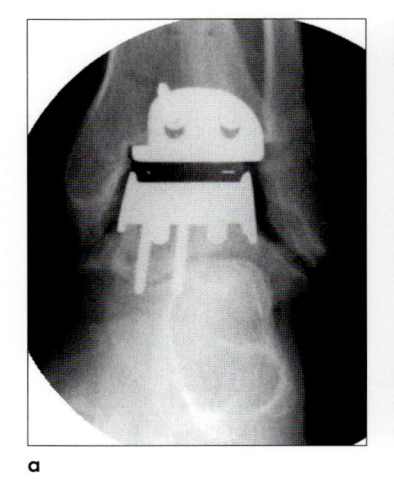

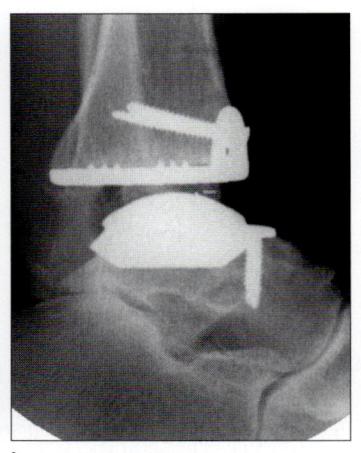

Fig. 8.32. Final check of the implants.
The position of the implants is checked by fluoroscopy: on anteroposterior view, alignment of the hindfoot, and position of the implants (that is, the bone-implant contact) (**a**); on lateral view, alignment of the tibia and talus, and position of the implant (that is, the bone-implant contact) (**b**)

then inserted while protecting the articulating surface of the talar component with the trial insert. Finally, the polyethylene mobile bearing is inserted (Fig. 8.31) and, after removing the self-retaining retractor, the gained range of motion and stability is checked clinically. The tibial component is additionally stabilized by two screws until osseointegration has occurred. The screws are inserted to become positioned on the top of the gliding hole on the tibial shield, so as not to hinder the potential settling process of the tibial component during the first weeks [4]. Screws can optionally be used for additional fixation of the talar component (Fig. 8.31). Fluoroscopy is used to check the final position of the implants (Fig. 8.32).

8.5 Wound Closure

The retinaculum and tendon sheet are closed over one suction drain (Fig. 8.33), and the skin is closed using interrupted sutures (Fig. 8.34). The incision is then covered with a compressive dressing (Fig. 8.35), and a well-padded short leg splint (Fig. 8.36) is used to keep the foot in a neutral position.

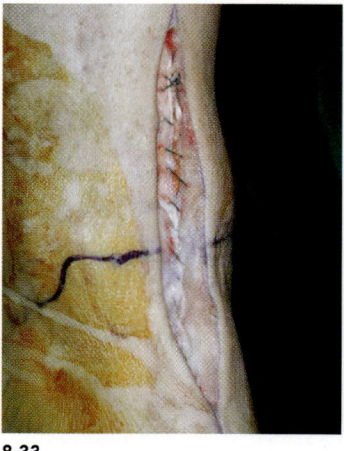

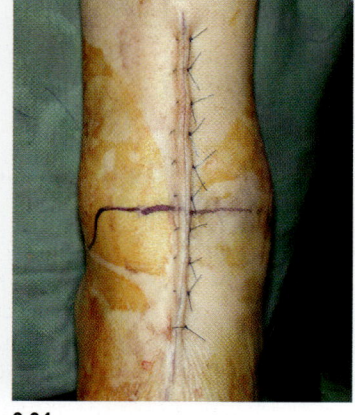

Fig. 8.33. Closure of the retinaculum.
The retinaculum is closed over a drain

Fig. 8.34. Wound closure.
The skin is closed by interrupted sutures

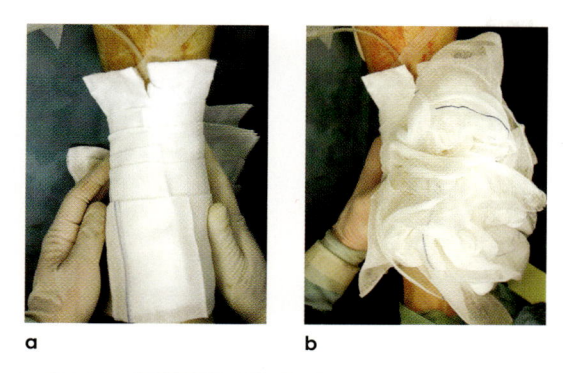

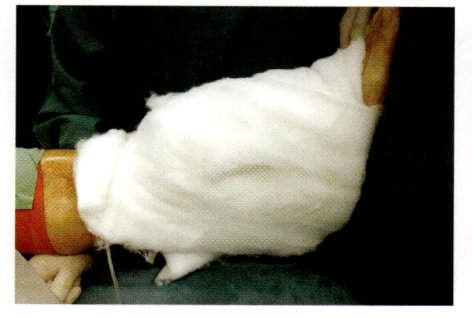

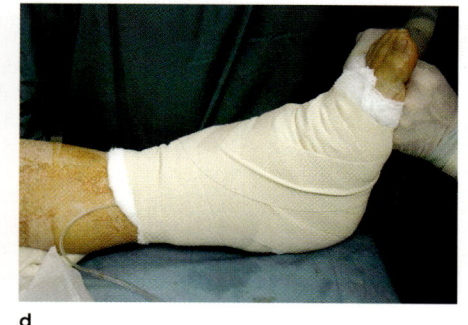

Fig. 8.35. Compressive dressing.
Compressive dressing is applied step by step: first layer with smooth wound contact (**a**); second layer for high absorption (**b**); cotton wool (**c**); and compressive bandage (**d**)

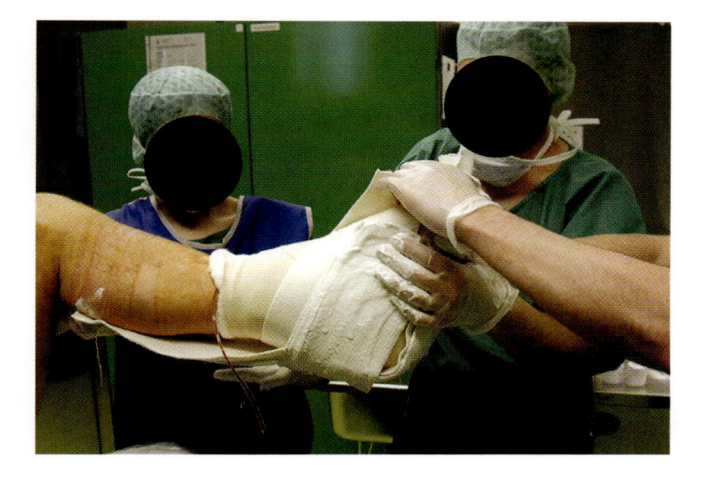

Fig. 8.36. Short leg splint.
A short leg splint is applied to keep the foot in neutral position

8.6 Additional Surgeries

In the case of malalignment, ligamentous instability, and concomitant osteoarthrosis of hindfoot joints, additional surgeries are considered prior to prosthetic implantation; whereas, heel cord lengthening may be considered at the end of the ankle replacement surgery.

8.6.1 Lateral Ligament Reconstruction

Varus deformity that is associated with lateral ligamentous instability can be managed with direct anatomic lateral reconstruction, with or without medial release of the deltoid ligament, particularly for chronic instability (see Chap. 7, Sect. 7.3.7: Hindfoot-Ankle Instability) [7].

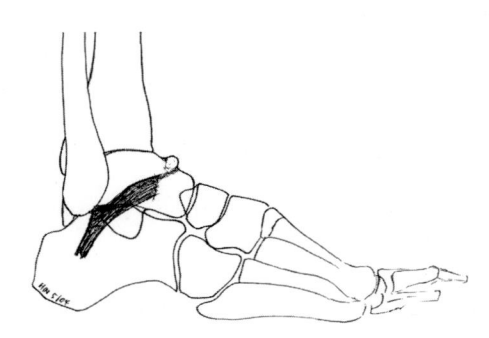

8.37 a

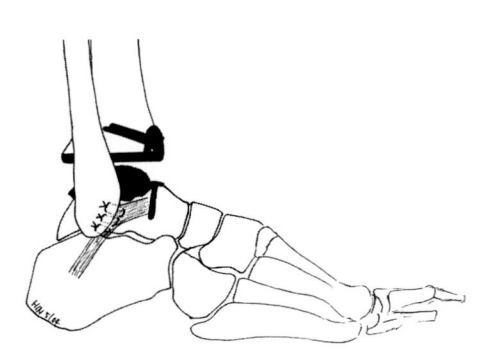

8.37 b

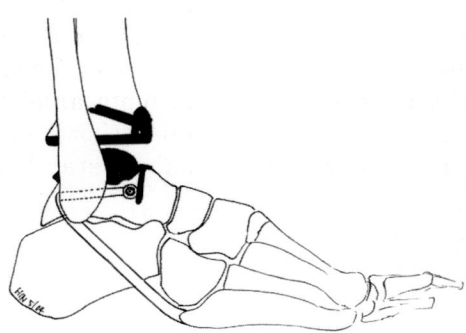

8.37 c

Fig. 8.37. Lateral ligament reconstruction.
Varus-supination deformity with lateral ankle instability typically results in anterolateral subluxation of the talus out of the mortise, and posterior dislocation of the fibula, respectively (**a**). The lateral ankle ligaments (for example, the anterior talofibular and calcaneofibular ligaments) are mostly disconnected from the distal fibula. If the remaining lateral ankle ligaments are substantially preserved, their continuity to the fibula is reconstructed by transosseous sutures, thereby stabilizing the talus within the ankle mortise (**b**). If the remaining lateral ankle ligaments are insufficient for being reconstructed, then the short peroneal tendon is dissected as proximally as possible (that is, where the muscle belly starts) and re-routed through a tunnel to the anterior aspect of the fibula, to be attached under tension to the talar neck (**c**)

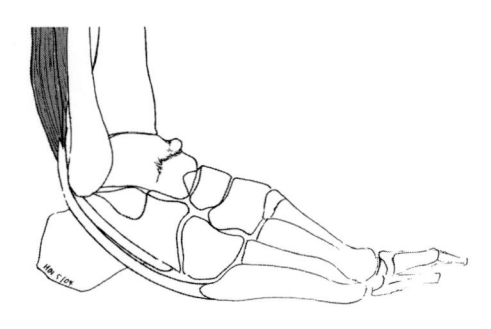

8.38 a

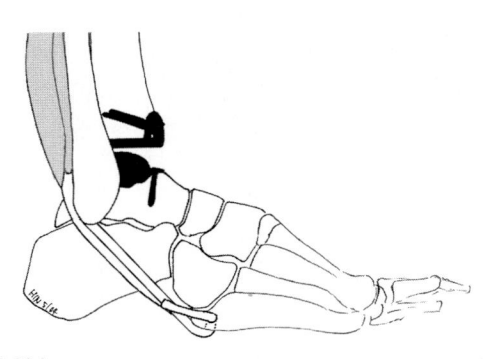

8.38 b

Fig. 8.38. Peroneal tendon transfer.
Abnormal tightness of the long peroneal tendon is typically observed in long-standing varus-supination deformity with lateral ankle instability, thus causing plantar flexion of the first metatarsal (**a**). The long peroneal tendon is dissected through a small incision over the cuboid and then tenodesed to the base of the fifth metatarsal (**b**)

8.6 Additional Surgeries

The anterior talofibular ligament may be reconstructed anatomically with local structures, if possible (that is, the Broström technique). In the case of anterior subluxation of the talus (for example, with total loss of anterior talofibular ligament function), plasty of the anterior talofibular ligament is necessary. The short peroneal tendon is split (in a modification of the Evans procedure) and then routed from posterior to anterior through a drill hole in the lateral malleolus, to be attached under tension to the lateral talar neck (Fig. 8.37).

8.6.2 Peroneal Tendon Transfer

If abnormal tightness of the long peroneal tendon is observed, it is tenodesed through a small incision over the cuboid to the base of the fifth metatarsal, with or without medial release of the deltoid ligament, particularly for chronic instability (see Chap. 7, Sect. 7.3.7. Hindfoot-Ankle Instability) (Fig. 8.38). Alternatively, the long peroneal tendon can be sutured to the short peroneal tendon through a lateral incision at the ankle joint level, for instance while fusing the anterior syndesmosis (as is required when using the AGILITY™ ankle.)

8.6.3 Dorsiflexion Osteotomy of the First Metatarsal

If a plantar-flexed first ray is present (that is, having a neutral position that is plantar flexed relative to the lesser metatarsals), a dorsiflexion osteotomy of the base of the first metatarsal is performed through a second small incision (see Chap. 7, Sect. 7.3.7. Hindfoot-Ankle Instability) (Fig. 8.39).

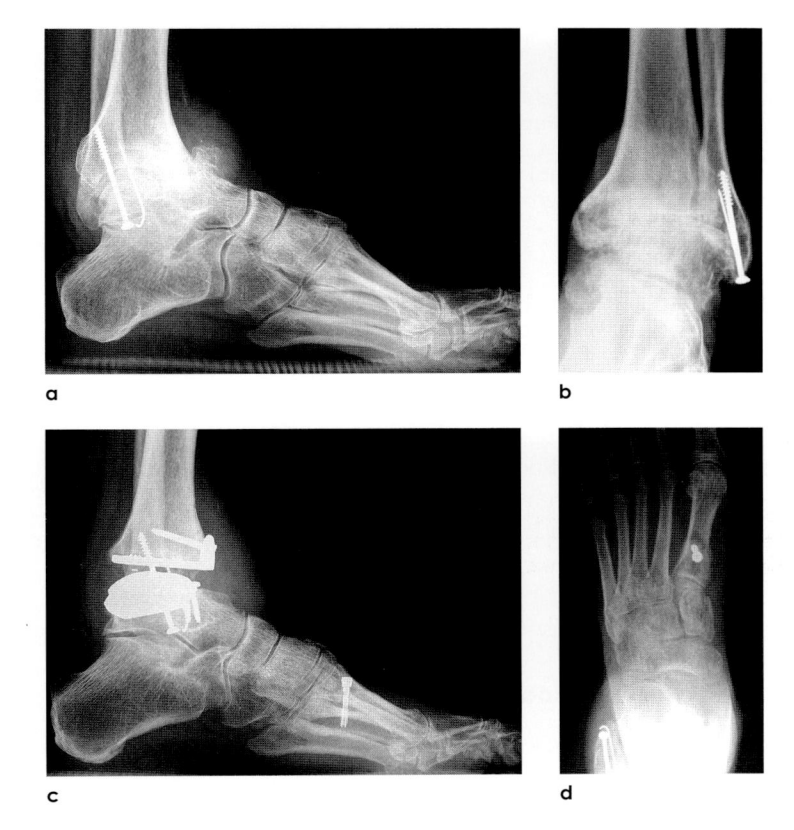

Fig. 8.39. Dorsiflexion osteotomy of the first metatarsal. If abnormal plantar flexion of the first metatarsal (**a**) causes varus-supination deformity of the hindfoot (**b**), dorsiflexion osteotomy of the first metatarsal is performed through a small dorsomedial incision (**c, d**)

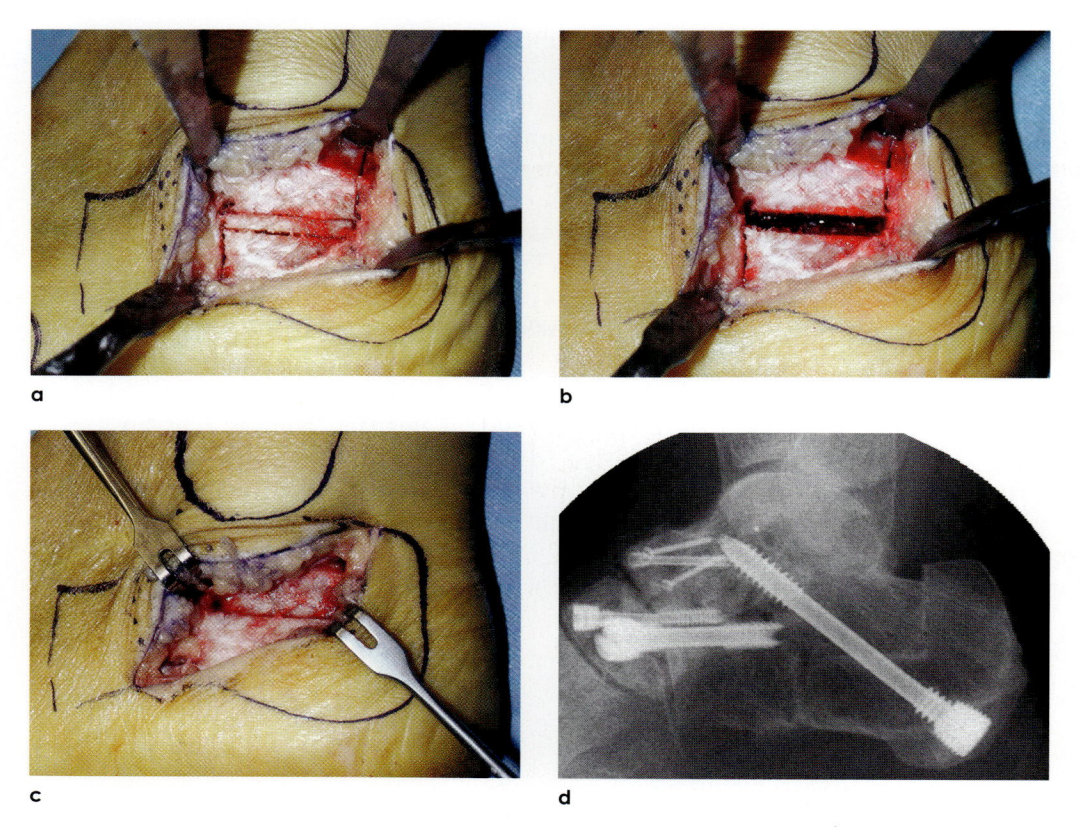

Fig. 8.40. Valgisation osteotomy of the calcaneus.
If abnormal varus deformity of the calcaneus causes supination forces through eccentric pull of the triceps surae, a valgisation osteotomy is considered. The calcaneus is exposed through a lateral incision just posterior to the peroneal tendons, and a Z-shaped osteotomy is performed (**a**). A second horizontal osteotomy is performed convergent to the first to create a wedge that is removed (**b**). The calcaneal tuber is slid laterally to the desired position, and everted to close the horizontal osteotomy (**c**). Fixation is obtained using a compression screw inserted percutaneously from the heel (**d**)

8.6.4 Valgisation Osteotomy of the Calcaneus

If the heel remains in varus after ligament reconstruction, the heel might be corrected to minimize the varus moment about the ankle. Through a lateral incision just posterior to the peroneal tendons, a lateral Z-shaped calcaneal osteotomy is performed, which allows the calcaneal tuber to be slid laterally and tilted into a physiological valgus (see Chap. 7, Sect. 7.3.7. Hindfoot-Ankle Instability) (Fig. 8.40).

8.6.5 Medial Ligament Reconstruction

In the case of a valgus ankle, the incompetent medial ligaments are reconstructed by restoring and tensioning the deltoid-spring ligament complex (see Chap. 7.3.7. Hindfoot-Ankle Instability) (Fig. 8.41) [9].

8.6.6 Medial Sliding Osteotomy of the Calcaneus

If the hindfoot remains in valgus after the ankle and forefoot are realigned (see Chap. 7, Sect. 7.3.7. Hindfoot-Ankle Instability), then a medial sliding osteotomy of the calcaneus is performed through a lateral incision just posterior to the peroneal tendons, and the tuber is slid medially at least 1 cm (Fig. 8.42).

8.6.7 Hindfoot Fusion

The management of adjacent joint arthritis (subtalar and transverse tarsal joints) in the presence of

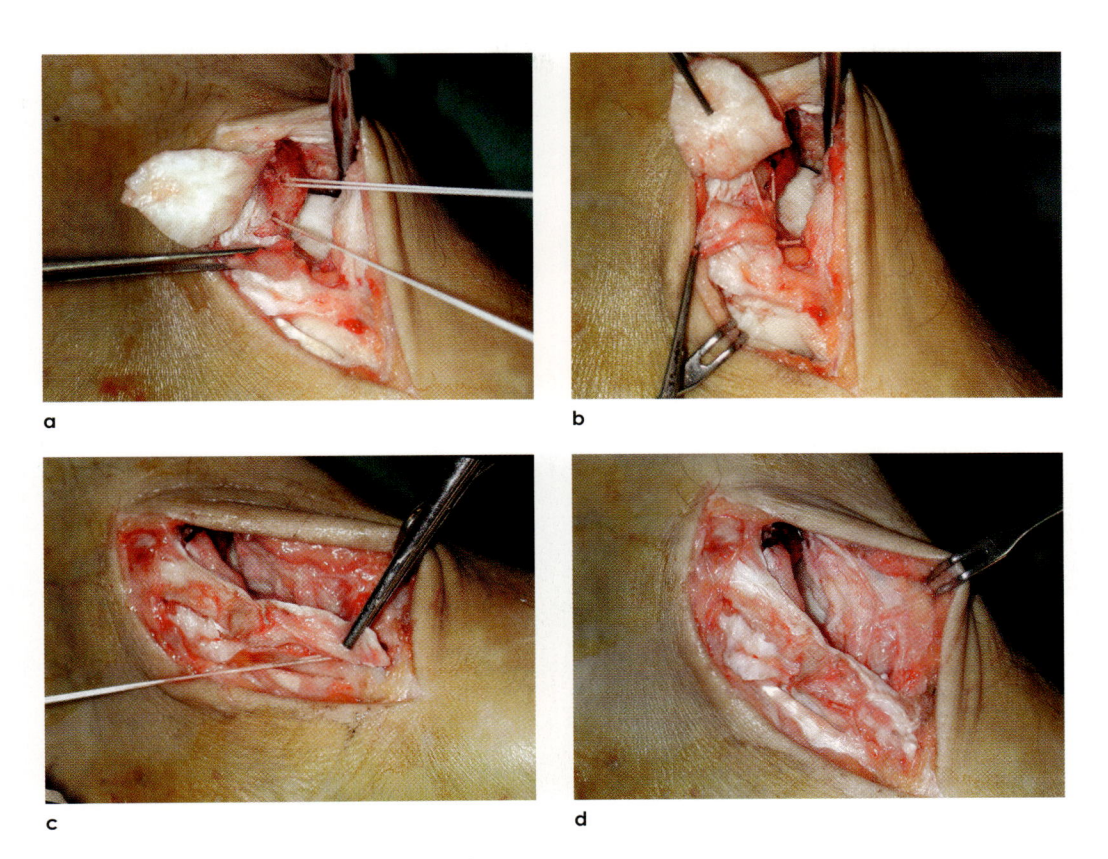

Fig. 8.41. Medial ankle ligament reconstruction.
If abnormal medial ankle instability is present, causing supple pronation deformity of the hindfoot and/or valgus tilt of the talus within the ankle mortise while weight-bearing, reconstruction of the medial ankle ligament is considered. The superficial proximal part of the deltoid is dissected distally to expose the deep layer, which is dissected proximally, and the anterior aspect of the fibula is seen (**a**). One or two anchors are inserted into the distal fibula (**b**). While the foot is held in supination and varus, the deep layer of the deltoid is reattached to the fibula using the bone anchors, and the superficial layer is reattached distally (**c**). Additional sutures are used for final reconstruction of a strong ligament structure (**d**)

an arthritic ankle is still a matter of considerable debate (see Chap. 7, Sect. 7.3.5. Adjacent Joint Arthritis). If necessary, it is proposed to proceed with subtalar (Fig. 8.43), talonavicular (Fig. 8.44), or triple arthrodesis (Fig. 8.45) before total ankle arthroplasty in order to obtain a rigid plantigrade foot. However, the surgeon should be aware that concomitant fusions of the hindfoot may affect the long-term outcome of the total ankle replacement.

8.6.8 Heel Cord Lengthening

If more than 5° of dorsiflexion cannot be achieved even after removing the posterior ankle joint capsule (Figure 8.20), then lengthening of the gastrocnemius-soleus complex should be considered (see Chap. 7, Sect. 7.3.8. Heel Cord Contracture). This can be performed at the musculotendinous junction or by Achilles tendon lengthening. In some instances, tenolysis of the posterior tibial tendon through a separate incision should be considered (Fig. 8.46) [1].

8.7 Conclusions

Proper incision technique and careful handling of the soft-tissue mantle are of utmost importance for successful total ankle arthroplasty. With a few

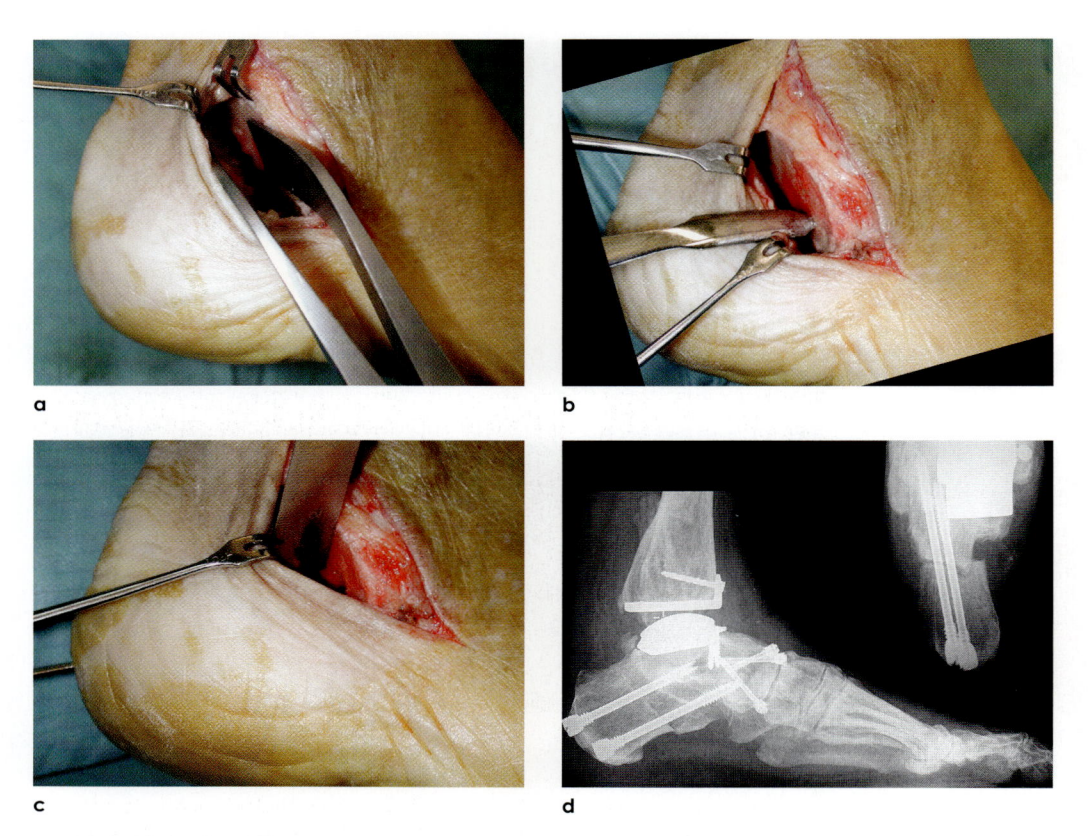

Fig. 8.42. Medial sliding osteotomy.
If abnormal valgus of the hindfoot causes pronation forces through eccentric pull of the triceps surae, a medial sliding osteotomy is considered. The calcaneus is exposed through a lateral incision just posterior to the peroneal tendons, and an oblique osteotomy is performed. A lamina spreader is used to mobilize the tuber fragment (**a**). A Hohmann retractor is used to slide the calcaneal tuber medially to the desired extent (**b**). One or two Kirschner wires are inserted from posteriorly to stabilize the tuber against the calcaneal body. The achieved medial displacement can then be measured (**c**), and the overhanging bone removed using a luer. Fixation is achieved by inserting one or two compression screws over the Kirschner wires. This X-ray shows the situation six weeks after surgery (**d**)

exceptions, current total ankle systems use an anterior approach between the anterior tibial and extensor hallucis longus tendons. Once the arthritic ankle joint is exposed, the osteophytes have to be removed and the fibrotic capsule sufficiently released in order to make the ankle joint as normal as possible. This makes it possible to recognize potential malalignment and/or instability, and to address such concomitant problems prior to the ankle replacement.

When considering the bony cuts, it is extremely important to respect the individual anatomy of the patient, particularly the tibiotalar angle in the coronal plane. In addition, correct positioning of the talar component in the sagittal plane is mandatory in order to have a well-balanced ankle after replacement. Heel cord lengthening is seldom necessary when the entire fibrotic capsule has been removed.

8.7 Conclusions

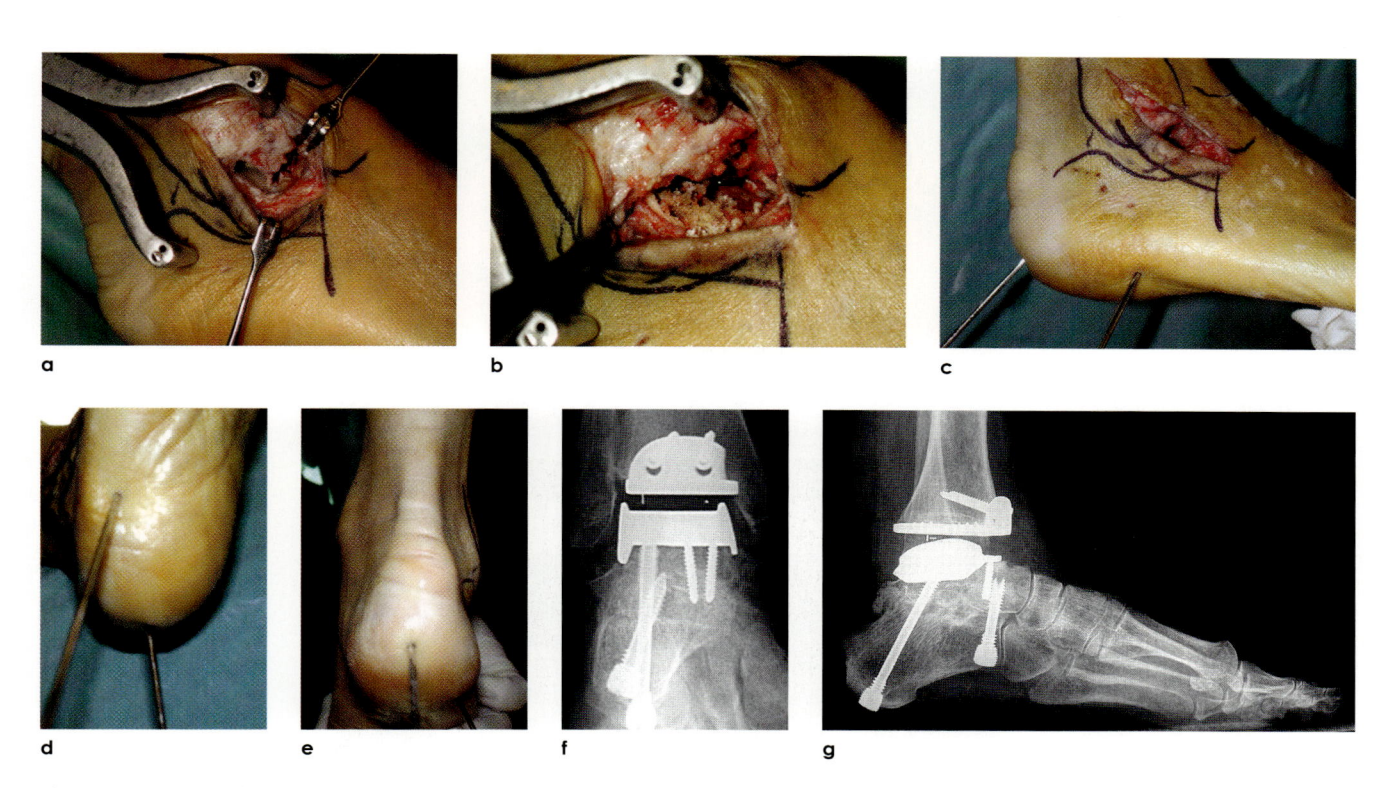

Fig. 8.43. Subtalar fusion.
The subtalar joint is exposed through a lateral approach. The Hintermann™ Distractor is used to distract the subtalar joint and to get an interior view (**a**). After removing the remaining cartilage, a drill is used to break the sclerotic subchondral bone (**b**), and the spreader is removed. Once the desired position for the arthrodesis is achieved, two Kirschner wires are inserted from posteriorly (**c**) and distally (**d**), and hindfoot alignment is checked while elevating the leg from the table (**e**). After six weeks, radiological assessment under full weight-bearing shows a well-aligned hindfoot and achieved fusion on anteroposterior (**f**) and lateral (**g**) views

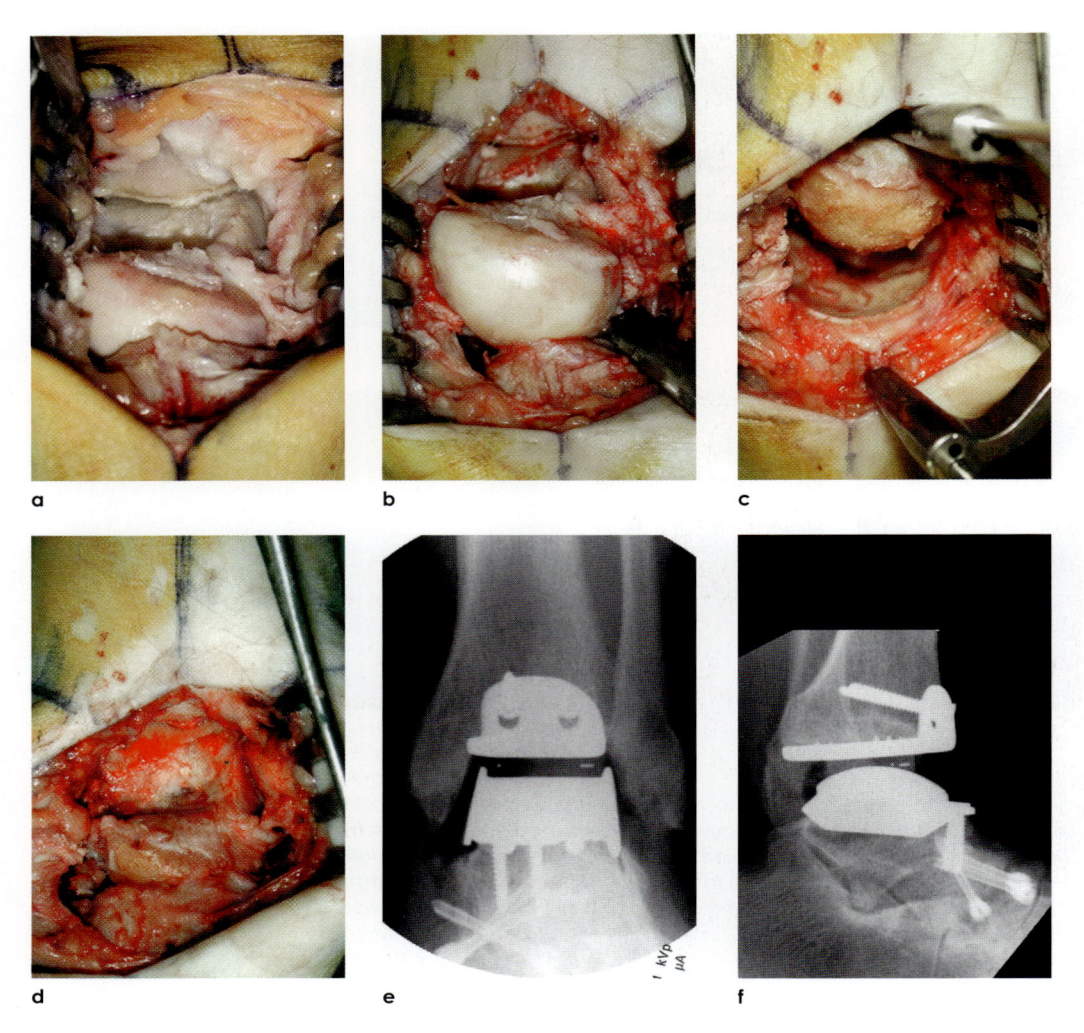

Fig. 8.44. Talonavicular fusion.
The talonavicular joint is exposed through the longitudinal anterior approach that is used for implantation of the ankle prosthesis (**a**). The Hintermann™ Distractor is used to distract the navicular joint (**b**). The talar (**c**) and then the navicular (**d**) joint surfaces are carefully cleaned of cartilage, being careful to preserve the contours of the surfaces. The postoperative radiographs show a well-aligned hindfoot and achieved fusion on anteroposterior (**e**) and lateral (**f**) views

8.7 Conclusions

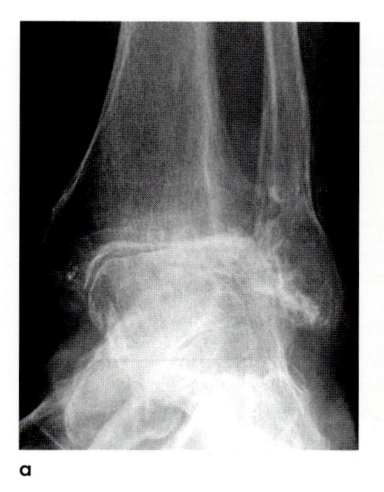

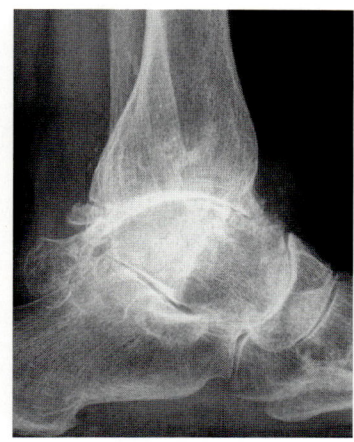

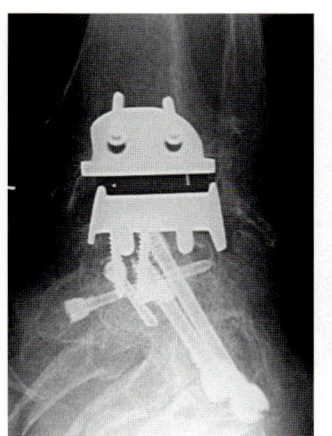

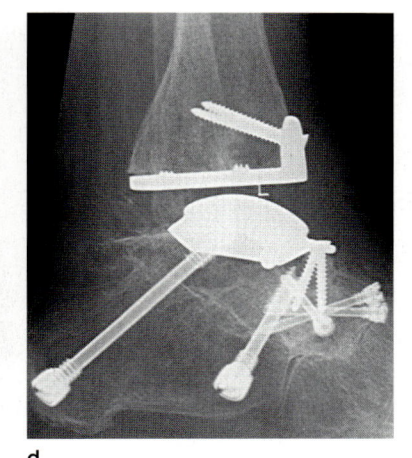

Fig. 8.45. Triple fusion.
This patient (female, 66 years) with rheumatoid arthritis exhibits a valgus and pronation deformity with involvement of the ankle, subtalar, and talonavicular joints. There is severe osteoarthritis of the ankle with valgus malalignment of the talus (**a**), together with significant arthritic changes in the subtalar and talonavicular joint (**b**). As a result, triple arthrodesis is considered at the time of total ankle replacement. The subtalar joint is fused using a lateral approach, in the same way as for an isolated subtalar fusion (Fig. 8.43), and the talonavicular joint is fused as shown in Fig. 8.44. The calcaneocuboid joint is not fused in order to preserve some mobility in the lateral column of the foot. After eight weeks, radiological assessment shows a well-aligned hindfoot and achieved fusion on anteroposterior (**c**) and lateral (**d**) views

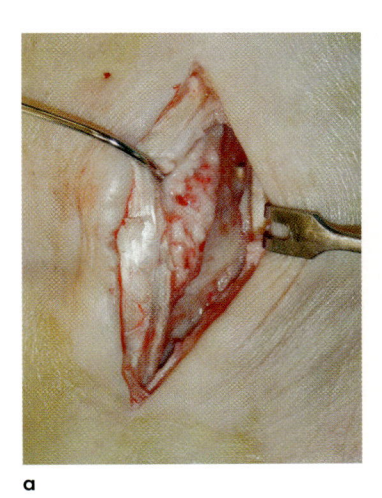

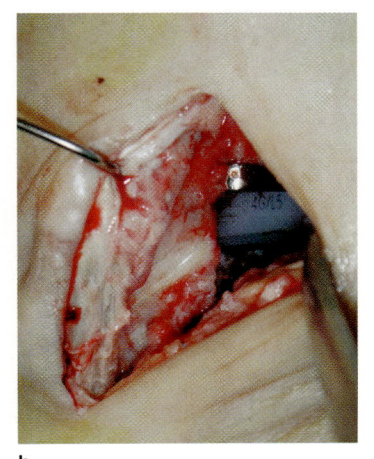

Fig. 8.46. Posterior tibial tendon and posteromedial capsule release.
Nine months after total ankle replacement (for osteoarthrosis eight years after open fracture of the lateral and medial malleoli), this patient (female, 54 years) presented with tenderness and painful swelling along the posterior tibial tendon, combined with dorsiflexion limited to 5°. The tendon is exposed through a posteromedial approach and identified behind the medial malleolus. After extensive debridement and release of the scar tissues, the tendon is dislocated and the flexor digitorum tendon is seen (**a**). While a Hohmann retractor is inserted to keep the posterior structures away from the capsule of the ankle, arthrotomy of the ankle is performed and the capsule resected, allowing the implanted prosthesis to be seen (**b**)

References

[1] Bonnin M (2002) Prothèse total de la cheville. In: Techniques chirurgicales: orthopédie-traumatologie (Encyl Med Chir, ed). Editions scientifiques et médicales, Paris, chap 44, pp 903–907

[2] Bonnin M, Judet T, Colombier J, Piriou P, Gravaleau N, Buscayret F (2004) Mid-term results of the first 98 consecutive SALTO total ankle arthroplasties. In: Proc. AAOS Congress, San Francisco, USA

[3] Buechel FF, Buechel FF, Pappas MJ (2002) Eighteen-year evaluation of cementless meniscal bearing total ankle replacements. AAOS Instruct. Course Lect., chap 16, pp 143–151

[4] Carlsson A (2004) Radiostereometric analysis of the double coated S.T.A.R. total ankle prosthesis. A 4-year follow-up of 5 cases with rheumatoid arthritis. In: Proc. 5th EFAS Congress, Montpellier, France

[5] Conti SF, Wong YS (2001) Complications of total ankle replacement. Clin Orthop 391: 105–114

[6] Conti SF, Wong YS (2002) Complications of total ankle replacement. Foot Ankle Clin 7: 791–807

[7] Gould JS, Alvine FG, Mann RA, Sanders RW, Walling AK (2000) Total ankle replacement: a surgical discussion. Part II. The clinical and surgical experience. Am J Orthop 29: 675–682

[8] Hintermann B, Valderrabano V (2003) Total ankle replacement. Foot Ankle Clin 8: 375–405

[9] Hintermann B, Valderrabano V, Boss AP, Trouillier HH, Dick W (2004) Medial ankle instability – a prospective study of 54 cases. Am J Sports Med 32: 183–190

[10] Hintermann B, Valderrabano V, Dereymaeker G, Dick W (2004) The HINTEGRA ankle: rationale and short-term results of 122 consecutive ankles. Clin Orthop 424: 57–68

[11] Inman VT (1991) The joints of the ankle, 2nd ed. Williams & Wilkins, Baltimore, pp 31–74

[12] Knupp M, Hintermann B (2004) The surgical tibiotalar angle – a radiological study. Foot Ankle Int (submitted)

[13] Kofoed H (1998) Medium-term results of cementless Scandinavian total ankle replacement prosthesis (LINK S.T.A.R.) for osteoarthrosis. In: Current status of ankle arthroplasty (Kofoed H, ed), chap 24. Springer, Berlin, pp 116–120

[14] Kofoed H, Lundberg-Jensen A (1999) Ankle arthroplasty in patients younger and older than 50 years: a prospective series with long-term follow-up. Foot Ankle Int 20: 501–506

[15] Lin S, Drzala M (1998) Independent evaluation of Buechel-Pappas 2nd generation cementless total ankle arthroplasty; intermediate-term results. In: Proc. American Orthopaedic Foot and Ankle Society Specialty Day Meeting, New Orleans, USA

[16] Mendolia G (1998) Ankle arthroplasty – The Ramses prosthesis. In: Current status of ankle arthroplasty (Kofoed H, ed), chap 21. Springer, Berlin, pp 99–105

[17] Pyevich MT, Saltzman CL, Callaghan JJ, Alvine FG (1998) Total ankle arthroplasty: a unique design. Two to twelve-year follow-up. J Bone Joint Surg Am 80: 1410–1420

[18] Rudigier J, Grundei H, Menzinger F (2001) Prosthetic replacement of the ankle in posttraumatic arthrosis. Europ J Trauma 2: 66–74

[19] Takakura Y, Yanaka Y, Sugimoto K, Tamai S, Masuhara K (1990) Ankle arthroplasty. A comparative study of cemented metal and uncemented ceramic prostheses. Clin Orthop 252: 209–216

[20] Valderrabano V, Hintermann B, Dick W (2004) Scandinavian total ankle replacement: a 3.7-year average follow-up of 65 patients. Clin Orthop 424: 47–56

[21] Wood PLR (2002) Experience with the STAR ankle arthroplasty at Wrightington Hospital, UK. Foot Ankle Clin 7: 755–765

Chapter 9

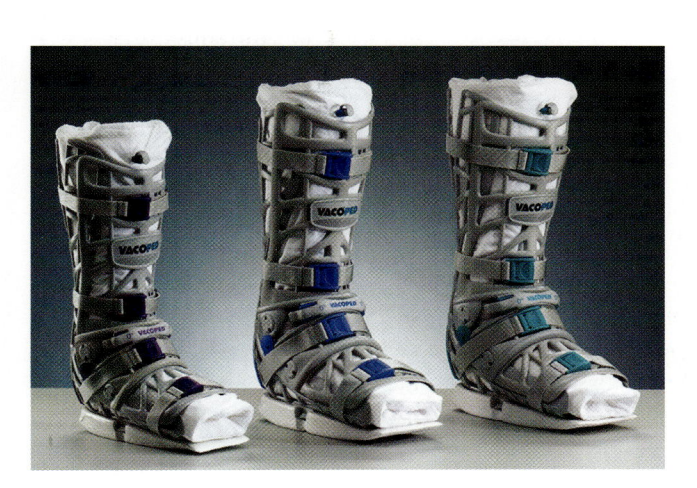

POSTOPERATIVE CARE AND FOLLOW-UP

As a principle, the ankle should be protected postoperatively against uncontrolled movements to promote wound healing and to permit stable bone ingrowth to the implants. The design of the ankle, implantation technique, additional surgeries, and associated foot disorders may each play a significant role in determining the postoperative regimen. This section summarizes the author's postoperative treatment concept.

9.1 Postoperative Care

Weight-bearing to tolerance is begun on the first postoperative day, with intermittent elevation when nonambulatory. When the wound condition is suitable, typically after two to four days, the initial short leg splint is replaced by a brace (Vacuped®, Oped, Cham, Switzerland; Fig. 9.1) that protects the ankle against eversion, inversion, and plantar

Fig. 9.1. Vacuped®.
The Vacuped® (oped, Cham, Switzerland) is available in three sizes. As the vacuum is applied, the air cushion is stabilized while maintaining a proper and stable fit to the foot and ankle (see text)

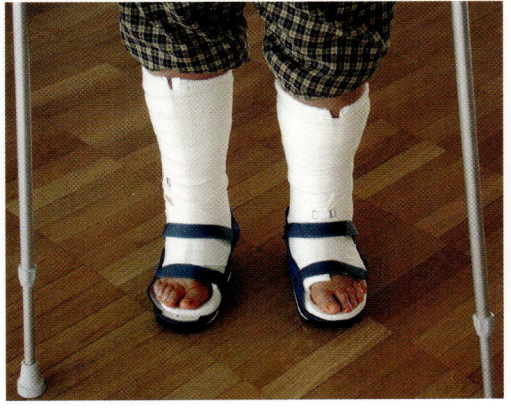

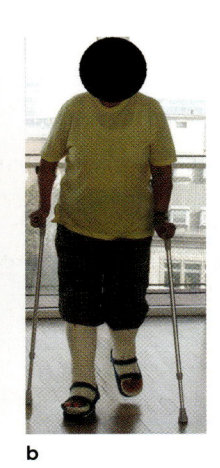

Fig. 9.2. Short weight-bearing cast.
Short weight-bearing casts were used for this patient (female, 66 years, second postoperative day) because of lateral ligament reconstruction on both ankles during bilateral total ankle replacement. These temporary casts with anterior openings (**a**) allow for some weight-bearing (**b**), but will be replaced by stronger, circular casts when local swelling is gone

flexion movements for six weeks. For patients with poor bone quality, and/or who have undergone additional surgeries such as realignment, ligament reconstruction, and/or joint fusions, a short weight-bearing cast (Fig. 9.2) is used for six weeks, and a brace is used for an additional four to six weeks. Stable shoes and support stockings are then recommended for two to six months until the swelling has subsided and ankle strength has returned. Thereafter, comfortable footwear is worn during activities of daily living. Custom-molded shoes or corrective orthotic insoles may be prescribed for associated complex foot disorders.

9.2 Rehabilitation Program

A stretching program is commenced immediately after surgery. The patient is asked to bear as much load as possible on the operated foot, and then to bring the knee successively anteriorward until the heel starts to lift up off of the floor (Fig. 9.3). The patient is advised to perform this exercise once or twice a day. Lymphatic drainage is started after removal of the sutures, usually two weeks after surgery. If a short leg cast is used, lymphatic drainage and stretching exercises are started after removal of the cast. Active range-of-motion exercises are begun six weeks after surgery. The rehabilitation program additionally includes exercises to improve muscular strength and muscular control of foot movement, with gradual return to full activities as tolerated.

9.3 Follow-up Examination

Regular clinical and radiological controls may help to identify problems at an early stage, and thus prevent failures. To date, the author sees his postoperative patients at six weeks, at four months, and at one year, and yearly thereafter for clinical and radiological control. An extensive standardized protocol is used at one year, and thereafter for each yearly control.

9.3.1 Clinical Assessment

Patients are asked to indicate their current level of function (as compared with preoperative function) in activities of daily living and in specific activities (sports and climbing stairs, for example) (Table 9.1), as well as their level of satisfaction with the procedure.

The clinical examination includes a careful assessment of the alignment of the ankle with the patient standing, and the range of motion and stability of the ankle with the patient sitting and standing. The range of motion is determined clinically using a goniometer along the lateral border of the leg and foot. Alignment, stability, and motion are compared with the uninvolved side.

The patient then is asked to rate his or her pain on a scale of 0 to 10 points, with no pain giving 0 points, and maximal pain giving 10 points. Then the AOFAS Hindfoot Score is calculated [3].

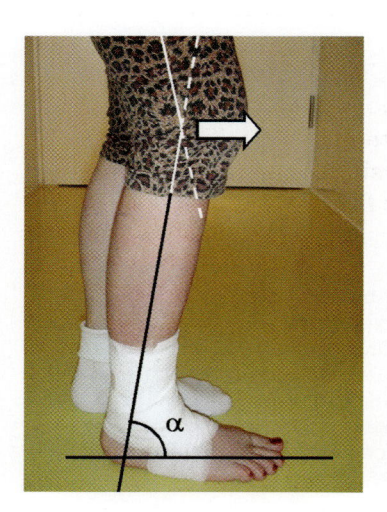

Fig. 9.3. Stretching program.
The knee is brought anteriorward (knee flexion) until the heel starts to lift up off of the floor (female, 49 years, second postoperative day; see text)

9.3 Follow-up Examination

Table 9.1. Clinical score

Grade	Pain	Limitation of Recreational Activities	Limitation of Daily Activities	Requirement for Support	Wearing of Fashionable Shoes
Excellent	None	None	None	None	Yes
Good	Mild, occasional	Some	None	None	Some
Fair	Moderate, frequent	Yes	Yes	One cane	None
Poor	Severe, nearly always	Severe	Severe	Walker or brace	Orthopedic shoes

9.3.2 Radiographic Measurements

Postoperative radiographic examinations are best taken with the aid of fluoroscopy in order to obtain standardized and true anteroposterior and lateral views of both components. Image intensification is used to obtain straight anteroposterior and lateral views of the tibial component. This allows the evaluation of migration or loosening on serial radiographs (Fig. 9.4).

Angular and linear values are defined to delineate alignment and component migration (Fig. 9.5: α-angle, β-angle, γ-angle, distances "a" and "b," diameter of potential lysis) and measured digitally with a special metric software system (Imagic Access®, PIC Systems AG, Glattbrugg, Switzerland).

Loosening of the tibial component is defined as a change in position of greater than 2° of the flat base of the component in relation to the long axis of the tibia. For example:
- with the HINTEGRA® ankle [2]; angles "a" and "b" in Fig. 9.5b, and/or as a progressive radiolucency of more than 2 mm in either the anteroposterior or the lateral view, and
- with the S.T.A.R. ankle [1, 4]; angles "a" and "b" in Fig. 9.6b, and/or as a subsidence into the tibial bone of greater than 2 mm (distance "a" in Fig. 9.6a).

Loosening of the talar component as seen on the lateral radiograph is defined as subsidence into the talar bone of greater than 5 mm. For example:
- with the HINTEGRA® ankle [2]; distances "a" and "b" in Fig. 9.5b, or a change in position of greater than 5° relative to the line drawn from the top of the talonavicular joint to the tuberosity of the calcaneus (angle γ in Fig. 9.5b), and
- with the S.T.A.R. ankle [1, 4]; distances "b" and "c" in Fig. 9.6b, or a change in position of greater than 5° relative to the line drawn from the top of the talonavicular joint to the tuberosity of the calcaneus (angle γ in Fig. 9.6b).

Evaluation of a minor change in position of the talar component on the anteroposterior radiograph is very difficult, and it is not possible to evaluate radiolucencies beneath the talar component on either view.

True foot and ankle motion are measured by lateral views under fluoroscopy, while the patient is standing on a footplate (Fig. 9.7). The footplate is plantar flexed and dorsiflexed as much as possible, until the tibia tends to follow foot motion.

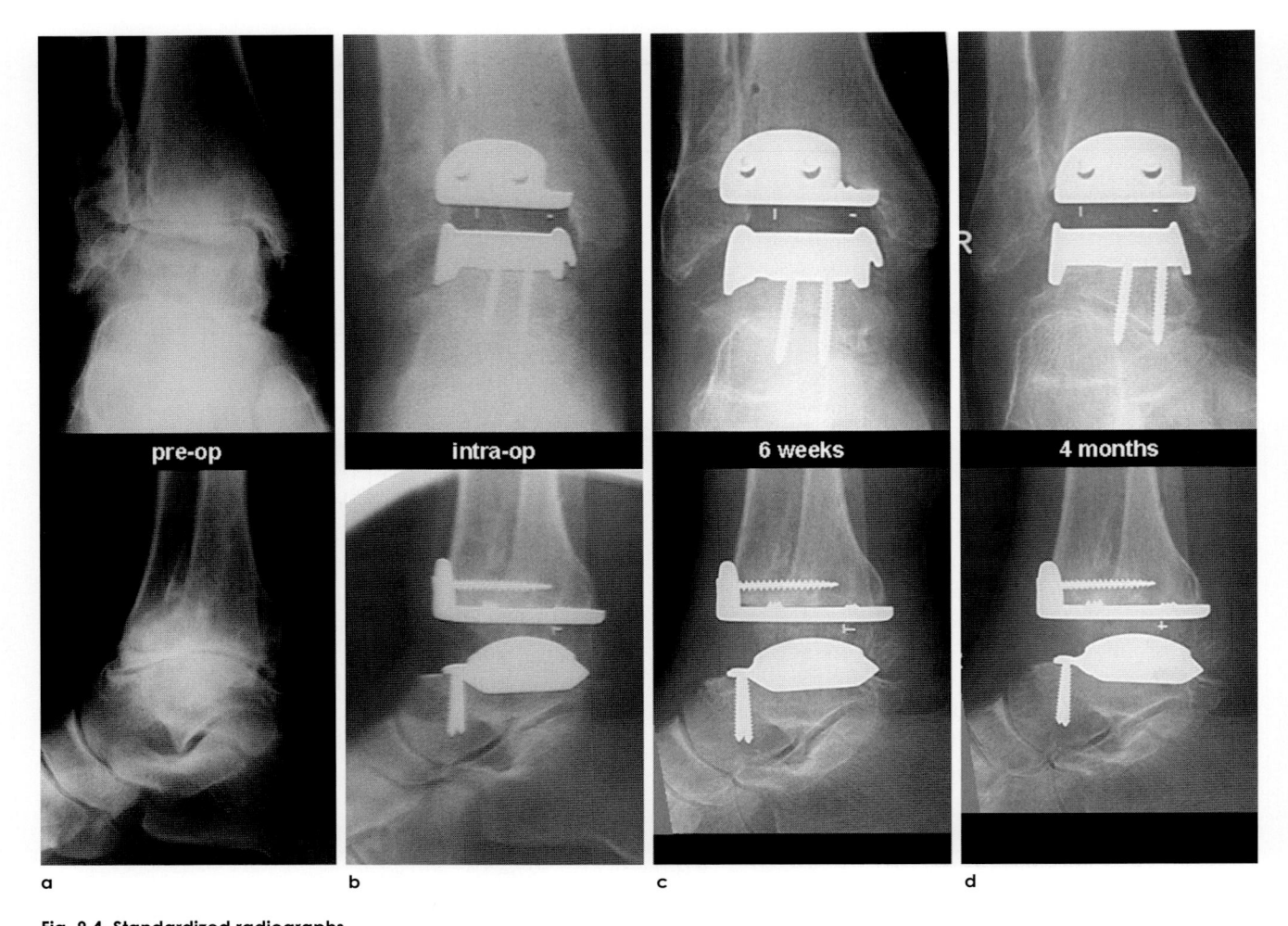

Fig. 9.4. Standardized radiographs.
Post-traumatic osteoarthrosis after ankle fracture (male, 59 years, smoker): Standardized anteroposterior and lateral views (**a**) are obtained using image intensification to show the position of the implants and the bone-implant interface similarly for all follow-up controls (**b–h**)

9.3 Follow-up Examination

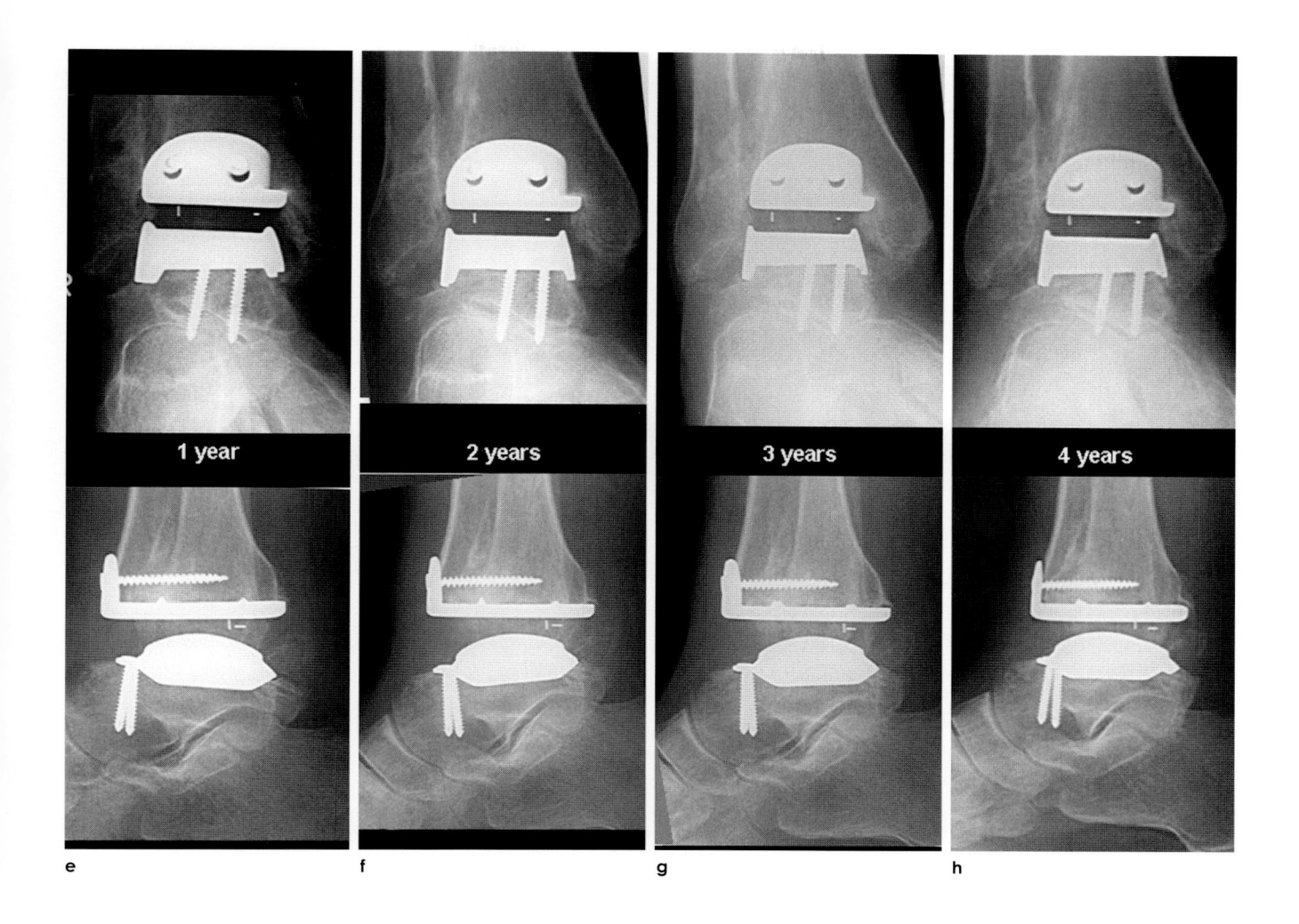

1 year	2 years	3 years	4 years
e	f	g	h

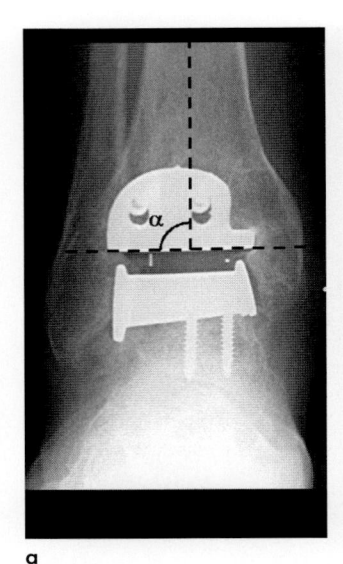

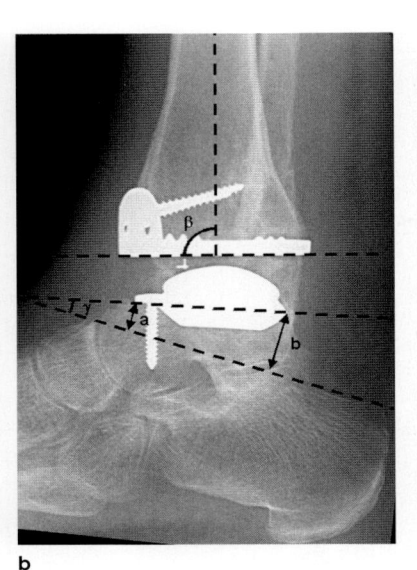

Fig. 9.5. Reference lines – HINTEGRA® ankle.
The following reference lines and angles are used to evaluate stability and loosening of the tibial and talar components [2]:
a: α = the angle, on anteroposterior view, between the longitudinal axis of the tibia and the articulating surface of the tibial component;
b: β = the angle, on lateral view, between the longitudinal axis of the tibia and the articulating surface of the tibial component; γ = the angle, on lateral view, between a line drawn through the anterior shield and the posterior edge of the talar component and a line drawn between the dorsal aspect of the talonavicular joint and the tuberosity of the calcaneus; "a" = the perpendicular distance, on lateral view, from the most anterior part of the talar component to a line drawn between the dorsal aspect of the talonavicular joint and the tuberosity of the calcaneus; and "b" = the perpendicular distance, on lateral view, from the most posterior part of the talar component to the same line described under "a" (female, 43 years; two-year follow-up)

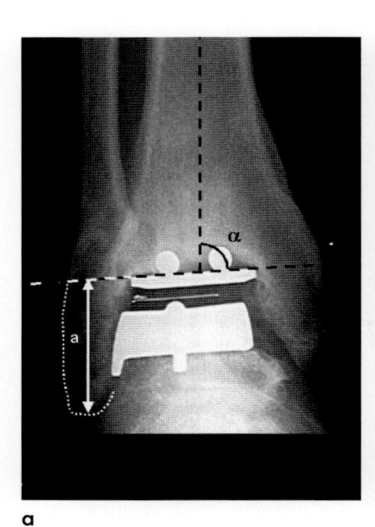

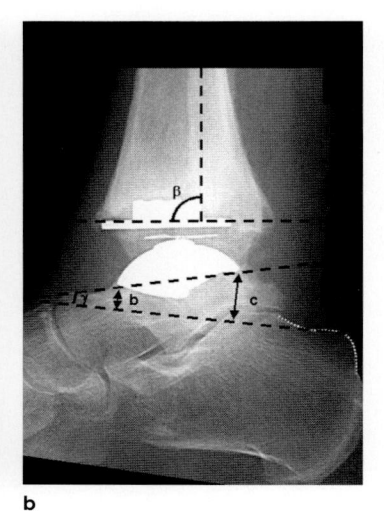

Fig. 9.6. Reference lines – S.T.A.R. ankle.
The following reference lines and angles are used to evaluate stability and loosening of the tibial and talar components [1, 4]:
a: α = the angle, on anteroposterior view, between the longitudinal axis of the tibia and the articulating surface of the tibial component; "a" = the perpendicular distance, on anteroposterior view, between the tip of the lateral malleolus and a line drawn through the base of the tibial component;
b: β = the angle, on lateral view, between the longitudinal axis of the tibia and the articulating surface of the tibial component; γ = the angle, on lateral view, between a line drawn through the anterior shield and the posterior edge of the talar component and a line drawn between the dorsal aspect of the talonavicular joint and the tuberosity of the calcaneus; "b" = the perpendicular distance, on lateral view, from the most anterior part of the talar component to a line drawn between the dorsal aspect of the talonavicular joint and the tuberosity of the calcaneus; and "c" = the perpendicular distance, on lateral view, from the most posterior part of the talar component to the same line described under "a" (male, 52 years; five-year follow-up)

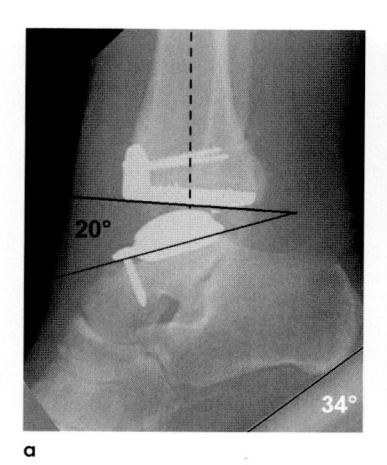

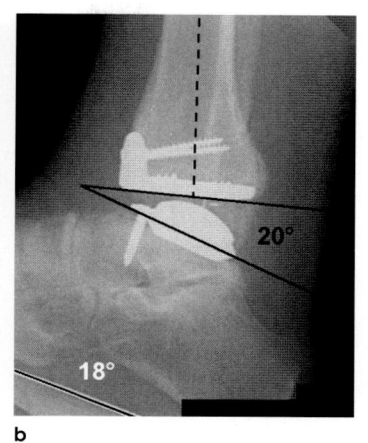

Fig. 9.7. Foot and true ankle motion.
Radiographs show range of motion as measured for plantar flexion (**a**) and dorsiflexion (**b**). "True ankle motion" (the motion within the prosthetic system), and "foot motion" (the total motion of the hindfoot with respect to the tibial long axis – dashed lines) (male, 68 years; one-year-follow-up)

9.4 Conclusions

The replaced ankle should be protected postoperatively against uncontrolled movements to promote wound healing and to permit stable bone ingrowth to the implants. Most implants allow for weight-bearing, as tolerated, within one to two weeks after surgery. As a principle, the main rehabilitation program starts after six weeks, including stretching exercises, lymphatic drainage, active range-of-motion exercises, and exercises to improve muscular strength and muscular control of foot movement, with gradual return to full activities as tolerated. Regular clinical and radiological controls may help to identify problems at an early stage, and thus prevent failures. A standardized clinical and radiographic examination is recommended.

References

[1] Anderson T, Montgomery F, Carlsson A (2003) Uncemented S.T.A.R. total ankle prosthesis. Three to eight-year follow-up of fifty-one consecutive ankles. J Bone Joint Surg Am 85: 1321–1329
[2] Hintermann B, Valderrabano V, Dereymaeker G, Dick W (2004) The HINTEGRA ankle: rational and short-term results of 122 consecutive ankles. Clin Orthop 424: 57–68
[3] Kitaoka HB, Alexander IJ, Adalaar RS, Nunley JA, Myerson MS, Sanders M (1994) Clinical rating systems for the ankle-hindfoot, midfoot, hallux, and lesser toes. Foot Ankle Int 15: 349–353
[4] Valderrabano V, Hintermann B, Dick W (2004) Scandinavian total ankle replacement: a 3.7-year average follow-up of 65 patients. Clin Orthop 424: 47–56

Chapter 10

WHAT IS FEASIBLE IN TOTAL ANKLE ARTHROPLASTY?

There has been a vast change in the treatment approach for managing ankle osteoarthritis over the past decade. Not only has the surgical treatment armamentarium expanded, but the viable options are now more numerous, and total ankle arthroplasty is emerging as an alternative to ankle arthrodesis. It is apparent that there are several arthroplasty designs to choose from, and each has its staunch advocates. The complications experienced by total ankle arthroplasty patients in the early days of the procedure remain a concern, but one which fortunately seems to be overcome by gaining a more thorough understanding of the prostheses, the literature, and the execution of the surgery. As the available knowledge of total ankle arthroplasty increases, more interest is given to the question of how far total ankle arthroplasty can go, and what is feasible. This section attempts to summarize some of the author's experience with regard to the possibilities and limitations of total ankle arthroplasty.

10.1 Reconstruction of the Malaligned Ankle

Restoring and maintaining proper bony alignment and muscle balance in the limb is essential if there is to be any chance for long-term survival of a total ankle arthroplasty. If proper alignment is not achieved, the talar component can tilt in the mortise, leading to unacceptably high pressures in the polyethylene insert, (which results in increased polyethylene wear; see Fig. 11.3, Chap. 11: Complications of Total Ankle Arthroplasty), excessive shear forces at the bone-implant interface (which increases the risk of component loosening), and excessive tension of the ligaments (which creates secondary instability; see Fig. 11.7, Chap. 11: Complications of Total Ankle Arthroplasty).

10.1.1 Varus Malalignment

Recurrent sprains and chronic lateral ankle instability may develop into ankle osteoarthritis over time. Ankles with anterior talofibular ligament incompetence seem to end up anteriorly extruded (Fig. 10.1), whereas those with incompetence of the calcaneofibular ligament seem to experience more ankle varus (Fig. 10.2). In either case, most of these feet exhibit some hindfoot varus and a high arch, and a plantar-flexed first ray is common. Identifying the location of the bony deformity is imperative.

In the first case (extruded varus ankle, Fig. 10.1), a dorsiflexion osteotomy of the first ray (see Fig. 8.39, Chap. 8: Surgical Techniques) and a peroneal longus tendon transfer to the base of the fifth metatarsal (see Fig. 8.38, Chap. 8: Surgical Techniques) were done during total ankle replacement. Calcaneal osteotomy and lateral ligament reconstruction were not deemed necessary. At four months, the foot looks well aligned and stable, and the patient is extremely satisfied with the obtained result. Apparently, accommodation of the first metatarsal and strengthening the abduction and pronation power of the peronei were sufficient to correct the deformity and to normalize the varus moment about the ankle, in spite of not repeating a ligamentoplasty (because of three previously performed and failed ligamentoplasties). There were no changes until the most recent follow-up at three years.

In the second case (concentric varus ankle, Fig. 10.2), however, only a medial ligament release was performed at the time of surgery, while the forefoot deformity was not corrected. At four months, the varus deformity persisted with a continuous feeling of instability. Therefore, a dorsiflexion osteotomy of the first metatarsal and a lateral sliding osteotomy (see Fig. 8.40, Chap. 8: Surgical Techniques) were

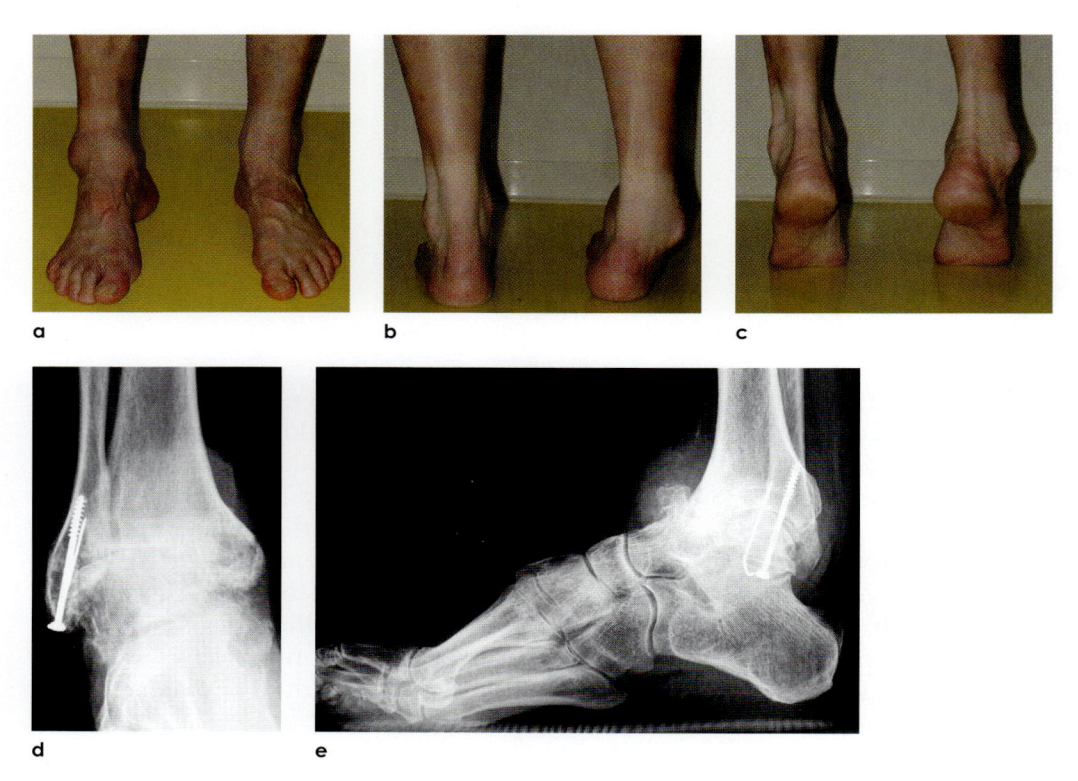

Fig. 10.1. The extruded varus ankle.
This 67-year-old man developed ankle osteoarthritis many years after recurrent sprains. There was an anterolateral swelling and tenderness (**a**), and a varus malalignment of the heel, together with an externally rotated tibia and posteriorly dislocated fibula, respectively (**b**) that was partially corrected while in tip-toe position (**c**). The weight-bearing X-rays show the varus deformity to be caused by erosion of the medial tibial plafond (**d**), a high arch with plantar-flexed first ray, and incompetence of the anterior talofibular ligament and consequent anterior extrusion of the talus (anterolateral dislocation of the talus out of the ankle mortise); the integrity of the subtalar joint was preserved (**e**). The pedobarography (Emed-System, Novel, Munich, Germany) shows increased pressure beneath the head of the first metatarsal (**f**). During total ankle replacement, exposure of the ankle showed the erosion of the medial tibial plafond, and cartilage wear on medial talus (**g**). Four months after surgery (which included dorsiflexion osteotomy of the first metatarsal, peroneal longus transfer, and total ankle replacement), there is still some periarticular swelling and a slight varus malalignment of the heel, but no extrusion of the talus nor external rotation of the tibia (**h–j**). On the mortise view, the hindfoot is well aligned (**k**), and the lateral view shows the talus correctly positioned within the mortise (that is, having correct tibiotalar alignment and position of the fibula), and a well-balanced medial arch (**l**). The anteroposterior view of the loaded foot also shows proper alignment (**m**). The hardware in the distal fibula is from previous lateral ligament reconstruction, and was left in place while asymptomatic

performed. After this, the ankle remained well aligned and stable until the most recent follow-up at two years.

The Author's Recommendation
The arthritic varus ankle is not a single entity. All contributing pathologic processes have to be identified and addressed during surgery. Special attention must be paid to the subtalar joint: if its integrity is preserved, repositioning and stabilization of the talus within the ankle mortise, as well as restoration of peroneal brevis strength are mandatory to attain a well-aligned and stable hindfoot. If the integrity of the subtalar joint is destroyed (which causes instability), restoration of triceps strength by calcaneal osteotomy is mandatory, and, if not sufficient to achieve a well-aligned and stable hindfoot, even a subtalar fusion is advised. Associated deformities such as a plantar-flexed first ray should be corrected as well.

10.1 Reconstruction of the Malaligned Ankle

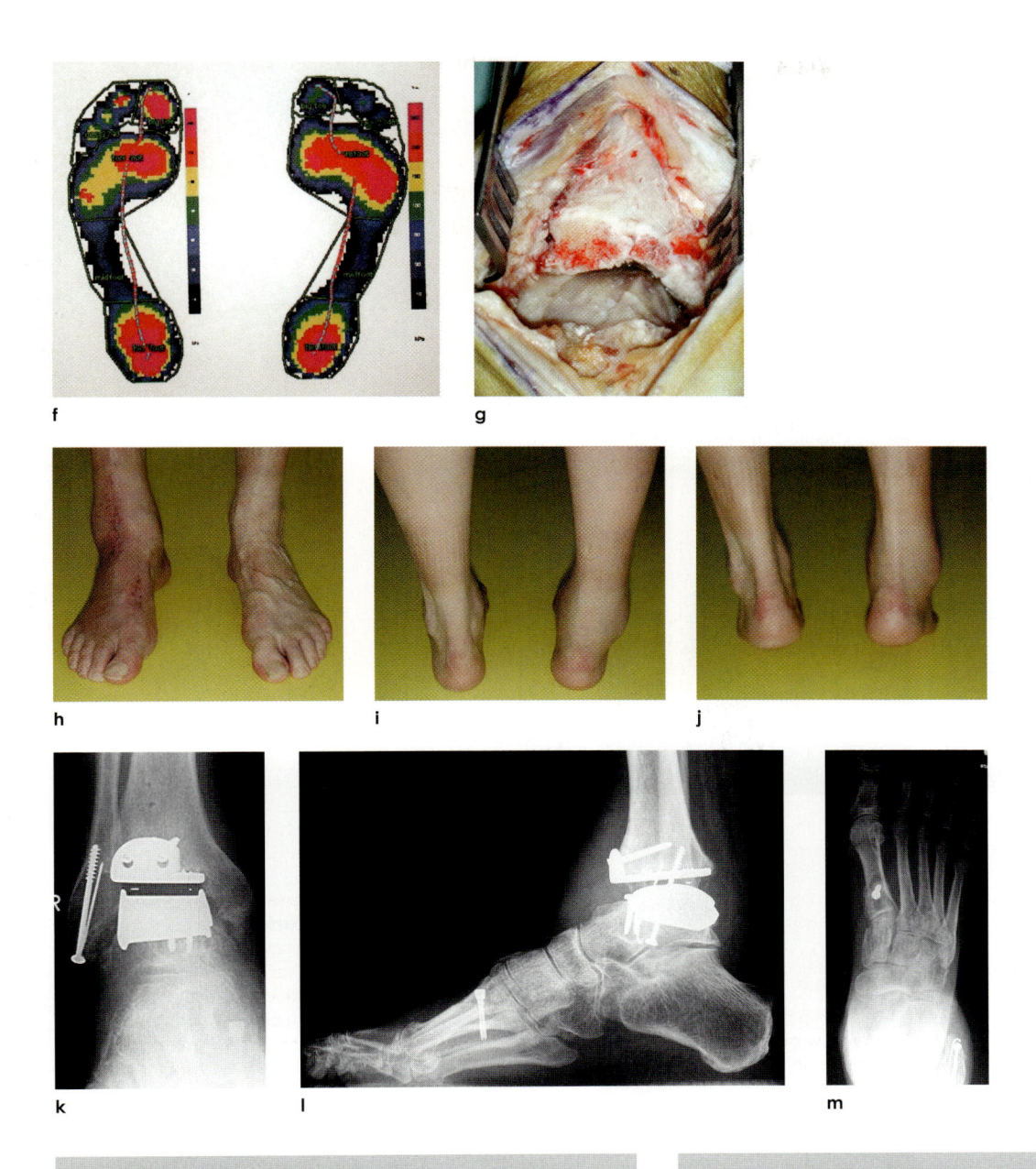

In summary, replacement of an arthritic varus ankle is thought to be successful as long as all associated problems have been properly addressed during surgery. A varus tilt of the talus greater than 30° is probably borderline for achieving sufficient correction and balancing of the ankle, and thus a contraindication for total ankle arthroplasty. Although not yet proven, the use of an ankle system that provides intrinsic stability against inversion moments may have a better prognosis with respect to recurrent varus deformity, but may also potentially experience more polyethylene wear and higher shear forces at the bone-implant interface. Proper aligning and balancing of the whole foot and ankle is, therefore, mandatory for success with any ankle prosthesis. Total ankle arthroplasty performed without attention to the deforming forces in the foot may result in varus tilting of the talus and early failure.

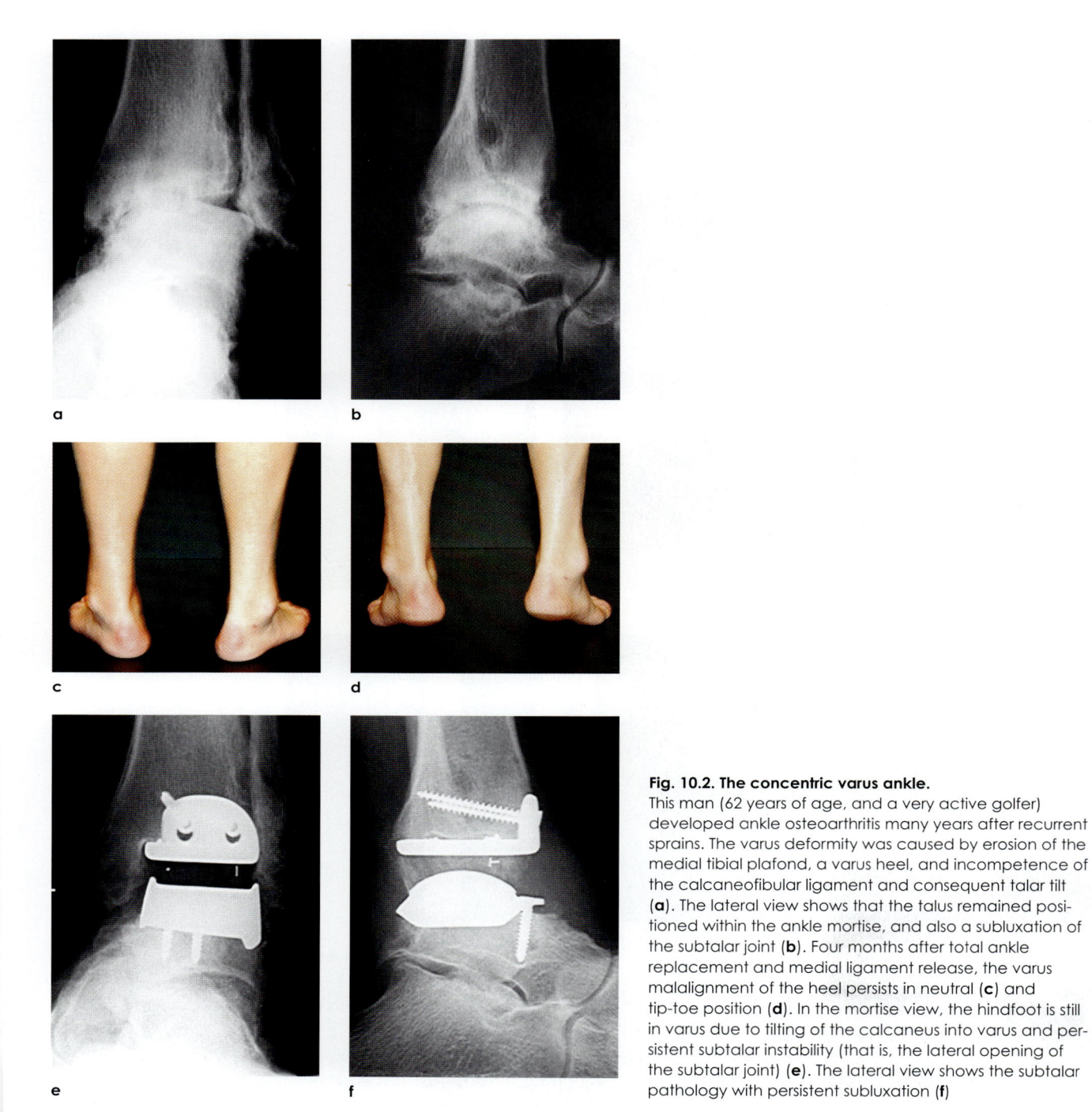

Fig. 10.2. The concentric varus ankle.
This man (62 years of age, and a very active golfer) developed ankle osteoarthritis many years after recurrent sprains. The varus deformity was caused by erosion of the medial tibial plafond, a varus heel, and incompetence of the calcaneofibular ligament and consequent talar tilt (**a**). The lateral view shows that the talus remained positioned within the ankle mortise, and also a subluxation of the subtalar joint (**b**). Four months after total ankle replacement and medial ligament release, the varus malalignment of the heel persists in neutral (**c**) and tip-toe position (**d**). In the mortise view, the hindfoot is still in varus due to tilting of the calcaneus into varus and persistent subtalar instability (that is, the lateral opening of the subtalar joint) (**e**). The lateral view shows the subtalar pathology with persistent subluxation (**f**)

10.1 Reconstruction of the Malaligned Ankle

10.1.2 Valgus Malalignment

Occasionally, a valgus ankle may develop after a severe trauma (for example, an ankle fracture involving the syndesmosis) because the lateral tibial plafond wears away while the deltoid ligament remains tight (Fig. 10.3). Patient complaints are typically related to subfibular pain due to bony

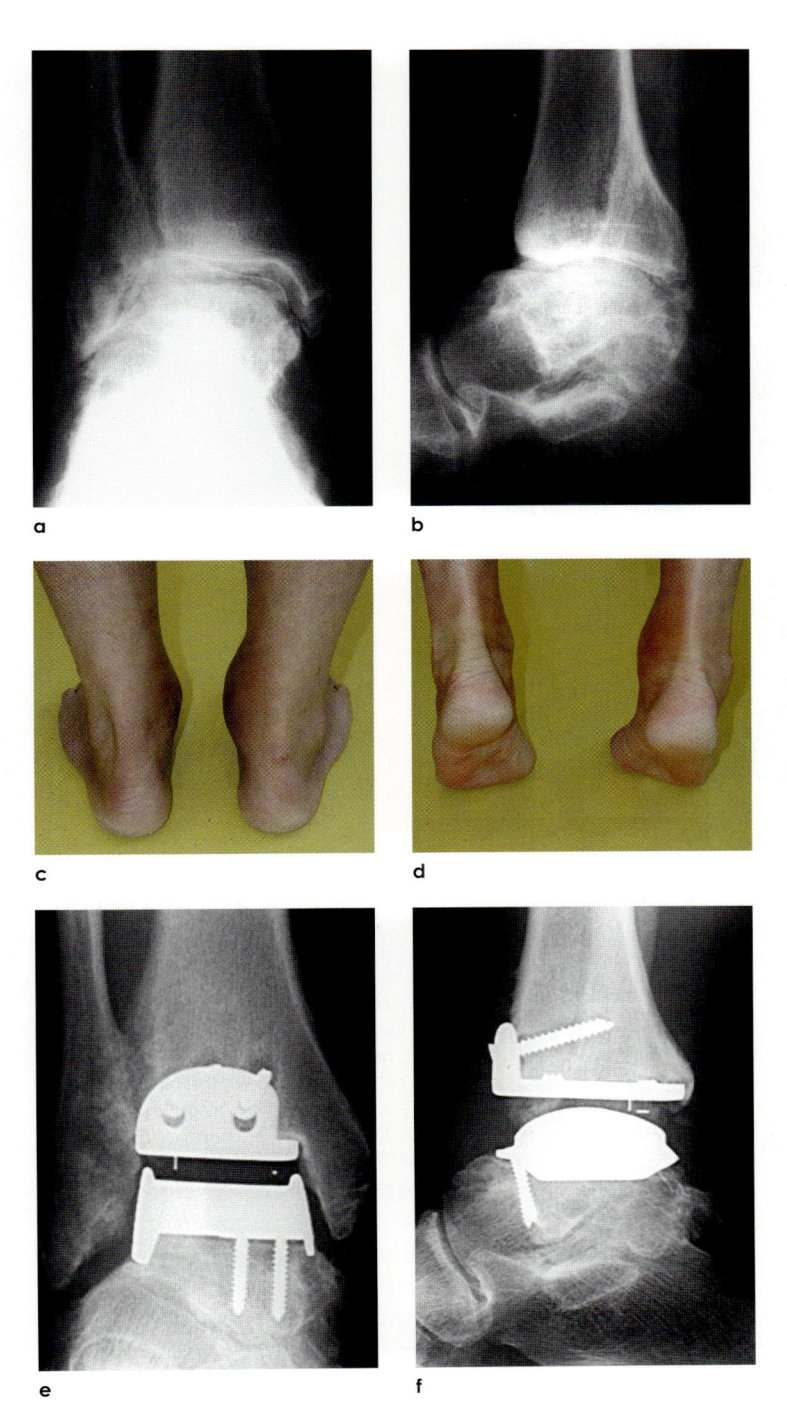

Fig. 10.3. The valgus ankle.
This 64-year-old man developed ankle osteoarthritis in his right ankle 22 years after a severe sprain and conservative treatment. The mortise view shows the valgus tilt of the talus caused by some erosion of the lateral tibial plafond, and severe osteoarthritic changes of the talofibular joint secondary to bony impingement (**a**). The lateral view evidences osteophyte formation on the talar side, and some anterior dislocation of the talus out of the ankle mortise (**b**). At a follow-up of two years, there is still some periarticular swelling on the medial aspect of the ankle, but the foot and ankle are well aligned and stable in neutral (**c**) and tip-toe position (**d**). Weight-bearing X-rays show a well-aligned and stable ankle in both the mortise view (**e**) and lateral view (**f**)

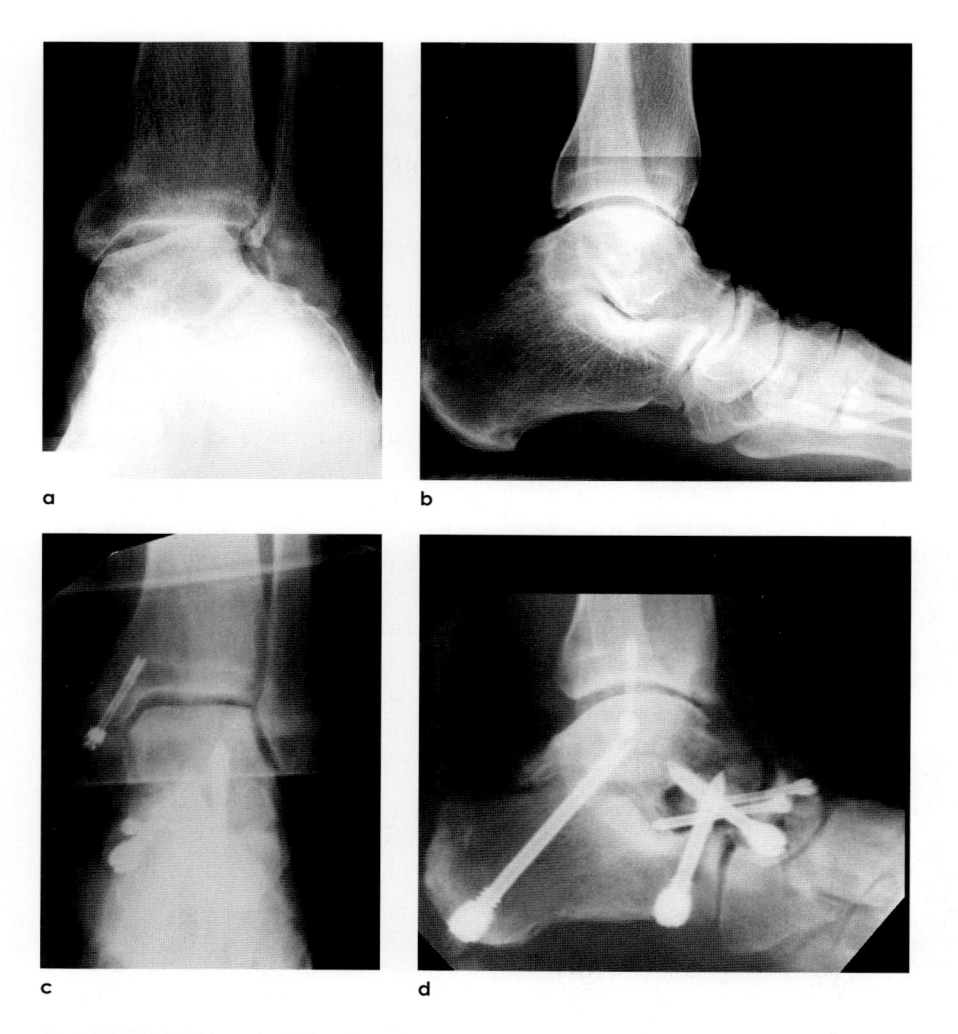

Fig. 10.4. The collapsed valgus hindfoot.
This 58-year-old man had a long history of a "fallen arch," but his pain worsened recently when his ankle tilted into valgus. The deltoid ligament was attenuated from chronic loss of medial column support and progressive forefoot supination (**a**). The lateral view (**b**) shows the breakdown of the medial arch. A triple fusion and medial ligament reconstruction were done in a first step (**c** and **d**; intraoperative views). Because of significant pain relief, total ankle replacement, in a second step, was postponed; it remains, however, a viable option once osteoarthritis of the ankle has progressed

impingement. As the ankle joint collapses, the ligaments become slack, especially on the lateral side. Therefore, minimal bone should be resected during total ankle replacement, and while distracting the ankle, the joint is stabilized and the hindfoot becomes realigned through implantation of the prosthesis.

Recurrent sprains may stretch the deltoid ligament over time, allowing the talus to tilt into valgus (Fig. 10.4). Similarly, a valgus ankle may be the result of a progressive collapse of the arch in an adult flatfoot that is associated with a collapse of the medial column (that is, the talonavicular or spring ligament, navicular-cuneiform, and first tarsometatarsal) joints. As the arch is lost, the ankle tilts more into valgus. Because the lack of deltoid support is a contraindication for ankle replacement, the basic principle of arthroplasty in the valgus joint is to regain bony and ligamentous medial column support first, by means of a medial sliding osteotomy of the calcaneus or by lateral column lengthening, which restores and tensions the deltoid-spring ligament complex (see Chap. 8: Surgical Technique).

> **The Author's Recommendation**
> The arthritic valgus ankle is not a single entity. All contributing pathologic processes have to be identified and addressed during surgery. If a valgus tilt of the talus has occurred secondary to bone wear on the lateral tibial plafond, but the deltoid ligament is intact, total ankle replacement can be performed without any restriction, and usually no additional surgery is necessary. If the deltoid ligament has worn out and become incompetent, then bony and ligamentous medial column support must be regained first. Achieving this first provides significant pain relief, and total ankle replacement can be postponed longer. With respect to this observation, a two-step procedure is probably better in all cases where the degenerative changes of the tibiotalar joint are minimal (specifically, where no subchondral cyst formation has occurred).
>
> In summary, replacement of an arthritic valgus ankle is considered to be successful as long as all associated problems have been properly addressed during surgery. A valgus tilt of the talus greater than 15° secondary to an incompetence of the deltoid ligament is probably borderline for achieving sufficient correction and balancing of the ankle, and thus a contraindication for total ankle arthroplasty. Although not yet proven, the use of an ankle system that provides intrinsic stability against eversion moments may have a better prognosis with respect to recurrent valgus deformity, but may also potentially experience more polyethylene wear and higher shear forces at the bone-implant interface. Proper aligning and balancing of the whole foot and ankle is, therefore, mandatory for success with any ankle prosthesis. Medial sliding of the heel (see Fig. 8.42, Chap. 8: Surgical Techniques) is particularly effective in normalizing the forces within the foot and ankle. Total ankle arthroplasty performed without attention to the deforming forces in the foot, however, may result in valgus tilting of the talus and early failure.

10.1.3 Sagittal Plane Malalignment

Sagittal plane malalignment occasionally occurs after malunion of a distal tibial fracture or supramalleolar osteotomy. If, in the presence of a recurvatum malalignment (Fig. 10.5), total ankle replacement was performed without bony correction, the anterior tibial component might be overloaded to the point of exceeding bony resistance, thus resulting in posterior tilt. Another concern is that the polyethylene inlay might not be fully covered by the tibial component, which, in turn, could cause increased wear and breakage. Thus, a correction osteotomy should be performed at the center of rotation and angulation of the deformity before total ankle replacement to enable the surgeon to properly balance the prosthesis.

> **The Author's Recommendation**
> Correction osteotomy of the tibia and fibula must be performed prior to total ankle replacement. If the deformity to be corrected is located in the distal tibial metaphysis, a one-step procedure may be appropriate. If the deformity is located more proximally, however (see Fig. 7.7, Chap. 7: Preoperative Considerations for Total Ankle Arthroplasty), a two-step procedure should be considered in order to minimize complications related to postoperative swelling and wound healing.
>
> In summary, sagittal plane malalignment can be efficiently addressed by correction osteotomy at the level of the deformity (center of rotation and angulation). As the loading axes become normalized, total ankle replacement may be successful.

10.2 Reconstruction of the Post-Traumatic Hindfoot and Ankle

Post-traumatic osteoarthrosis of the ankle may be the result of malunion, instability, and/or bone loss

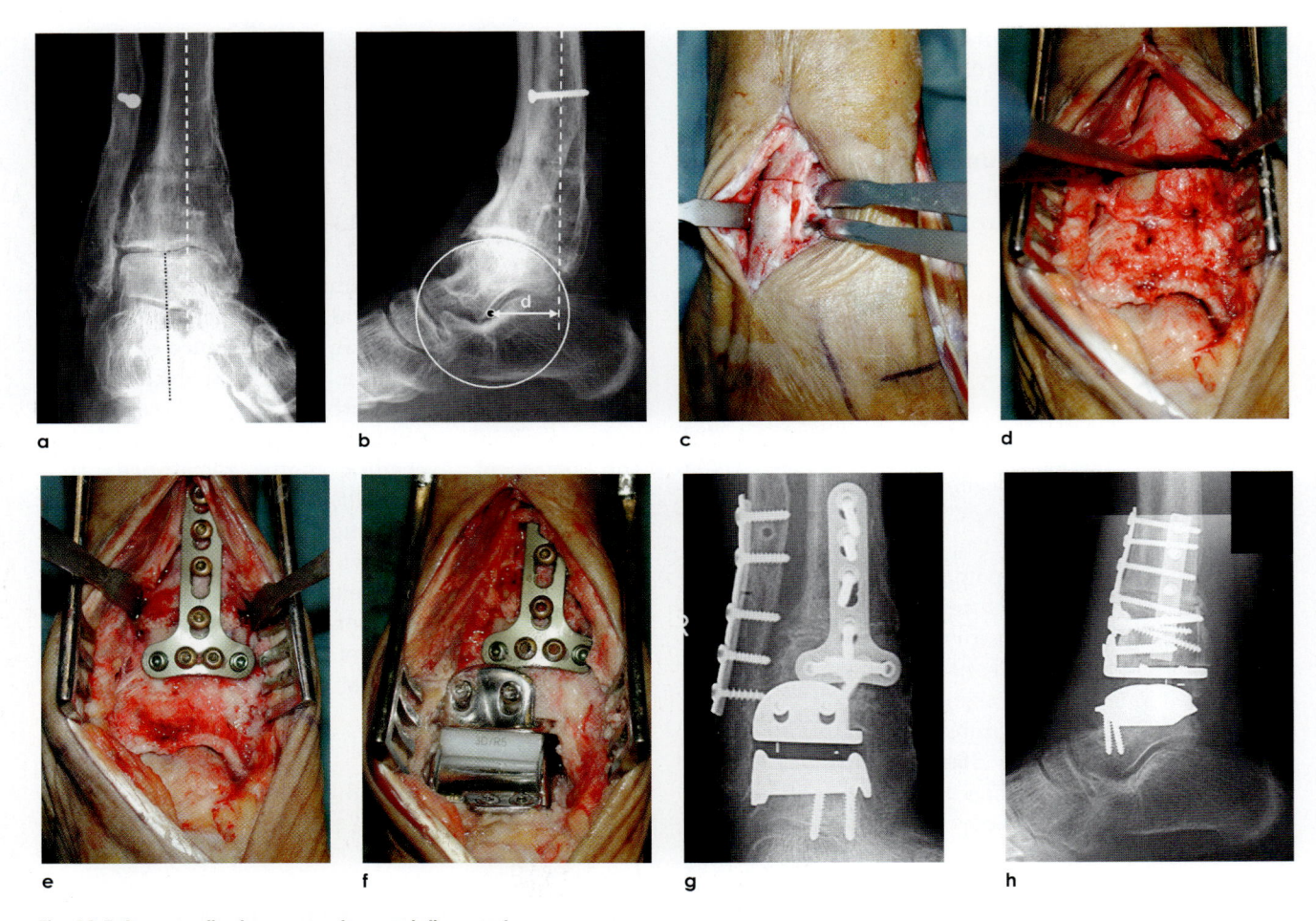

Fig. 10.5. Supramalleolar recurvatum malalignment.
This woman (66 years of age) had a supramalleolar osteotomy 12 years ago for painful varus osteoarthritis after several sprains, with delayed union and recurvatum malunion. As the tibiotalar joint is eccentrically loaded, the degenerative process is located in the medial compartment (**a**), whereas the recurvatum malalignment results in overload and wear of the anterior tibiotalar joint (**b**). A fibular osteotomy was done first through a lateral incision (**c**). Then, supramalleolar tibial osteotomy was done through the standard anterior approach to the ankle (**d**). A tricortical bone graft was inserted and internal fixation using a 3.5-mm plate was achieved (**e**). Thereafter, total ankle replacement was performed (**f**). At eight weeks, the implants were stable but the tibial osteotomy was not yet completely healed (**g**), so the patient was advised to continue with partial weight-bearing. The lateral view shows a well-aligned ankle (**h**).

(either insufficient bone support secondary to incomplete restoration of bony geometry during reconstructive surgery, and/or breakdown of the bone secondary to decreased mechanical resistance or avascular necrosis). A major concern is damage to the soft-tissue mantle. Therefore, an extensive preoperative investigation (including weight-bearing radiographs of both feet and ankles, CT scan, bone scan, and MRI) is mandatory to identify potential problems for total ankle replacement.

10.2.1 Fibular Malunion

If a malunion of the fibula is the underlying cause of an ankle deformity, then the fibula should be repositioned at the time of total ankle replacement. This is particularly true for a malunion with recurvatum malalignment that causes extrusion of the talus out of the ankle mortise (Fig. 10.6), and, to some extent, for a malunion with overlength of the fibula. An underlength fibula, how-

10.2 Reconstruction of the Post-Traumatic Hindfoot and Ankle

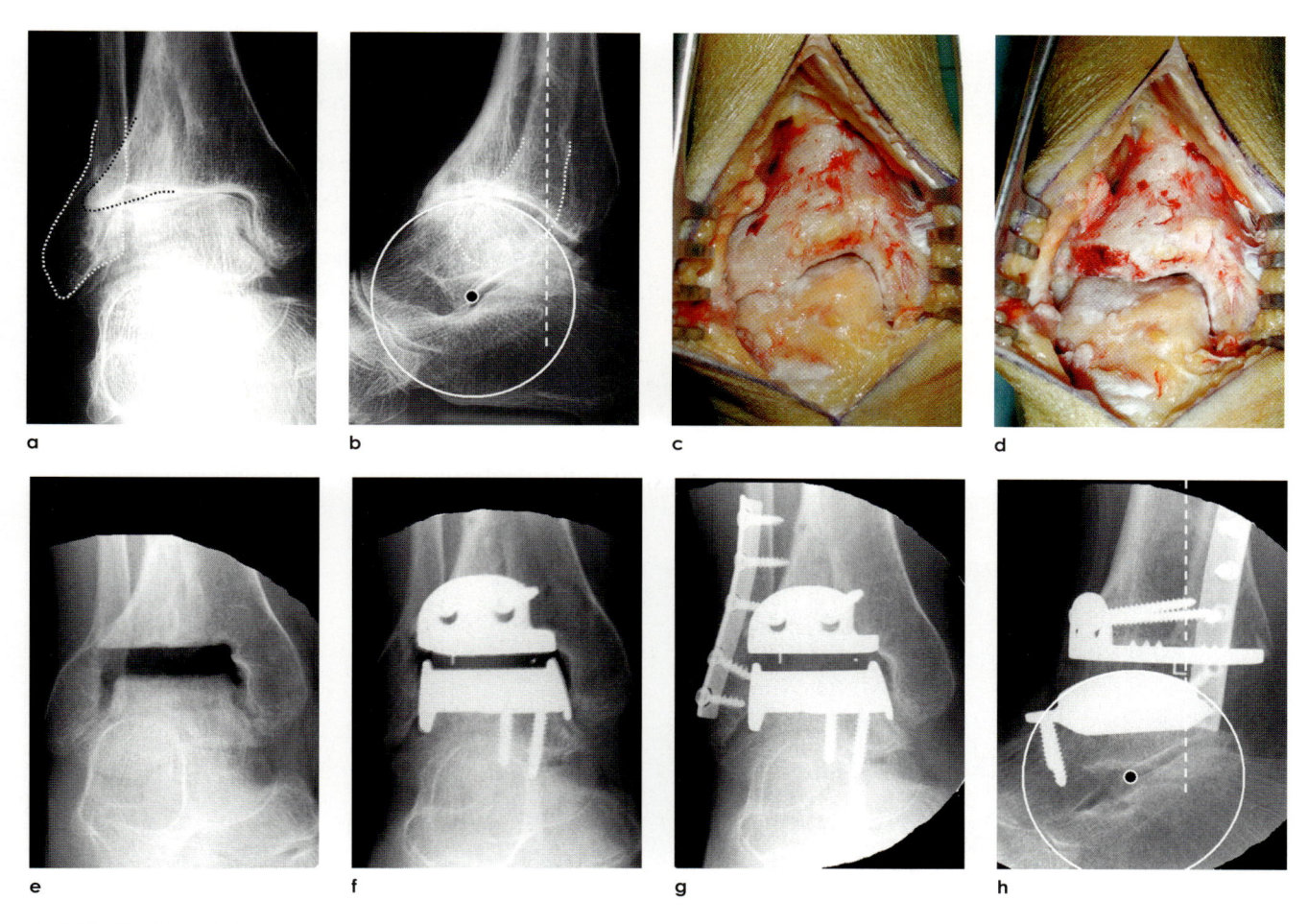

Fig. 10.6. Fibular malunion.
This 59-year-old woman developed ankle osteoarthritis 26 years after a conservatively treated ankle fracture. The mortise view shows a huge anterolateral osteophyte of the tibia that overhangs the talus significantly (**a**). The lateral view shows a marked extrusion of the talus out of the ankle mortise with posterior dislocation of the longitudinal axis of the fibular shaft. The tip of the fibula is, however, properly located close to the center of rotation of the talus (**b**). Surgical exposure of the ankle evidences the lateral tibial osteophyte (**c**) and, after its removal, the persisting anterolateral extrusion (that is, anterior extrusion with some internal rotation of the talus with respect to the ankle mortise) of the talus (**d**). After performing the resection cuts on the tibia, the talar cuts are done with respect to its center of rotation (that is, independent of its extruded position so that accurate resurfacing will be achieved) (**e**). Thereafter, the prosthesis is implanted and the fibula osteotomized (**f**). The fibula is then stabilized in an appropriate position through a lateral incision, as evidenced by fluoroscopy on anteroposterior (**g**) and lateral (**h**) views

ever, is not usually a problem for total ankle replacement.

The Author's Recommendation
Although uncommon, malunion of the fibula may represent a major problem during total ankle replacement as it hinders attempts to make the ankle normal. In such a case, the fibula is best osteotomized after performing the main resection cuts on the tibia and talus. Once the prosthesis is implanted, the fibula can be accurately repositioned and fixed so that the ankle is as close as possible to normal. Probably the most difficult issue in such a case is the abnormal position of the talus with respect to the tibia, which makes it impossible to use any resection jig that references

the anterior tibial border in determining the anteroposterior positioning of the talar cuts. The instruments for planning and performing the resection cuts must then include a feature that allows the surgeon to properly perform the resection cuts on the talus with regard to its center of rotation.

10.2.2 Tibiofibular Instability (Syndesmotic Incompetence)

Complex injuries to the ankle may cause syndesmotic incompetence, which may provoke lateral sliding of the talus within the unstable ankle mortise during loading. As a consequence, increased wear of the lateral tibial plafond occurs (even breakdown of the subchondral bone may occur), resulting in valgus tilting of the talus which, in turn, increases the lateral sliding of the talus and stress on the medial ligaments. An additional anterior extrusion of the talus may be particularly critical, as it leads to overloading of the weakest anterolateral area of the tibial plafond, which may break down under the imposed forces (Fig. 10.7). During ankle replacement, appropriate correction of the valgus malalignment should be achieved, and in some cases, even a tibiofibular fusion and/or medial ligament reconstruction should be considered to attain a well-aligned and stable ankle.

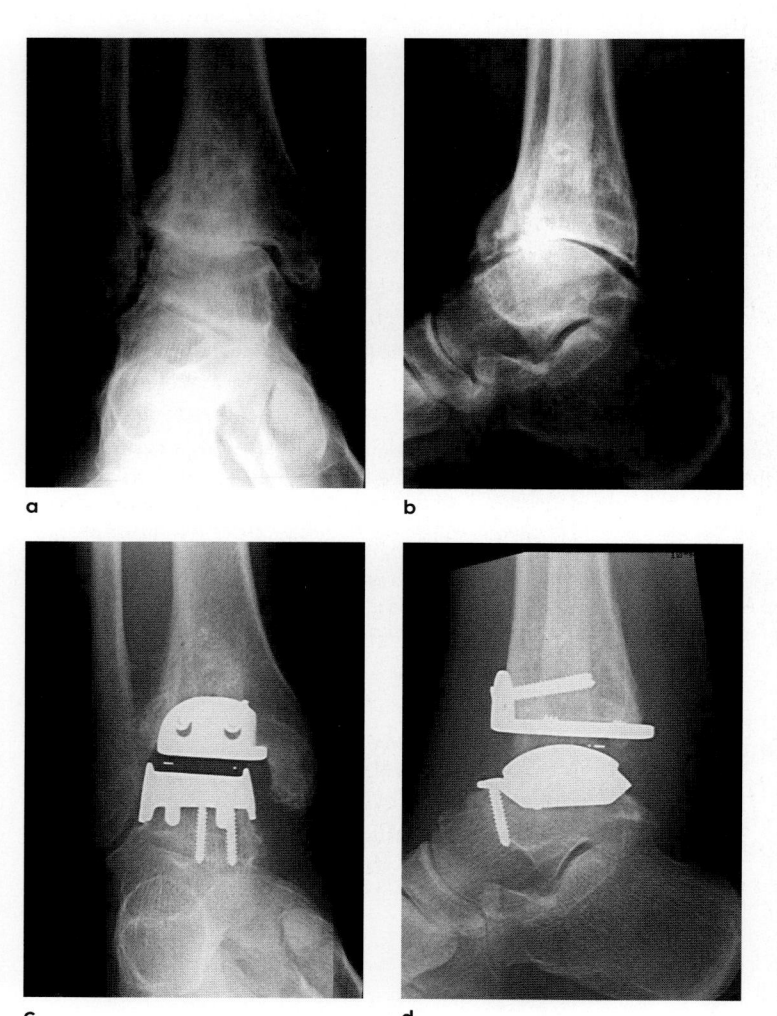

Fig. 10.7. Syndesmotic incompetence.
This 44-year-old man developed ankle osteoarthritis 23 years after sustaining a Weber Type C ankle fracture while in the army. The mortise view shows valgus tilting of the talus in the presence of wear on the lateral tibial plafond, while the deltoid ligament looks normal, and the tibiofibular space is widened (**a**). On lateral view, little anterior extrusion of the talus and wear on the anterior tibial plafond are seen (**b**). Obviously, tibiotalar alignment was not properly achieved during ankle replacement (a valgus angle of 4° persisted). At one-year follow-up, the patient was extremely satisfied. The anteroposterior weight-bearing X-ray (**c**) shows lateral translation of the talus within the mortise, with widening of the medial gutter (meaning that the deltoid ligament may have been stretched out to some extent), narrowing of the lateral gutter, but no widening of the tibiofibular space with regard to the preoperative situation. On the lateral view (**d**), the ankle looks well balanced. With regard to an improved long-term prognosis, a supramalleolar, medially based closing wedge osteotomy might be considered. At this time, however, the patient would not accept such treatment, as he has absolutely no pain and no loading limitations

> **The Author's Recommendation**
> Special attention should be paid to potential tibiofibular instability in a valgus malaligned ankle. Once the implant has been inserted, lateral and anterior sliding stress is applied to the heel to evaluate the competence of the syndesmotic ligaments. If fibular displacement is increased, but less than 5 mm, then intermediate tibiofibular fixation by one or two screws and plaster immobilization with partial loading of the ankle for six weeks is advised. If the displacement is greater than 5 mm, then tibiofibular arthrodesis is advised. Theoretically, reconstruction of the deltoid ligament may help to prevent lateral sliding of the talus, but in practice, reconstruction of the deep portion of the deltoid ligament may be extremely difficult to achieve. Of utmost importance, however, is the tibiotalar angle obtained by resecting the tibia, which should be planned to include some degree of varus overcorrection.
>
> Again, although not yet proven, the use of an ankle system that provides intrinsic stability against eversion moments may better resist against recurrent valgus deformity, but may also potentially experience more polyethylene wear and higher shear forces at the bone-implant interface. Proper aligning and balancing of the whole foot and ankle is, therefore, mandatory for success with any ankle prosthesis. Medial sliding of the heel (see Fig. 8.42, Chap. 8: Surgical Techniques) and, alternatively, lateral column lengthening, are particularly effective in normalizing the forces within the foot and ankle.

10.2.3 Calcaneal Malunion

A malunion of the calcaneus after fracture is probably the most frequent cause of post-traumatic deformity and malalignment of the hindfoot (Figs. 10.8 and 10.9). In particular, if the Böhler angle has not been restored, the talus becomes dorsiflexed. This overloads the anterior tibiotalar joint, causes a widening stress on the ankle mortise (because the anteriorly wider talus is pressed into the mortise), destabilizes the ankle joint (because the collateral ligaments slacken due to the collapse), and causes painful subfibular impingement (because the tip of the fibula presses against the widened lateral calcaneus). The surgeon, therefore, encounters several pathologies when a patient presents with a severely traumatized ankle. Tibiocalcaneal arthrodesis may be a viable solution, but technically challenging if the hindfoot geometry has to be restored and the transverse joints repositioned. Total ankle replacement may also be a viable alternative, as it may preserve the transverse joints from further damage and joint degeneration secondary to overload. To be successful, however, appropriate restoration of hindfoot geometry and stability is mandatory. As a principle, the malunion should be corrected first, and then the total ankle replacement can be performed.

> **The Author's Recommendation**
> Extensive diagnostic measures are necessary in order to identify all associated problems and fully understand the underlying deformity. Weight-bearing radiographs of the contralateral (unaffected) foot and ankle are of the highest value. Surgery should start with restoration of the hindfoot, which is often only successful when considering fusion of the subtalar joint, with or without graft interposition. If the soft-tissue mantle is not critically damaged by previous trauma, total ankle replacement may be considered during the same surgery. If the surgeon lacks experience, and/or if this first step has taken too long, local swelling may hinder subsequent wound healing, and total ankle replacement may better be considered during a second surgery, once the local swelling has subsided. This treatment concept has been extremely successful, particularly with respect to pain relief and patient satisfaction.

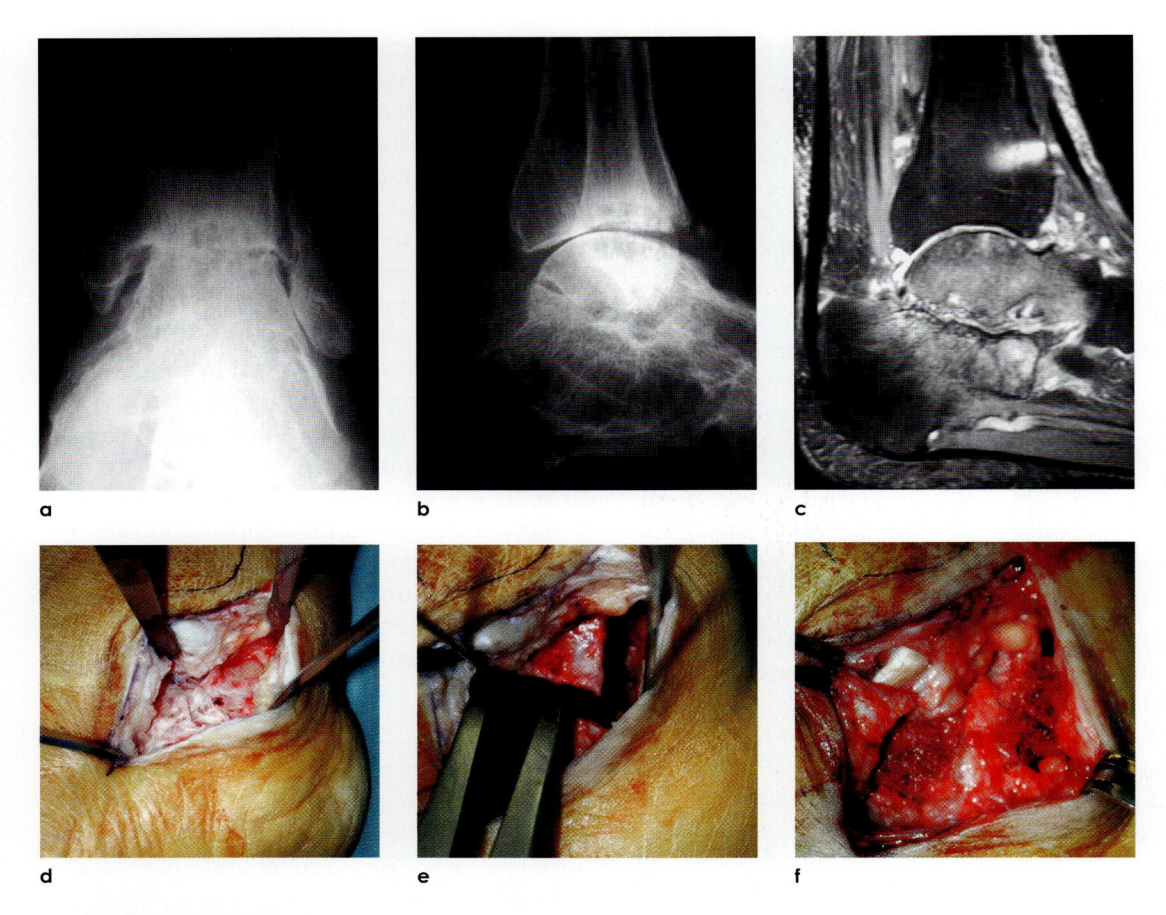

Fig. 10.8. Calcaneal malunion.
This woman (57 years of age), who suffers from rheumatoid arthritis, developed severe osteoarthritis in her left ankle 36 months after bilateral calcaneal fractures that were conservatively treated. The hindfoot looks well aligned in the coronal plane (**a**), but in the sagittal plane, there is evidence of a calcaneal malunion and ankylosis of the subtalar joint (**b**). The dorsiflexed position of the talus and the degenerative disease in the tibiotalar joint is more visible on MRI (**c**). The calcaneus is exposed directly behind the peroneal tendons (**d**), and a z-shaped osteotomy of the calcaneus is performed (**e**). After mobilizing and dislocating the tuber posteriorly (which lengthens the calcaneus), two bone grafts are inserted (**f, g**). Fixation is achieved using two screws, paying attention not to advance too far into the talus (**h**). Total ankle replacement is then performed through an anterior approach (**i**). At a follow-up of three years, the patient was extremely satisfied. The hindfoot was stable, and the range of motion was 45° (dorsiflexion 15°, plantar flexion 30°). The anteroposterior X-ray shows a well-aligned hindfoot with stable implants (**j**), and on lateral view as well (**k**). The talar component is positioned quite posteriorly, and it also evidences posterior tilt. If the intraoperatively obtained X-ray ([**l**], same X-ray as [**i**], but rotated) is taken as a reference, there has been only very little posterior tilt and subsidence, respectively, which may have occurred during the initial settling process

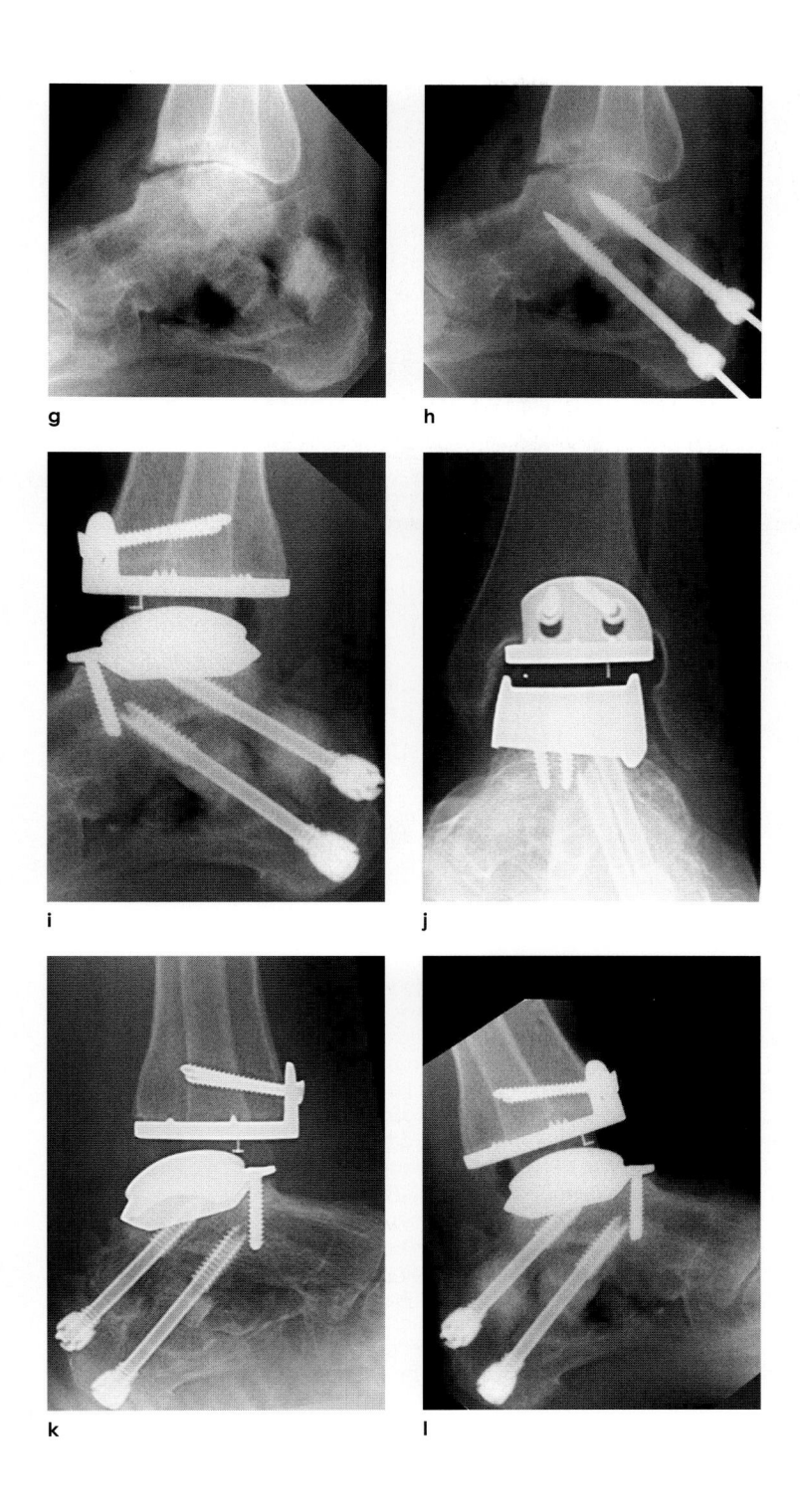

10.2 Reconstruction of the Post-Traumatic Hindfoot and Ankle

g

h

i

j

k

l

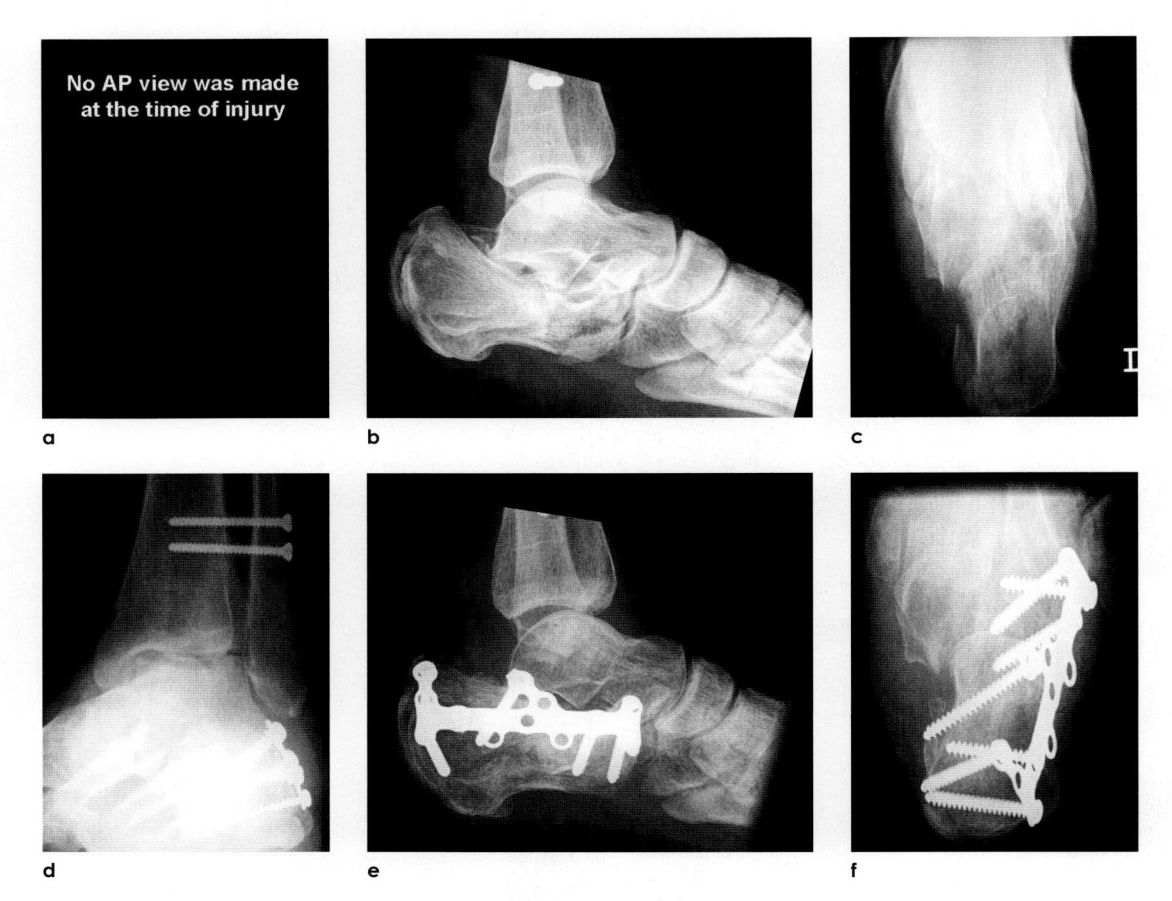

Fig. 10.9. Calcaneal malunion.
This 33-year-old woman developed severe ankle osteoarthritis 14 months after a complex crush injury while motorcycling. The tibiofibular disruption (a Maisonneuve-type injury) was immediately fixed using two screws; obviously, the diagnosis was made through fluoroscopy, and no X-ray is available (**a**). The depression fracture of the calcaneus (**b**) with involvement of the tuber (**c**) was fixed after 11 days, when swelling in the foot subsided. At two months, the ankle looks well aligned (**d**), but the calcaneus shows a persistent flattening of Böhler's angle (**e**) and subtalar malalignment (**f**). At 14 months, the patient complained of intense pain and a feeling of instability when loading her foot. The mortise view shows marked destruction of the tibiotalar joint (particularly in its lateral part), associated with some valgus tilt of the talus (**g**). The talus has further dorsiflexed due to the breakdown of the posterior subtalar joint, and destruction of the anterior tibiotalar joint has occurred (**h**). The axial view evidences a progressive subtalar disruption with lateralization of the calcaneus (**i**). First, the calcaneus was exposed through the old incision, and, after the hardware was removed, the former subtalar joint was carefully opened using chisels and spreaders (**j**). A tricortical bone graft was inserted and K-wires percutaneously positioned (**k**). After inserting canulated screws over the K-wires (paying attention not to advance too far into the talus), there is little valgus malalignment left (**l**). Exposure of the ankle joint through a second anterior approach evidences the achieved plantar flexion of the talus while the foot is kept in neutral flexion (**m**). The prosthesis was then implanted, paying attention to correct the remaining valgus malalignment caused by wear on the lateral tibial plafond (**n**). Fluoroscopy shows the achieved alignment at the end of surgery. At the two-month follow-up, achieved alignment and restoration of height were preserved (**o–q**). The patient was, however, advised not to weight-bear for another six weeks because of incomplete graft incorporation. The patient was allowed full weight-bearing and free mobilization (that is, without the protection of a brace or special shoes) after a further clinical and radiological assessment four months postoperatively. She returned to her professional activity as an employer (with mainly sedentary activities) after another month, and since then (now 26 months after surgical reconstruction), the recovery has been uneventful

g

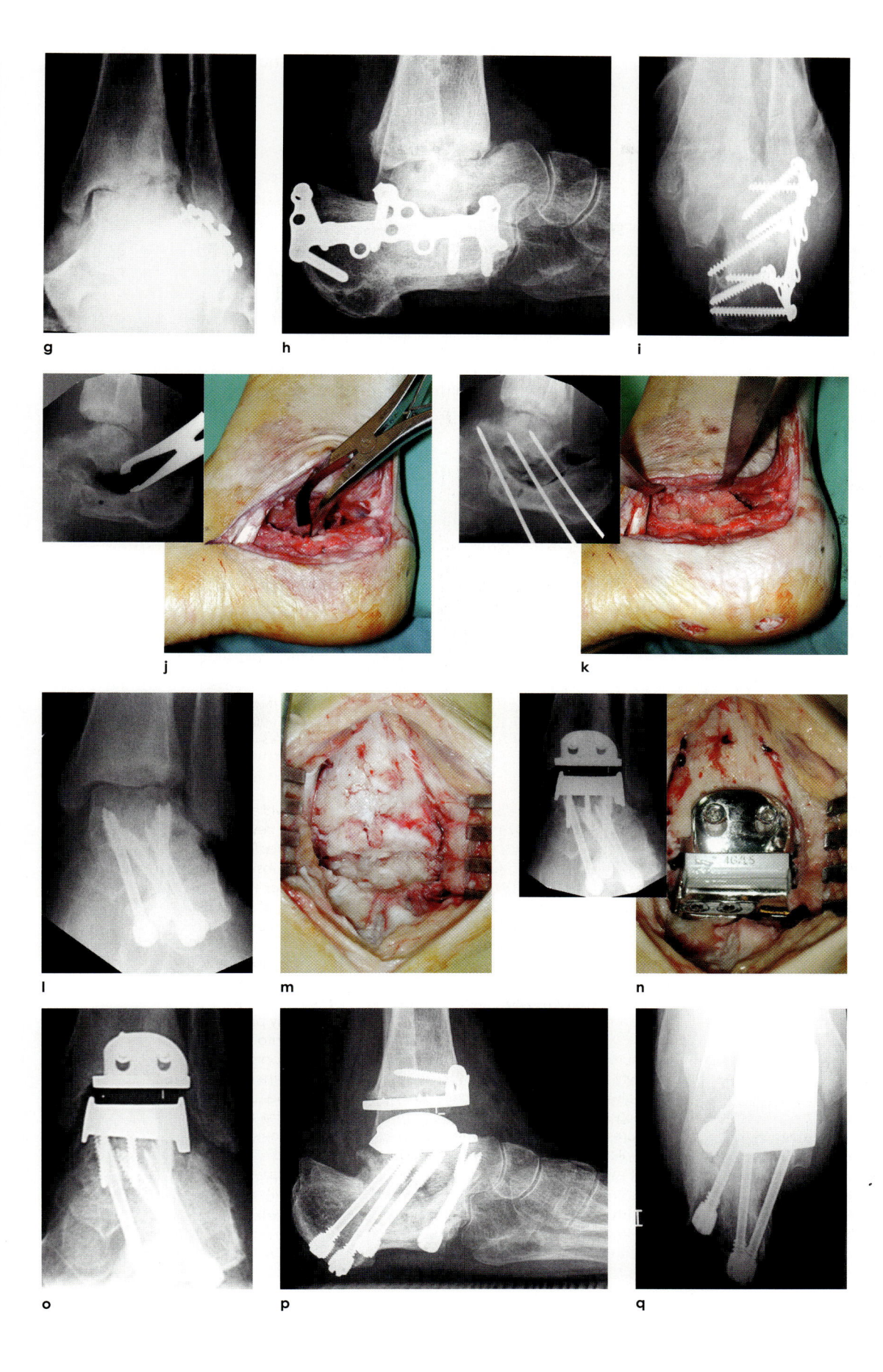

h

i

j

k

l

m

n

o

p

q

10.3 Specific Articular Pathologies and Disorders

While total ankle arthroplasty has emerged as a viable alternative to ankle arthrodesis, the indications and contraindications have not been elucidated in detail. This is particularly true for some specific articular pathologies and disorders. This section will discuss several of these conditions with respect to total ankle arthroplasty.

10.3.1 Systemic Inflammatory Arthritis

Because patients with rheumatoid or inflammatory arthritis often have progressive, symmetric involvement of the surrounding joints of the hindfoot and transverse tarsal joints over time, ankle arthrodesis potentially accelerates the degeneration of these adjacent joints. These patients will, therefore, be subjected to further arthrodesis. Given the generally poor functional results after pantalar arthrodesis, an alternative treatment (such as total ankle arthroplasty) that preserves some ankle joint motion is particularly favorable for these rheumatoid patients, who have generally low physical demands (Fig. 10.10). There is still, however, need for careful patient selection (see Chap. 7, Sect. 7.3.1. Rheumatoid Arthritis and Inflammatory Arthropathy).

Careful evaluation of all risk factors and extensive preoperative planning is particularly important. For instance, a triple arthrodesis together with total ankle arthroplasty may not be successful in the presence of a valgus deformity and instability at the ipsilateral knee joint with associated external rotation of the lower leg. In this case, the knee alignment and function must be restored first, followed by hindfoot reconstruction. If the associated problems are located distally to the ankle joint as with, for instance, flatfoot deformity (with or without forefoot abduction), then correction and stabilization can be performed before total ankle replacement during the same surgery.

> **The Author's Recommendation**
> Total ankle arthroplasty (with or without additional surgeries) is extremely beneficial for patients suffering from systemic joint disease. Since their connective tissues are generally weak as a result of long-term use of cortisone medications, appropriate restoration of foot and ankle alignment and stabilization are mandatory for success. With improved techniques and increased experience, a combined procedure that addresses all pathologies at once has become the standard. This is also the case for combined knee and ankle pathologies: first, total knee replacement is performed, and second, hindfoot reconstruction including total ankle arthroplasty is performed. This treatment concept has been found to be extremely beneficial for subsequent rehabilitation, and it is also cost effective.

Fig. 10.10. Systemic inflammatory arthritis.
This woman (63 years of age) with rheumatoid arthritis suffered from progressive, disabling arthritis and ankylosis of both feet and ankles. She underwent bilateral knee replacement 18 months ago, but because of the bilateral foot and ankle involvement, rehabilitation was extremely difficult and she was mainly confined to a wheelchair. The preoperative X-rays show bilateral valgus arthritis of the ankle joint (**a, b**), extensive arthritic changes in the subtalar and talonavicular joints, and a loss of the medial arch that is more pronounced on the left foot than on the right foot (**c, d**). The transverse metatarsal joints were more involved on the left foot, and there was (particularly on the left side) a talonavicular subluxation with forefoot abduction (**e**). One-stage bilateral surgery was performed, including a triple arthrodesis, first metatarsophalangeal arthrodesis, and total ankle arthroplasty. At the two-year follow-up, the patient was extremely satisfied and demonstrated free ambulation without pain. Radiographically, both ankles look well aligned, and the implants are stable (**f, g**). The triple arthrodesis healed in both feet (**h, i**); however, a breakdown at the navicular-cuneiform joint did occur on the left side. Both feet are well aligned (**j**). Notice that some of the hardware was removed 14 months after surgery. Although the first metatarsophalangeal arthrodesis on left side did not heal properly, the patient has no pain

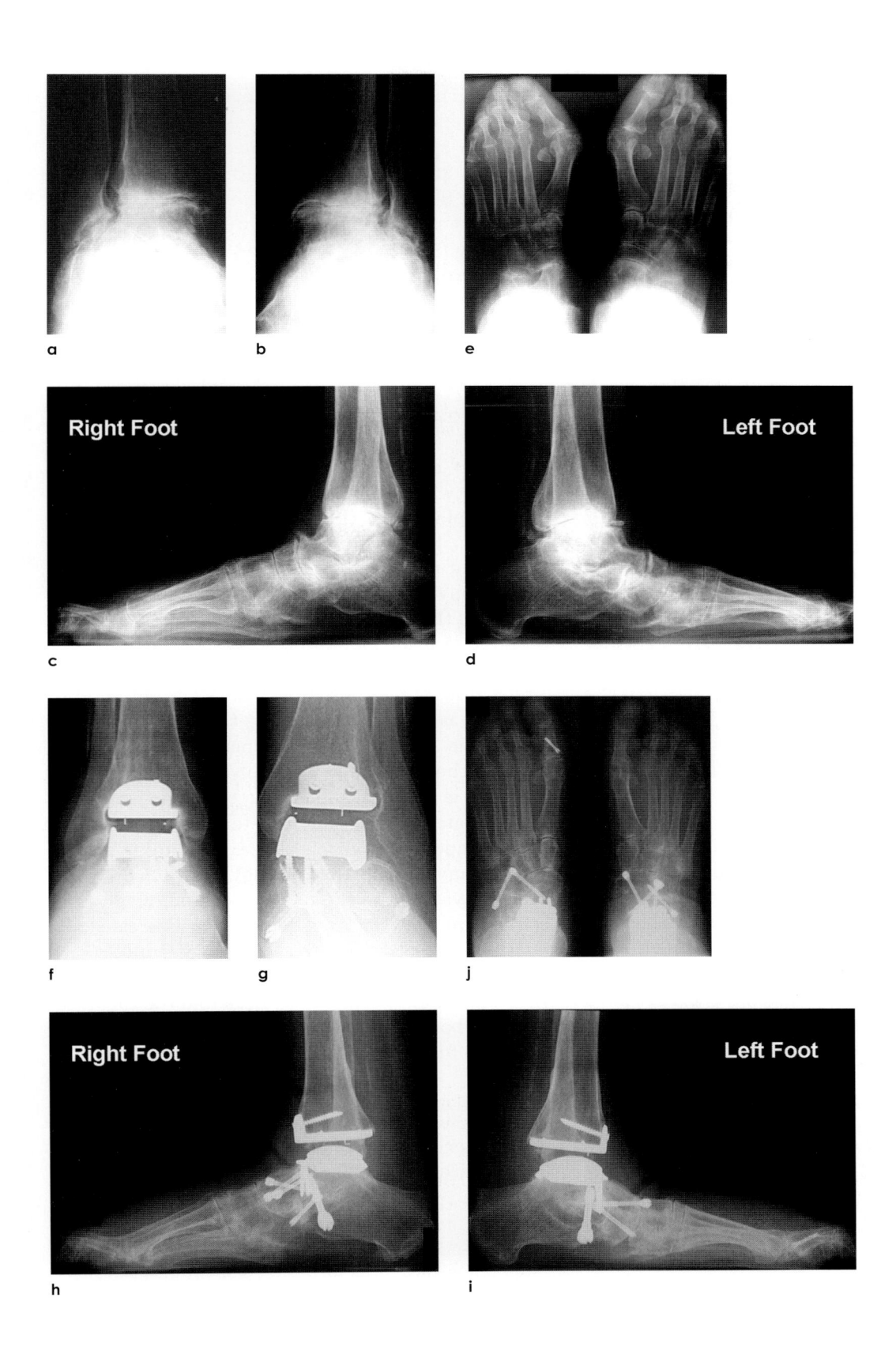

10.3 Specific Articular Pathologies and Disorders

151

a

b

c

d

e

f

g

h

i

j

10.3.2 Clubfoot Deformity

Clubfoot deformity can result in painful ankle osteoarthritis, particularly if the heel has been overcorrected into a pronation position and subtalar fusion has been performed. There are no conclusive answers in the literature to the question of whether total ankle arthroplasty may be a viable alternative to ankle arthrodesis in this case. A major concern, however, is the small, dysplastic talus, which makes the positioning of a talar implant extremely difficult. On the other hand, it remains unclear to what extent the dysplastic ankle joint (that is, a joint that has never developed regular gliding and rolling movements) may profit from a prosthetic resurfacing.

> **The Author's Recommendation**
> Total ankle replacement of an osteoarthritic ankle joint in a clubfoot deformity has not been found to be beneficial. Positioning the implants is extremely difficult, since bony support for the talar component may be insufficient. Because the obtained motion is, in most instances, highly disappointing, and pain relief is minimal, the author no longer replaces the ankle when there is a clubfoot deformity.

10.3.3 Post-Polio Foot Deformity

The paralytic deformity and instability of the foot and ankle that is typical of polio cases may cause osteoarthritis of the ankle. This is often the case when there is a loss of extensor function, which is usually accompanied by a loss of peroneal function. Therefore, the foot develops a progressive varus and equinus deformity. There are no conclusive answers in the literature to the question of whether total ankle arthroplasty may be a viable alternative to ankle arthrodesis or to other reconstructive measures in this case. The lateral instability of the hindfoot and loss of muscular function that occur as a result of polio are a major concern, however, and make the potential benefits of total ankle replacement very minimal.

> **The Author's Recommendation**
> Total ankle replacement of an osteoarthritic ankle joint in a foot affected by polio may not work. First of all, the ankle is insufficiently stabilized without muscular power, which puts the replaced ankle at risk of dislocation. Second, it does not make sense to select a motion-preserving method when muscular function is lacking. The author does not consider total ankle arthroplasty to be a valuable alternative to other therapeutic measures available for treating a post-polio foot deformity.

10.3.4 Avascular Necrosis

Avascular necrosis of the talus remains a question to debate with respect to the risk it presents for total ankle replacement (Figs. 10.11 and 10.12; see also Chap. 7, Sect. 7.2. Contraindications). Certainly, the extent of the necrotic process, as well as its location may limit the potential success of the procedure. If the necrotic process involves only the apex of the talar body, then flat resection of the talus may be an option to completely remove the necrotic area. The quality of the remaining bone stock of the talus, however, is crucial for the long-term support of the prosthesis. Conversely, if the necrotic process goes down to the subtalar joint, involving the entire talar body, it is almost impossible to locate sufficient viable bone stock for the long-term stability of any talar component. In such a case, total ankle arthroplasty may not be the optimal solution. A viable alternative may be the use of a custom-made talar component that is fixed directly to the calcaneal body, which provides the necessary support. An intermediate solution could be the use of a prosthetic design that uses the talar neck and the calcaneal tuber as bony support, as long as the subtalar joint has been fused before.

> **The Author's Recommendation**
> There is no doubt that avascular necrosis of a part or the whole talar body is very problematic with respect to long-term support of a talar component. Since younger patients usually present with secondary degenerative joint disease following avascular necrosis, it is often necessary

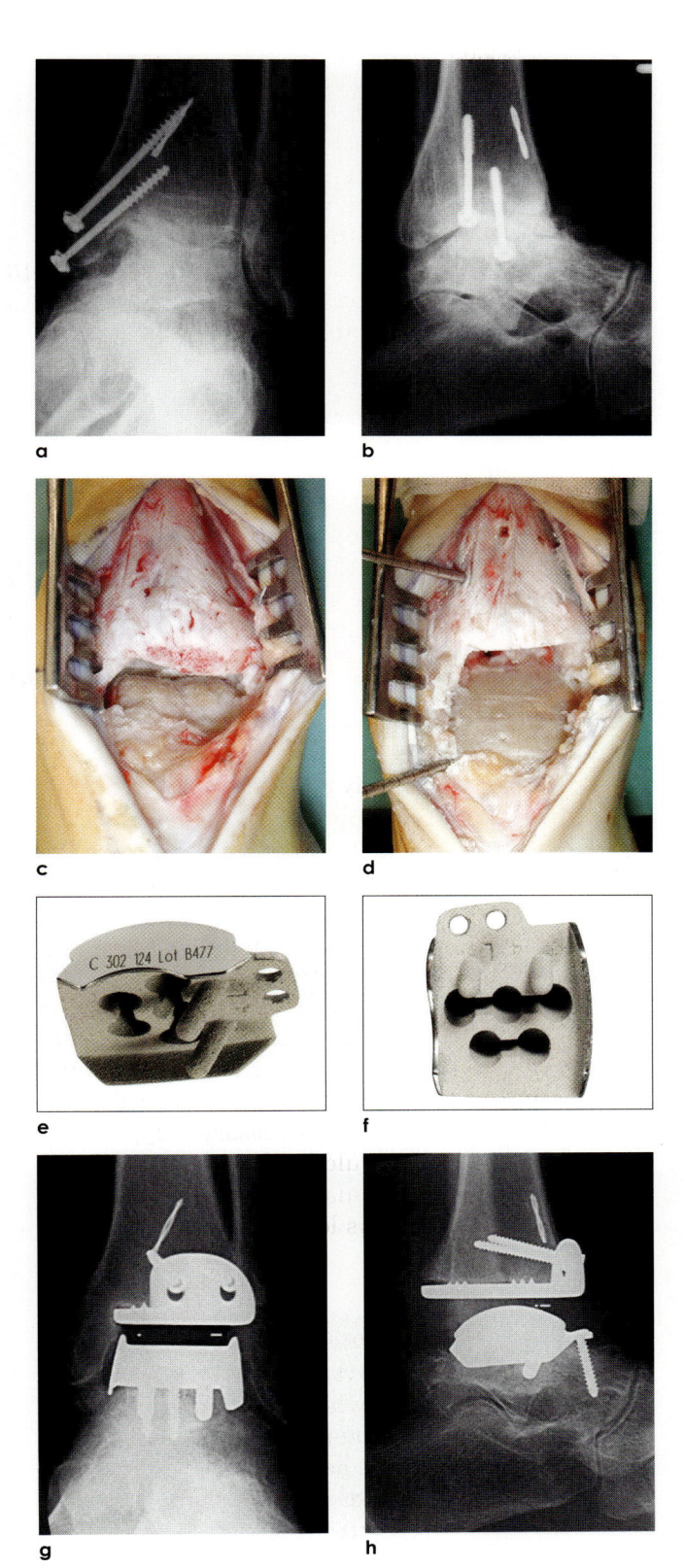

10.3 Specific Articular Pathologies and Disorders

Fig. 10.11. Avascular necrosis of the talus.
This man (43 years of age) had a mosaicplasty that was done through an osteotomy of the medial malleolus, and two further revisions including arthroscopic drilling and debridement. The X-rays show destruction of the upper part of the talar body, with incongruency and some anterior extrusion of the talus (**a, b**). Further investigation by MRI and CT scan revealed avascular necrosis involving only the upper part of the talus (less than 50%). Therefore, ankle arthroplasty was considered a viable, time-saving option until arthrodesis may become necessary. Intraoperative exposure showed the breakdown of the articular surface (**c**). Flat bone resection revealed a sclerotic resection surface (**d**), but after drilling several times, bleeding from the bone was visible, which was considered to indicate some vitality of the remaining bone. The HINTEGRA® revision talar component (which has a flat inferior surface) (**e, f**) was inserted. After four months, the X-rays show a well-aligned hindfoot with properly positioned implants (**g, h**)

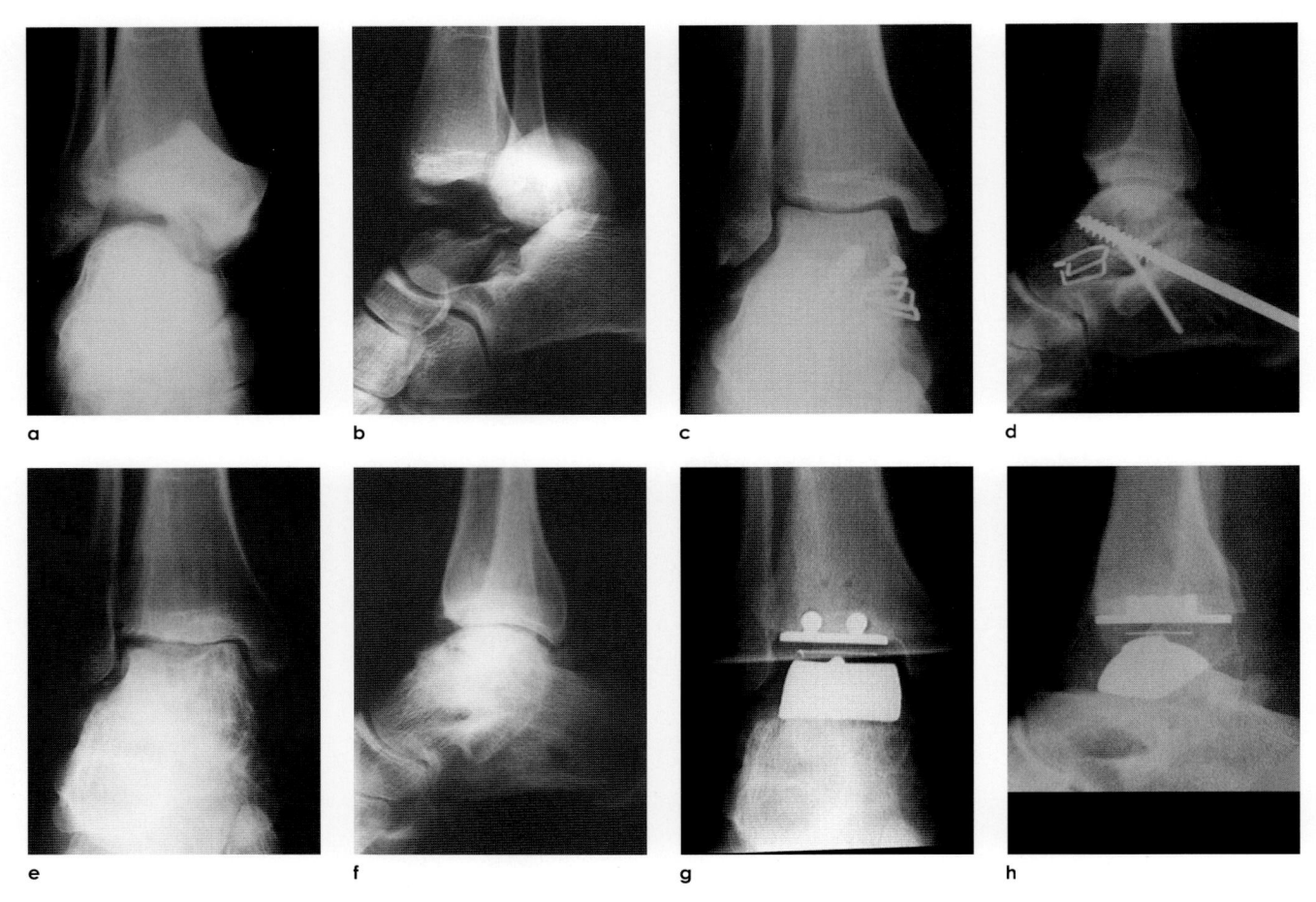

Fig. 10.12. Avascular necrosis of the talus.
This 34-year-old man sustained a complex fracture dislocation of the talus (**a, b**) that was reduced and treated by primary subtalar joint arthrodesis (**c, d**). Three years later, he presented with tremendous pain due to avascular necrosis (**e, f**). The patient absolutely refused ankle arthrodesis (because one of his best friends had had an ankle arthrodesis and was very unsatisfied), so total ankle replacement was performed in spite of the risk of failure. The postoperative X-rays showed a well-aligned hindfoot (**g**), but a slightly anteriorly positioned talar component after cutting down the bone at the talar neck by about 3 mm (**h**). For the first six years, the patient was extremely satisfied with the obtained result, but at the seven-year follow-up, he complained of intense pain on the lateral and medial sides of the ankle. The X-rays evidenced marked subsidence of the talar component due to breakdown of the talar body (**i, j**). The removal of the implant revealed necrotic bone on the talar side (**k**); therefore, the entire talar body was removed until vital bone of the calcaneal body was visible (**l**). A custom-made talar component (**m, n**) that included an anterior and posterior arm to be supported by the talar neck and calcaneal tuber, respectively, and a bulky body to replace the removed talar body was inserted. At the one-year follow-up, the patient was extremely satisfied, was pain free, and able to load his foot without limitations. The X-rays (**o, p**) show a well-aligned hindfoot with stable implants

to find a viable, functional solution. A flat talar component is used for superficial avascular necrosis (Fig. 10.11). In the case of more extensive avascular necrosis that does not involve the subtalar joint, a custom-made talar component that uses the talar neck and the calcaneal tuber for bony support (Fig. 10.12) may be useful. If the necrotic process involves the entire talar body, a custom-made talar component that uses the calcaneal body as bony support may be useful. It must be emphasized, however, that these treatment options are only considered for younger, highly compliant patients. With this restriction, all such cases to date have been successful.

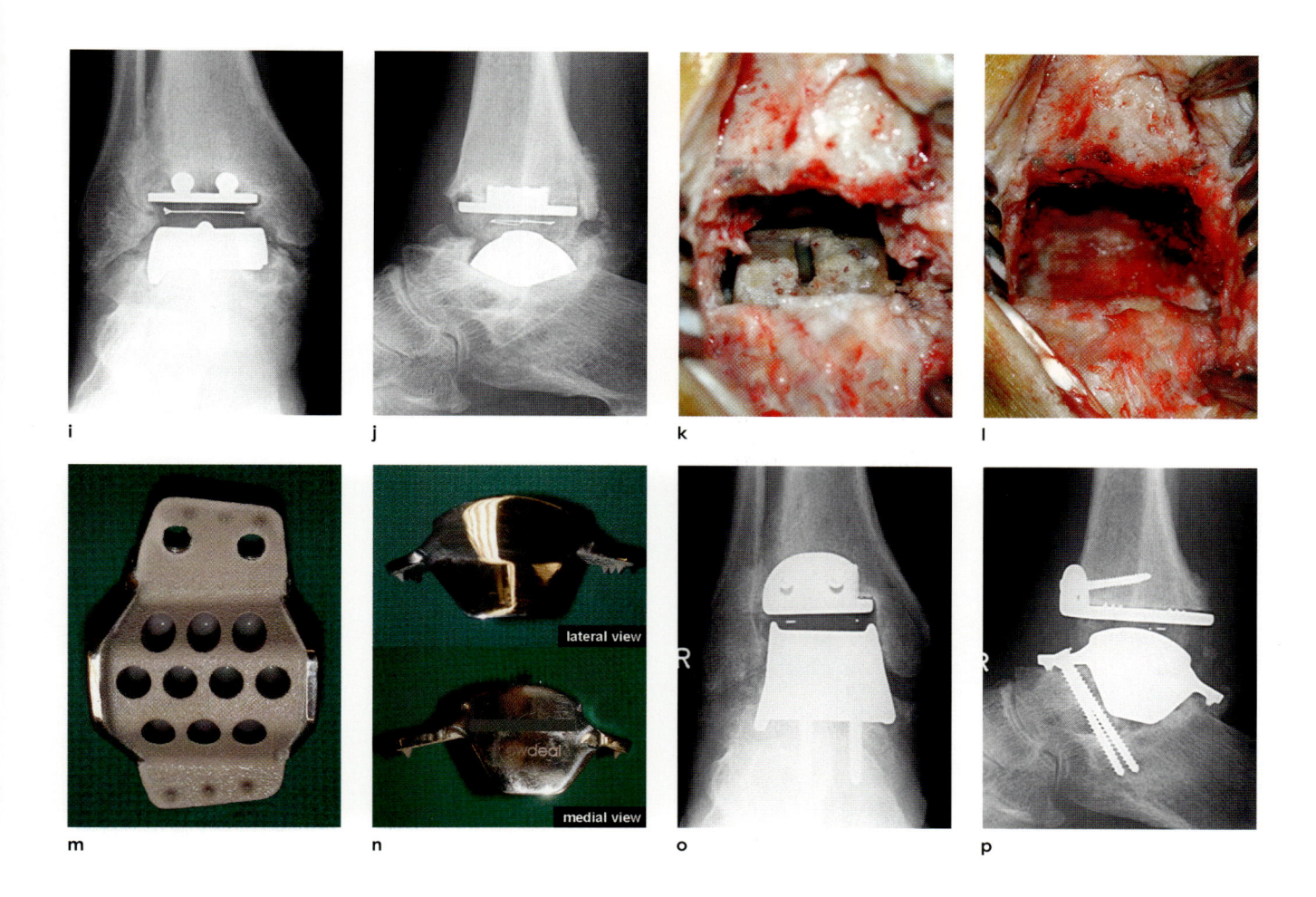

10.3 Specific Articular Pathologies and Disorders

i j k l

m n o p

10.3.5 Septic Arthritis

There is consensus that active or recent infection is a contraindication for total ankle arthroplasty or arthroplasty in general. There has been little discussion in the orthopedic literature, however, about ankle replacement in patients with previous infection of the ankle joint or the surrounding soft tissues (Fig. 10.13; see also Chap. 7, Sect. 7.3.2. Infection). Theoretically, there may be an increased risk of reinfection or reactivation of a subclinical infection after total ankle arthroplasty in these patients.

After septic arthritis of the ankle joint, the main

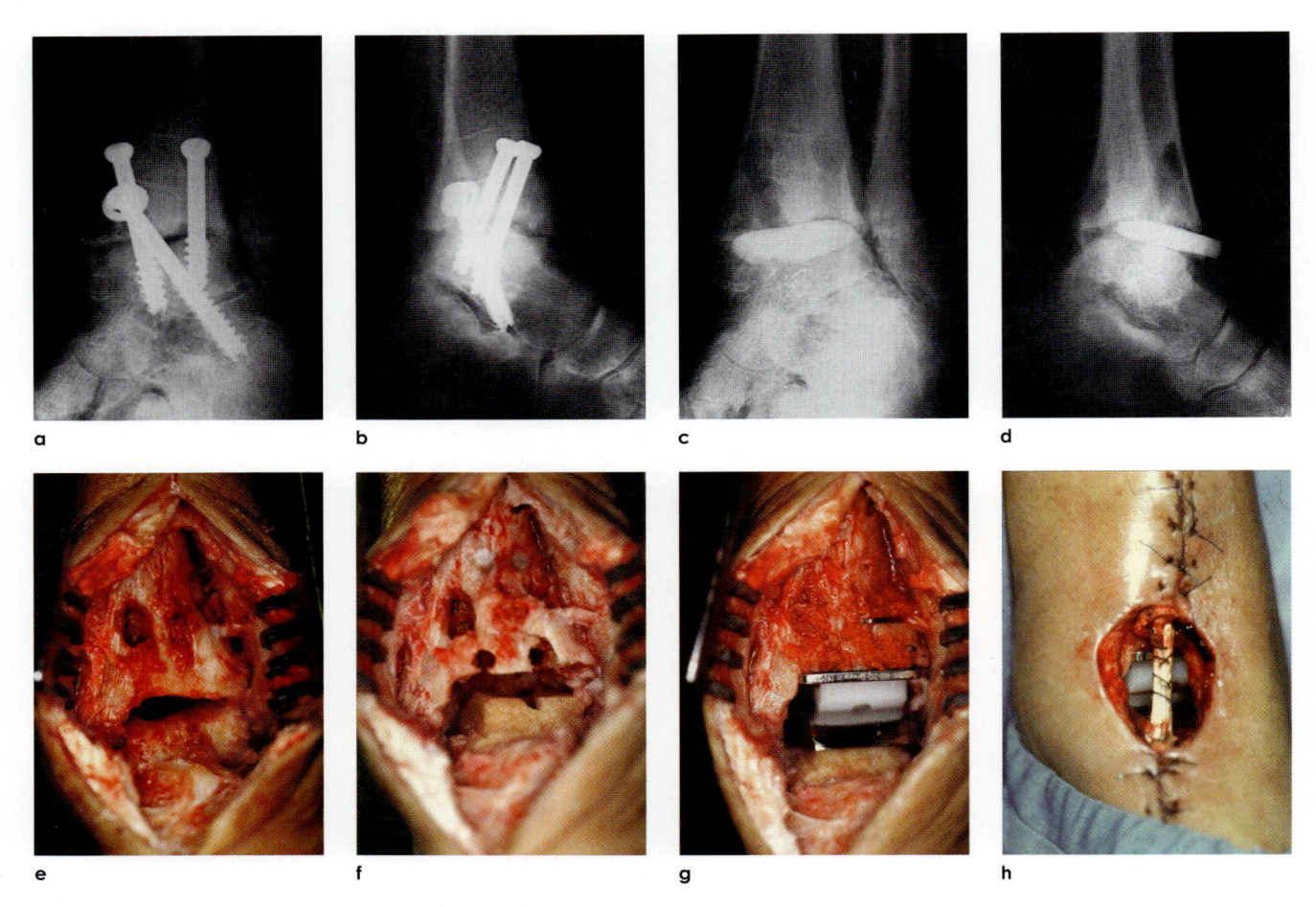

Fig. 10.13. Total ankle replacement after septic arthritis.
This woman (71 years of age) underwent ankle arthrodesis through anterior mini-arthrotomy and developed a deep wound infection with fistulation. The infection progressed despite four local debridements and systemic antibiotics. At the time of referral, seven weeks after initial surgery, there was an anterior wound defect to the bone, and the anterior tibial tendon was gone. The X-rays showed a gap at the former tibiotalar joint (**a, b**). The wound was extensively debrided, the hardware removed, and a gentamicin-loaded Palacos® spacer was inserted (**c, d**). Six weeks later, the spacer was removed, and bacteriologic analyses were taken. The bone looked quite normal (**e**), so resection cuts were performed (**f**) as required for the insertion of a S.T.A.R. ankle prosthesis (**g**). The fibula was additionally stabilized by a plate. The anterior tibial tendon was reconstructed by end-to-end sutures, but primary wound closure was not possible because of the pre-existing defect (**h**). In a second step three days later, the defect was covered by a vascularized flap from the upper arm (triceps), thereby also restoring the extensor retinaculum. The postoperative X-rays show a well-aligned ankle with properly positioned implants in the anteroposterior view (**i**); in the sagittal plane, however, the talar component was found to be positioned too posteriorly (**j**). The systemic antibiotics were continued for another three months. Five months after surgery, the fibula plate was removed, and subtalar fusion was performed because of progressive and painful subtalar arthritis. From this point, the recovery was uneventful, and the very active patient regained full and unlimited activities, including golfing. At the follow-up 6.6 years after total ankle arthroplasty, the foot was found to be well aligned and the implants stable (**k, l**), with active motion preserved (anteroposterior view: plantar flexion [**m**], dorsiflexion [**n**]; medial view: plantar flexion [**o**], dorsiflexion [**p**])

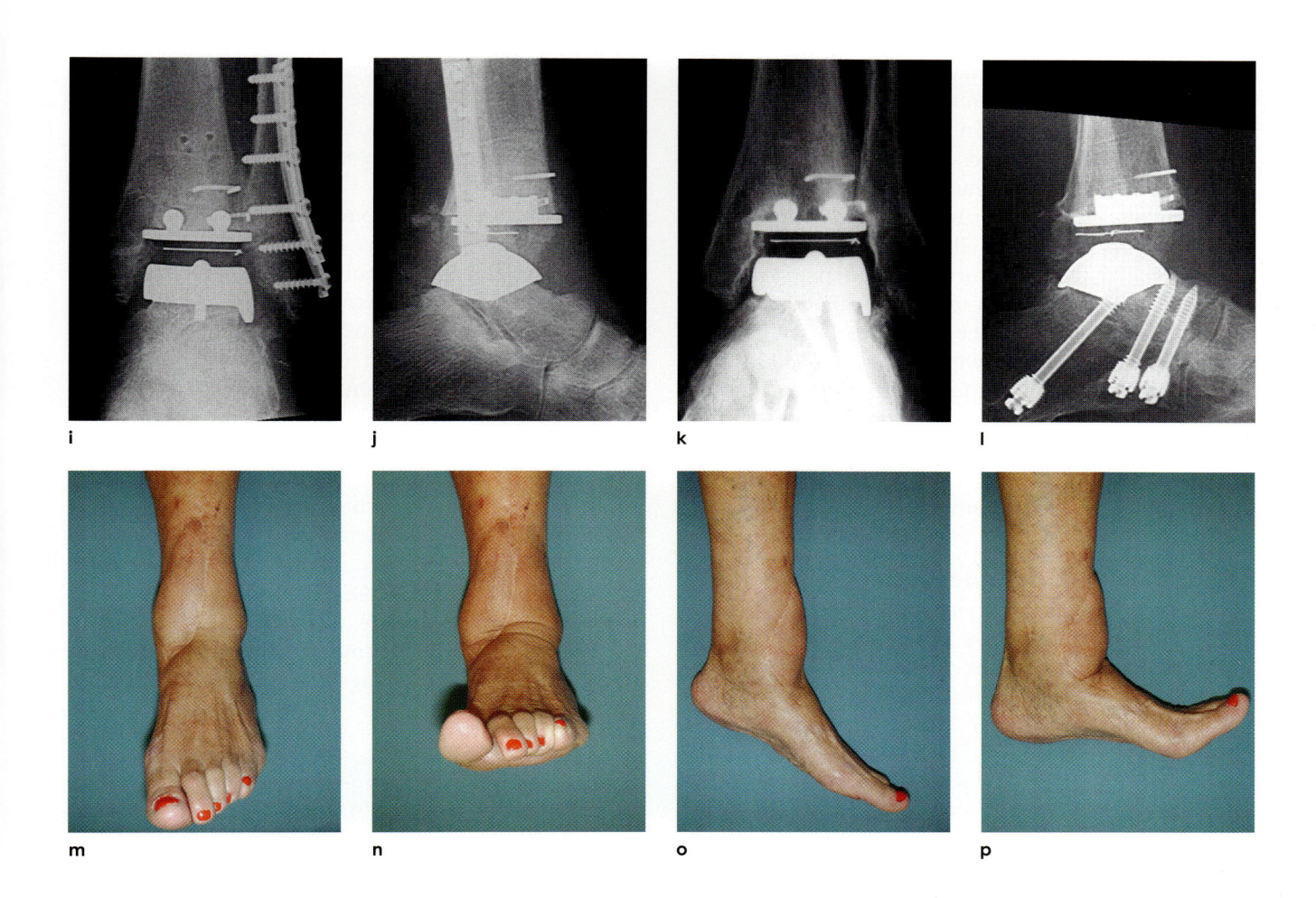

10.3 Specific Articular Pathologies and Disorders

i

j

k

l

m

n

o

p

problem is the development of secondary osteoarthritis in the subtalar joint, and very often, also in the talonavicular joint. In addition, the soft-tissue mantle is often scarred and gliding movement between the different tissues is highly compromised, resulting in general stiffness of the whole ankle joint complex. An isolated ankle arthrodesis may not sufficiently relieve pain, and, in most instances, an extensive arthrodesis must be considered. Total ankle replacement, together with an extensive hindfoot arthrodesis is, however, far better for the patient. If the risk of reinfection or reactivation of a subclinical infection can be minimized by careful preoperative investigation and appropriate perioperative antibiotic therapy, then total ankle arthroplasty may be considered.

The Author's Recommendation
Once an active infection and/or osteomyelitis have been excluded or appropriately treated, total ankle replacement is undertaken without any additional modalities. During surgery, however, bone biopsies are harvested for bacteriologic analysis, which allows (if necessary) specific long-term antibiotic therapy. To date, late infection has not been observed in any case after total ankle arthroplasty in a previously infected ankle. In four out of six cases, however, subtalar fusion, and in three of these four cases, an additional talonavicular fusion were necessary after isolated total ankle replacement to relieve pain.

10.4 Disarthrodesis

When a patient undergoes ankle arthrodesis, there is a significant likelihood that he or she will develop painful hindfoot arthritis, necessitating additional surgical treatment. An isolated ankle fusion may be treated by a pantalar fusion with its increased functional limitations and morbidity, such as the secondary degeneration of the neighboring joints. Therefore, an alternative treatment could be to take down the ankle arthrodesis and convert to a total ankle arthroplasty (Fig. 10.14). To date, however, there are no reports of this in the literature, and the question remains whether the conversion from ankle arthrodesis to total ankle arthroplasty is feasible, and what its potential benefit in the treatment of painful ankle arthrodesis with malunion, nonunion, or osteoarthrosis of adjacent joints might be.

In a recent prospective study, Hintermann et al (in review process) report on a consecutive series of 13 cases in which painful ankle arthrodeses were taken down and converted to total ankle arthroplasty using a current three-component ankle prosthesis. Twelve patients (13 ankles) had painful malunion (10 cases), nonunion (four cases), osteoarthrosis of the adjacent joints (nine cases), or stress fracture (one case). The first results were promising, and as far as comparison was possible, only slightly inferior to those of other reported series after primary total ankle arthroplasty: the regained range of motion was, on average, 23° (range, 8° to 40°), the obtained AOFAS Hindfoot Score was, on average, 64 points (range, 17 to 89 points), substantial pain relief was found in all but one patient (92%), and all but two patients (85%) were satisfied with the obtained result.

The Author's Recommendation
Based on the positive results of the first cases, take-down of painful ankle arthrodeses and conversion to total ankle arthroplasty must be considered, along with other options, a valid alternative. It particularly enables the removal of pathologic stress to the mid- and forefoot joints following malunion or secondary deformation due to degenerative joint disease (for example, the way that an ongoing osteoarthritic process of the subtalar joint tends to turn the foot into varus and equinus position). In addition, it may protect the tarsal joints from further degeneration. This surgery should, however, only be considered after extensive investigation, particularly with respect to the alignment in all planes and the quality of the soft-tissue mantle. Preoperative planning should include radiologic assessment of the contralateral ankle.

In order to make the first tibial resection cut at the appropriate level, it may be crucial during surgery to clearly identify the original height of the ankle by fluoroscopy. Too proximal a cut would result in implanting the prosthesis too far proximally in the weak cancellous bone of the tibial metaphysis (which may lead to early subsidence); whereas, too distal a cut would result in implanting the prosthesis too far distally in the talus (which may lead to extended weakening of the bone stock on talar side). In either case, if the prosthesis is implanted too distally or too proximally, proper ligament balancing may not be achieved, which, in turn, may increase the shear forces at the bone-implant interfaces (which may lead to subsidence), and stress to the malleoli (which may lead to pain and/or stress fractures).

Protection of the malleoli during surgery may be crucial for success. In most instances, the malleoli are damaged from the original arthrodesis, and the bone may have become weak because of stress protection by the tibiotalar fusion.

On the tibial side, the implant should fully cover the resection surface. First, it may protect the restored joint space from ossification. Second, it may optimize the load transfer at the bone-implant interface and thus protect the implant from subsidence into the weak bone until osseointegration and bone remodeling have occurred. On the talar side, the implant should have a large contact area with the bone, particularly in the sagittal plane. This may protect the implant from subsidence into the weak bone.

10.5 Revision Arthroplasty (for Failed Primary Arthroplasty)

Once a total ankle replacement fails, arthrodesis has been advocated as the treatment of choice. With the availability of a wide spectrum of implants, however, re-arthroplasty may become a viable alternative.

Failures of total ankle arthroplasties can be roughly classified as either:
- implant failures, where one or two components have loosened,
- implantation failures and/or progressive concomitant problems, where the implant components are stable, but associated problems such as recurrent deformity, instability, stiffness, or tendon dysfunction cause the arthroplasty to fail.

In the first case, where one or two components have become loose, the main problem might be bone loss due to subsidence of the implants. A potential problem on the talar side may also be avascular necrosis. In most instances, it is not possible to perform revision arthroplasty with the regular implants, as bone loss might prevent the achievement of solid fixation and ligament balancing. Special revision implants or custom-made implants, however, might replace the lost bone stock and allow a well balanced revision arthroplasty (Fig. 10.12; see also Fig. 11.16 in Chap. 11: Complications of Total Ankle Arthroplasty).

In the second case, where the implants are stable but other problems have caused the failure of the arthroplasty, accurate diagnosis is mandatory to identify the underlying causes. Then:
- malalignment may be addressed by osteotomies (see Fig. 11.10 in Chap. 11: Complications of Total Ankle Arthroplasty),
- deformities may be addressed by osteotomies and/or arthrodeses,
- instabilities may be addressed by ligamentoplasties, tendon transfers, and/or arthrodeses,
- stiffness may be addressed by capsular release and/or tendon release (see Fig. 11.14 in Chap. 11: Complications of Total Ankle Arthroplasty),
- tendon dysfunction may be addressed by tendon reconstruction and/or tendon transfer.

If revision arthroplasty is not considered to be a feasible option, ankle arthrodesis may be advised. Because of bone loss, however, isolated ankle arthrodesis is often difficult to achieve, and it may require huge tricortical bone grafts from the iliac crest, or allografts, and stable internal fixation (see Fig. 11.18, Chap. 11: Complications of Total Ankle Arthroplasty). If an isolated arthrodesis cannot be achieved, tibiocalcaneal arthrodesis is advised.

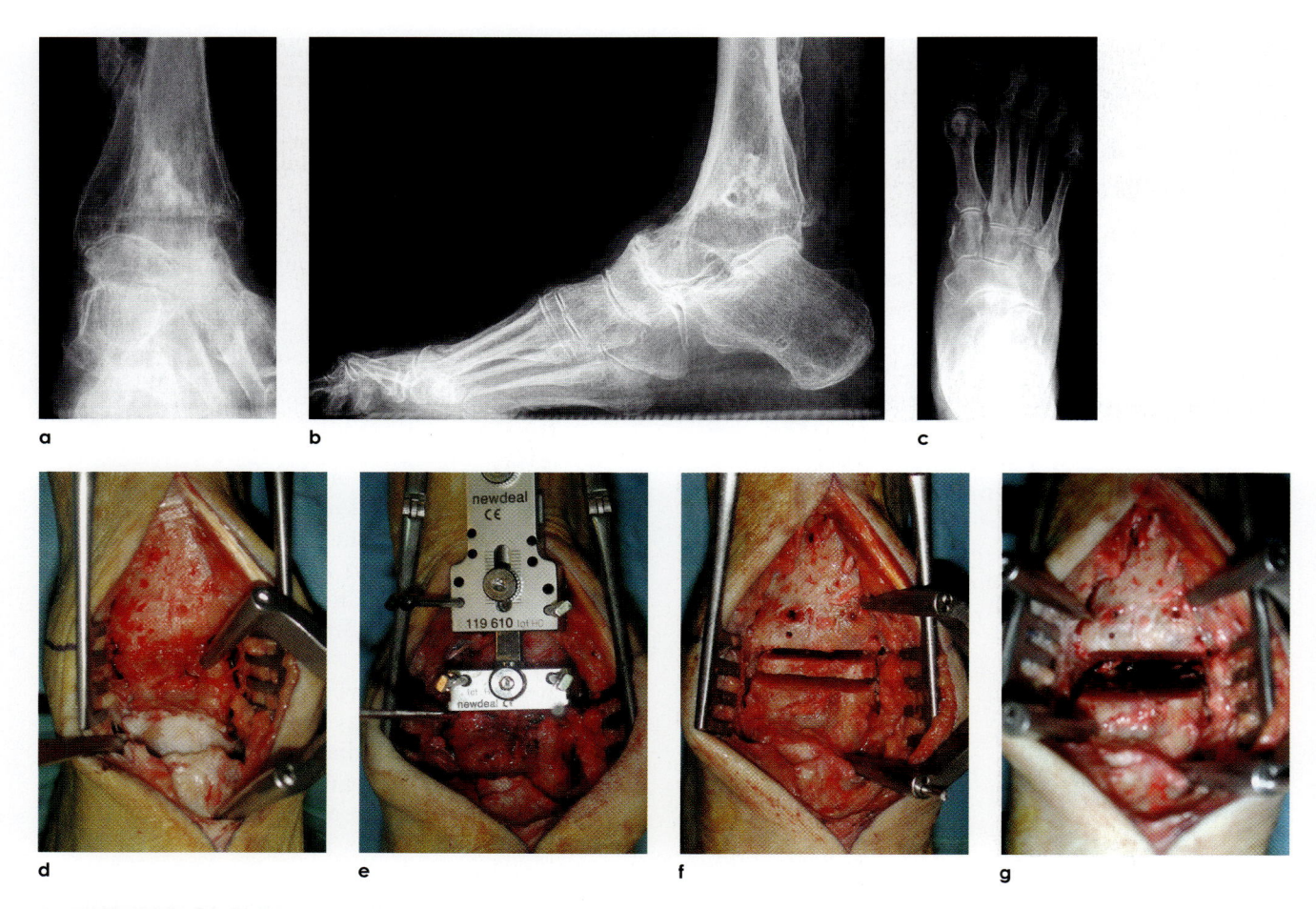

Fig. 10.14. Ankle disarthrodesis.
This 78-year-old woman, who underwent ankle arthrodesis 12 years ago for a post-traumatic osteoarthrosis 39 years after a tibial fracture (skiing accident), complained of intense pain that limited her activities to a minimum. The anteroposterior X-ray showed the ankle fused in a well-aligned position, with fibular osteotomy used for the arthrodesis (**a**). The lateral view of the ankle (**b**) and anteroposterior view of the foot evidenced advanced osteoarthrosis at the subtalar and talonavicular joints (**c**), but also degenerative disease in the transverse tarsal joints. First, the talonavicular joint was approached through the standard anterior approach to the ankle (**d**), and talonavicular arthrodesis was performed. Subtalar joint arthrodesis was achieved through an additional lateral approach (not shown). The tibial resection block was aligned (**e**) and the height of resection determined by fluoroscopy. K-wires were then used to protect the malleoli (**e**). After making the first tibial cut, the resection block was moved 6 mm distally and a second cut was made. Finally a medial and a lateral cut were done using the reciprocating saw (**f**). The osteotomized ankle was carefully mobilized with two Hintermann™ Distractors, and the posterior capsule was carefully resected until the flexor hallucis tendon was visible (**g**). The intraoperative anteroposterior (**h**) and lateral (**i**) fluoroscopic views show the ankle well aligned, as well as appropriate position of the fused subtalar and talonavicular joints. At a follow-up of two years, the ankle and hindfoot were still well aligned, with stable implants and healed arthrodeses (**j, k**). Using fluoroscopy, a dorsiflexion of 16° (**l**) and a plantar flexion of 16° (**m**) were measured ("true ankle motion"). Figures (**n**) through (**q**) show the obtained clinical function

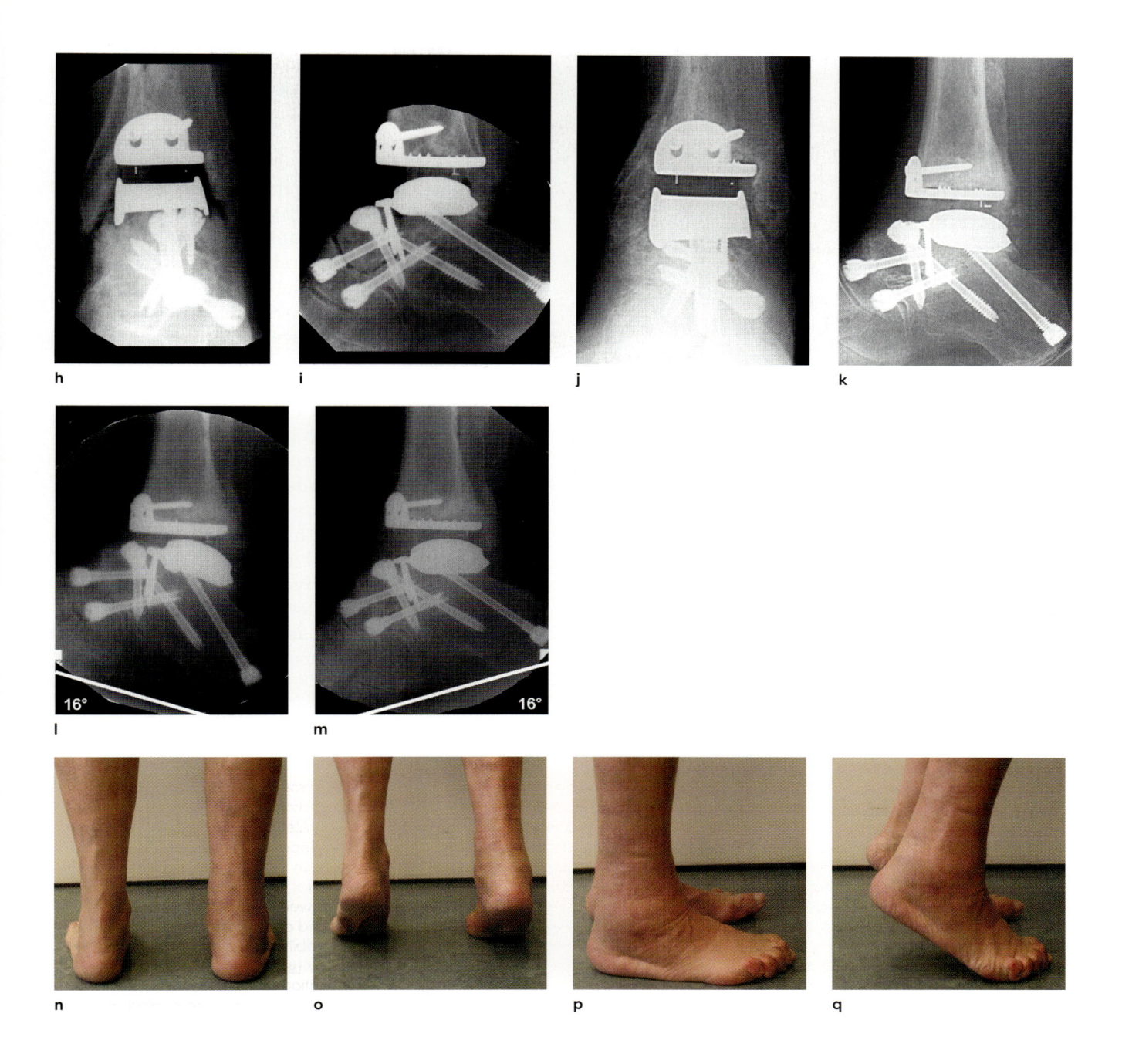

10.5 Revision Arthroplasty (for Failed Primary Arthroplasty)

h

i

j

k

l

m

n

o

p

q

> **The Author's Recommendation**
> If a total ankle arthroplasty has failed, the surgeon may have to decide whether a revision arthroplasty is feasible. An extensive analysis is mandatory to identify all associated problems. In the case of significant bone loss, particularly on the talar side, revision implants or custom-made implants might be necessary to achieve a stable, well-balanced and well-functioning arthroplasty. As it allows for early full weight-bearing and ambulation, revision arthroplasty may be superior to extensive arthrodesis which, in most instances, requires a long-standing cast immobilization. More experience is needed, however, to better define the possibilities and limitations of revision arthroplasty.

10.6 Conclusions

Aside from proper implantation technique, the success of total ankle arthroplasty depends mainly on achieved alignment, stability, and ligament balancing. Therefore, all associated problems must be carefully identified prior to surgery and addressed during surgery. As experience with the procedure increases, total ankle arthroplasty may become feasible in osteoarthritic ankles that were previously thought to be unsuitable candidates for ankle replacement.

Independent of the complexity of the deformity, instability, or malalignment, the main goal of total ankle arthroplasty remains the restoration of a normal, well-balanced, stable, and aligned ankle and hindfoot, where the ankle prosthesis is implanted to replace destroyed surfaces. It does not make sense to replace an ankle that never worked normally (for example, in clubfoot deformity), or where muscular function is lacking (for example, post-polio foot deformity, paralytic foot). Loss of bone stock is a problem that often cannot be solved using regular implants; however, revision implants or custom-made implants that rely on genuine bone support are a promising alternative to extensive salvage arthrodeses. If ankle arthrodesis results in painful malunion, forefoot overload, and/or degenerative disease of the neighboring joints, taking down the arthrodesis and converting it to arthroplasty may be a viable alternative to correction osteotomies and/or extensive fusion of the hindfoot.

Chapter 11

COMPLICATIONS OF TOTAL ANKLE ARTHROPLASTY

Complications such as postoperative stiffness, prosthesis subsidence, and residual deformity along with infection and wound healing problems jeopardize the successful outcome of total ankle arthroplasty. Adequate knowledge of the complex nature of the normal and arthritic ankle, careful preoperative planning, and strict attention to operative details are known to help minimize the incidence of these complications.

11.1 Characteristics of Ankle Osteoarthritis

Osteoarthritis of the ankle is different from other types of degenerative joint disease that the orthopedic surgeon routinely encounters in clinical practice. Hip and knee osteoarthritis, for instance, is predominantly of degenerative etiology in older patients. For osteoarthritis in general, a slow but progressive course is common for most patients, characterized by decreasing range of motion in the joint, development of contractures, excessive pain, pathological gait, and significantly decreased quality of life. The osteoarthritic joint typically loses its physiological pattern (axis, congruency, ligament balancing, etc.) and becomes stiff because of chronic inflammation. Although achieving a functional range of motion is always the goal of prosthetic joint surgery, regaining the physiological range of motion is not always possible. Achieving the range of motion needed for walking and daily activities, however, is rarely a problem.

11.1.1 Primary Osteoarthrosis of the Ankle

Primary osteoarthrosis is characterized by loss of joint cartilage, and hypertrophy of bone is predominant. The exact mechanisms have not been defined, but subchondral bone injury and mechanical stress contribute to the damage [22]. The radiographic hallmarks are joint space narrowing (which correlates with loss of joint cartilage), osteophyte formation, subchondral bone cysts, and subchondral sclerosis [22]. There is usually an absence of juxta-articular osteoporosis in this type of primary osteoarthrosis.

11.1.2 Post-Traumatic Osteoarthrosis of the Ankle

In contrast to the hip and knee, osteoarthrosis of the ankle is about 80% post-traumatic in origin [6, 17], and therefore occurs in patients younger than those with osteoarthrosis of the hip or knee. Patient expectations for recovery from and regaining activity after total ankle arthroplasty are high. Although there is essentially one bone above the ankle, there are 26 bones and even more joints below the ankle that can affect the alignment and functioning of a total ankle prosthesis. The soft-tissue envelope surrounding joints other than the ankle is generally thick, and is typically not altered by previous trauma. The normal soft-tissue envelope around the ankle is thin, however, and when there has been antecedent trauma and associated surgical repairs, it is often scarred and inelastic. These factors, combined with the period of immobilization subsequent to the trauma, lack of adequate physical therapy, chronic pain, and progressive periarticular osteophyte formation, often lead to significantly reduced range of motion (particularly for dorsiflexion) that may not always improve with replacement of the diseased ankle joint.

11.1.3 Rheumatoid Arthritis of the Ankle

In contrast to the success of hip and knee arthroplasty in rheumatoid patients, total ankle arthroplasty in patients with rheumatoid arthritis has many potential problems, including those related to wound healing, subsidence, and late aseptic loosening because of poor bone quality. Many patients with long-standing rheumatoid disease present with an acquired pes planovalgus et abductus deformity from subtalar inflammatory disease and consequent ligament incompetence (Fig. 11.1). Many have had either previous *in situ* hindfoot fusions (leaving them with a calcaneovalgus deformity), or have uncorrected hindfoot deformities at the time of total ankle arthroplasty. After undergoing total ankle arthroplasty, some patients develop both a pronation deformity of the foot and a valgus deformity of the knee. This may lead to a divergence between the mechanical and anatomic axes, with deleterious effects on the loading of the prosthesis, followed later by aseptic loosening and higher rates of failure.

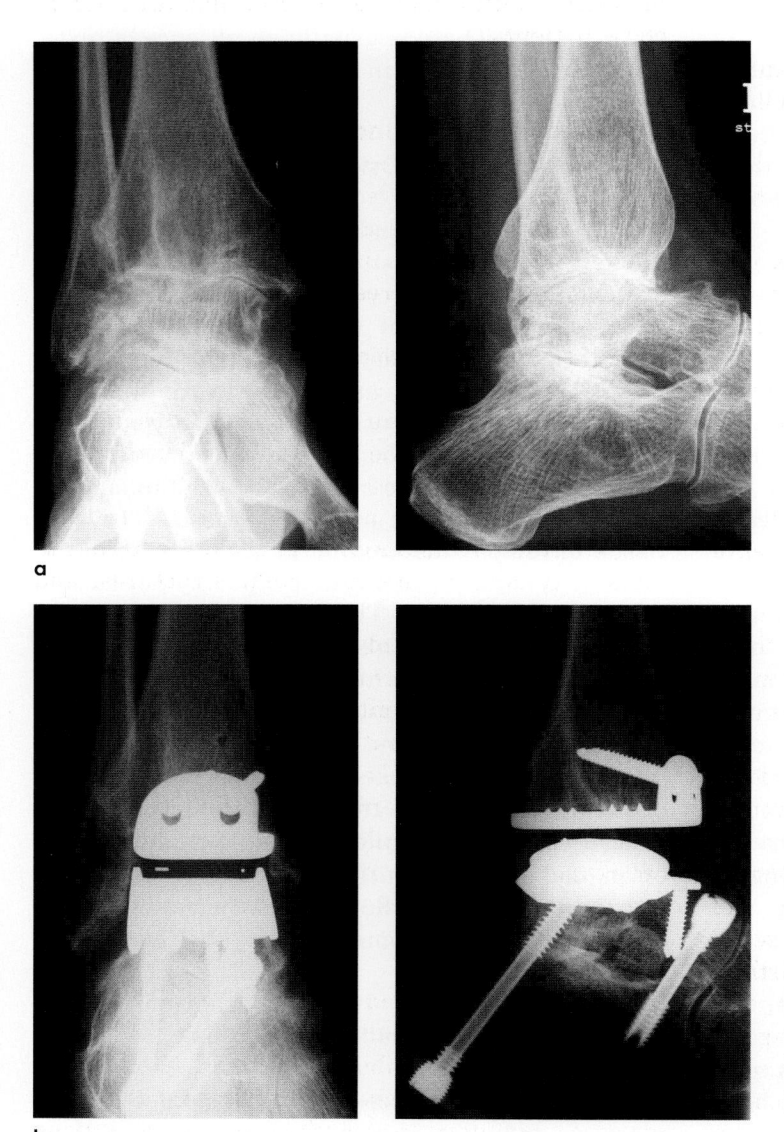

Fig. 11.1. Combination of total ankle replacement and subtalar arthrodesis.
Rheumatoid arthritis with fixed valgus deformity of the hindfoot, with arthritic changes mainly in the ankle and subtalar joint and significant osteolytic processes in the distal tibia (female, 45 years old) (**a**). The hindfoot was well aligned and stable when the plaster was removed six weeks after combined subtalar fusion and total ankle replacement (**b**). The patient was allowed to start bearing full weight in the plaster from the second day after surgery

11.2 Patient Selection

Careful patient selection is important for limiting complications and obtaining satisfactory results.

11.2.1 Age of the Patient

Age is a somewhat contentious issue in ankle replacement surgery (see Chap. 7, Sect. 7.3.10: Age Considerations). Clearly, older patients are better candidates for arthroplasty because of their reduced level of activity and the decreased likelihood that they will outlive the device.

Arguments against performing total ankle arthroplasty in younger patients include the following:
— Younger people tend to place more stress on their implants through higher impact activities, which can result in early failure of the implant.
— There are no long-term results that show second-generation arthroplasty survival rates, so it is not known how long they will last before requiring revision.
— There is little experience of revising failed arthroplasties, and the survival rate of the revisions is unknown.

On the other hand, arguments that support the use of total ankle arthroplasty in younger patients include the following:
— Most post-traumatic osteoarthritis of the ankle occurs in younger patients, so to exclude them from arthroplasty based on age alone is to withhold this treatment from most of the people who have this problem.
— There are long-term problems with ankle arthrodesis. Nearly all patients develop hindfoot or midfoot osteoarthritis within 15 to 20 years following their ankle arthrodesis, and then require fusion surgery [13, 18]. Theoretically, replacing the ankle in younger patients may delay the onset of this secondary hindfoot and midfoot osteoarthritis for many years. Then, when the prosthesis fails, an ankle fusion can be performed, giving the patient many more years of symptom-free use of his or her foot. With this "two-stage approach," a prosthesis system that requires minimal bone resection may be an enormous advantage with respect to the possibility of future ankle arthrodesis.

11.2.2 Weight of the Patient

Patient weight may also play an important role in prosthesis complications (see Chap. 7, Sect. 7.3.4: Weight Restrictions). Absolute weight may be less important than body mass index. Body mass index may be even more important in correlation with the size of the implanted prosthesis [15]. Premature prosthetic failure may result from implantation in obese patients.

11.3 Preoperative Conditions and Planning

Recognizing critical preoperative risk factors and doing careful preoperative planning are other important aspects of limiting complications and achieving satisfactory results [38].

11.3.1 Soft-Tissue Conditions

The more damage there is to the periarticular soft tissues of the ankle, the more potential there is for wound healing difficulties, chronic swelling, persistent stiffness, and lost range of motion [15]. In addition, chronic soft-tissue damage makes it harder to identify underlying neurovascular structures, and increases the likelihood that they may be damaged during surgery. Chronic soft-tissue damage is also associated with chronic soft-tissue discomfort, which ankle replacement surgery may not diminish (Fig. 11.2). Post-traumatic muscular insufficiencies coupled with relatively overpowered antagonists may be a very important issue in the outcome of a total ankle arthroplasty. The preoperative physical examination must include careful inspection of the cutaneous tissues, ligaments, tendons, and muscles.

11.3.2 Malalignment and Malunion

Large tibial bows or tibial malunions, fibular malunions, and hindfoot supination or pronation are major contributors to technical difficulties during

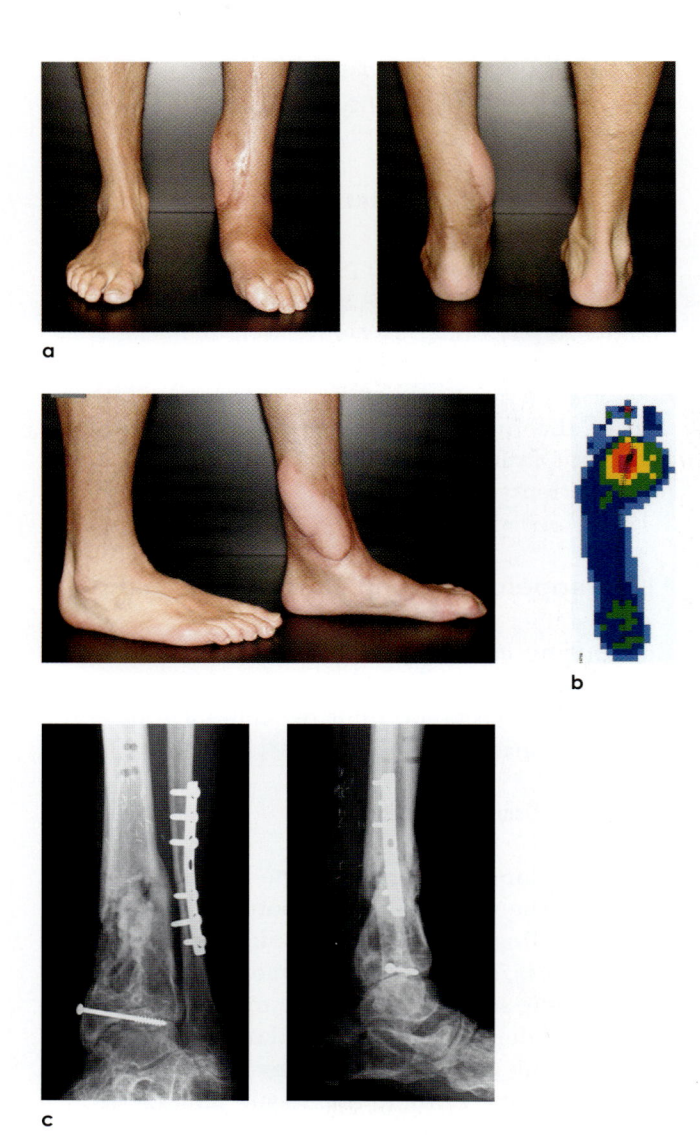

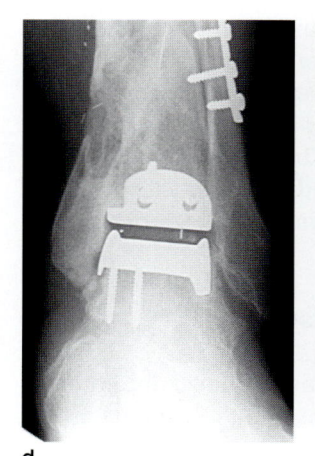

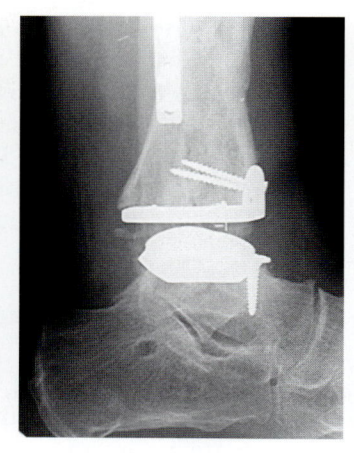

Fig. 11.2. Total ankle replacement for severe post-traumatic osteoarthrosis after open tibial pilon fracture.
Extensive soft-tissue damage four years after an open tibial pilon fracture that needed a free-vascularized flap for coverage (male, 49 years old) (**a**). The dynamic pedobarography (Emed-System, Novel, Munich, Germany) revealed an increased forefoot pressure because of soft-tissue contracture of the hindfoot (**b**). The distal tibia was solid, but the quality of the bone rather poor (**c**). Twelve months after total ankle replacement, the patient is extremely satisfied and reports almost complete pain relief (**d**). The hindfoot is stable and the dorsiflexion/plantar flexion obtained was 8° – 0° – 25°. At the time of surgery, heel cord lengthening was not done because more than 5° of dorsiflexion were achieved after extensive posterior capsular resection. The moderate varus position of the tibial component was accepted as given by the preoperative situation in order not to overstress the damaged medial soft-tissue structures

11.4 Implant- and Implantation-Related Complications

become problematic, however, if the talar component has a cylindrical shape, as this results in additional overstressing of the medial ligaments (Fig. 11.5) [41]. Medial (Fig. 11.6) or lateral (Fig. 11.7) malpositioning of the components may be complicated by the interplay between bone and soft-tissue tensioning, or cause fracture of the malleolus. Theoretically, posterior positioning allows the talar component to be seated on stronger posterior cortex, preventing potential subsidence while high-impact forces are applied during push-off. Such posterior positioning of the talus, however, exposes the weaker dorsal aspect of the tibial metaphysis to higher impact forces, which, in turn, may result in posterior tilt and subsidence of the tibial implant (Fig. 11.8). In addition, a posteriorward moment acts on the talar component, pushing it posteriorly during dorsiflexion of the foot, and potentially resulting in posterior tilt and subsidence (Fig. 11.9). Anterior positioning, by contrast, exposes the anterior aspect of the tibial metaphysis to higher impact forces, potentially resulting in anterior tilt and subsidence of the tibial implant (Fig. 11.10). In addition, anteroposterior malpositioning always leads to anisometric loading of collateral ankle ligaments, which results in painful restriction of motion and instability during dorsiflexion/plantar flexion of the foot.

Placement of the implants in a malaligned position may also have an adverse effect on implant longevity, though it is unclear what degree of coronal malalignment will lead to early failure. In the polyethylene insert of a total knee arthroplasty, malalignment leads to increased peak contact stresses [28], which, in turn, leads to increased polyethylene wear and clini-

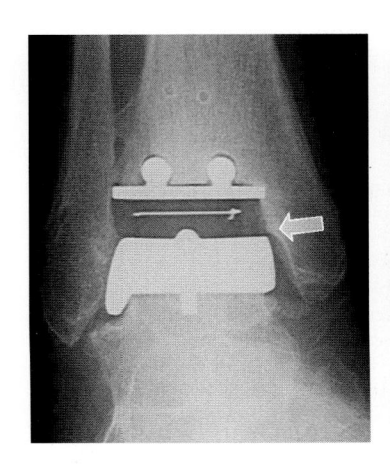

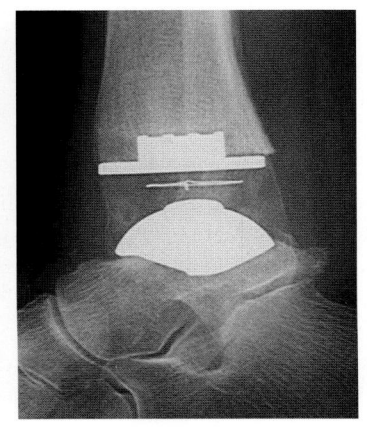

Fig. 11.4. Effect of excessive bone resection.
Excessive bone resection on the tibial side caused seating of the tibial component on soft metaphysial bone (the arrow indicates the original joint line), and the use of a large polyethylene insert was necessary (female, 58 years old). The increased size of the prosthesis is thought to increase the moments, thus shear forces at the bone-implant interface are increased

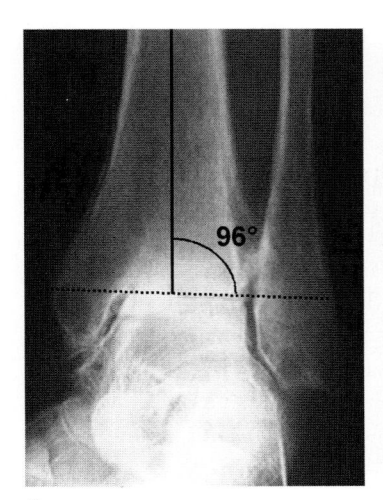

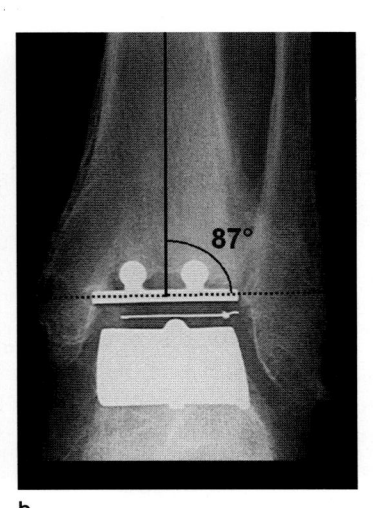

Fig. 11.5. Persistent medial ankle pain after total ankle replacement.
Varus ankle osteoarthrosis with a tibiotalar angle of 96° preoperatively (male, 62 years old) (**a**). Valgus alignment of the jig during surgery resulted in a tibiotalar angle of 87° (**b**), which may explain the persistent medial pain of the patient. Another reason may be the medial ossifications revealed in the X-ray after 12 months, which in the author's opinion are the result of chronic overstressing of the medial ligaments due to the cylindrical talar component of the S.T.A.R. prosthesis having too wide a medial radius. This malpositioning may be particularly problematic in non-anatomically shaped talar designs in general

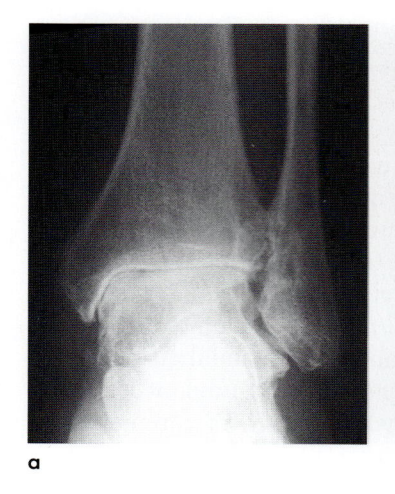

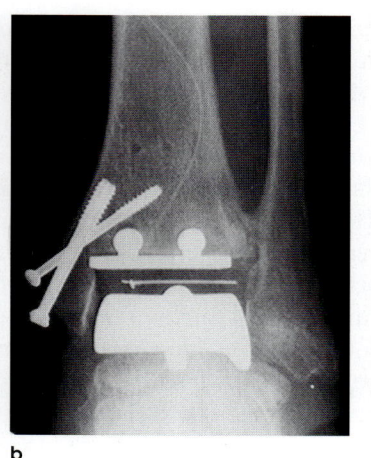

Fig. 11.6. Intraoperative fracture of the medial malleolus during implantation of a total ankle replacement.
The bone stock was well conserved in this patient, who suffered post-traumatic osteoarthrosis secondary to an ankle fracture (female, 64 years old) (**a**). However, wide bone resection and malpositioning of the tibial component too cranially and medially led to weakening of the medial shoulder of the distal tibia, and resulted in an intraoperative fracture. The fracture healed uneventfully within six weeks after screw fixation (**b**)

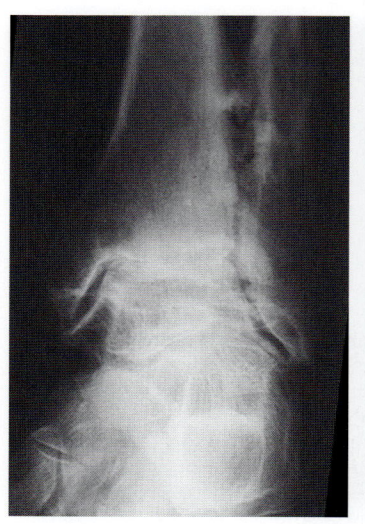

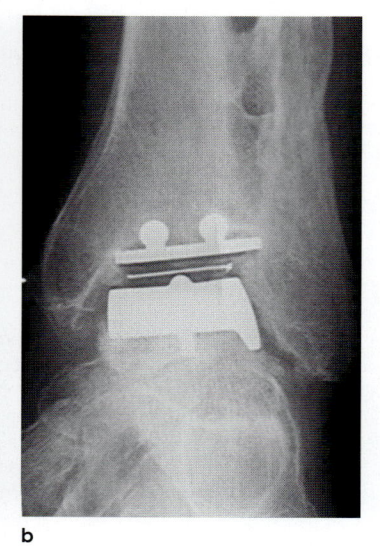

Fig. 11.7. Malpositioning of total ankle replacement with secondary valgus malalignment.
The hindfoot was well aligned in this patient, who suffered post-traumatic osteoarthrosis secondary to an ankle fracture (male, 56 years old) (**a**). Malpositioning of the tibial component too laterally (**b**) led, however, to some subsidence into the lateral weak bone of the distal metaphysis, which resulted in valgus malalignment of the whole hindfoot and painful subfibular impingement. Spontaneous tibiofibular synostosis may have been beneficial for overall stability of the ankle (at 30 months)

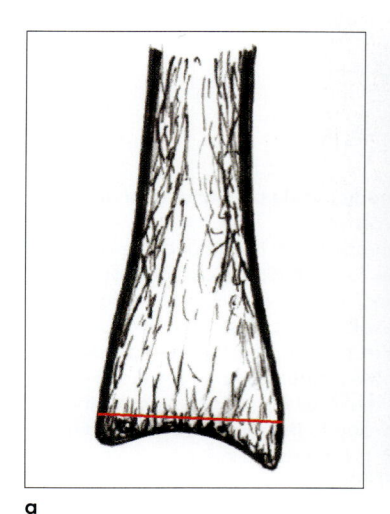

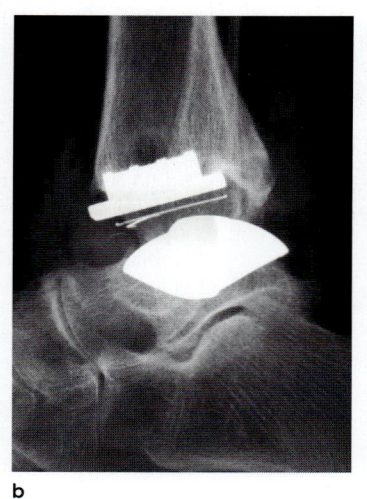

Fig. 11.8. Tilting of both components due to undersized tibial component and posterior malpositioning of the talar component.
Flat resection of the tibia removes the subchondral bone more extensively posteriorly than anteriorly, exposing a bony surface of the tibial metaphysis that is weaker on the dorsal aspect (**a**). The dorsal tibial metaphysis did not provide sufficient bony support for this undersized tibial implant (**b**), which caused posterior subsidence and tilting of the implant. In this case, posterior malpositioning of the talar component may have contributed to this component movement because of the increased impact forces on the posterior tibial component

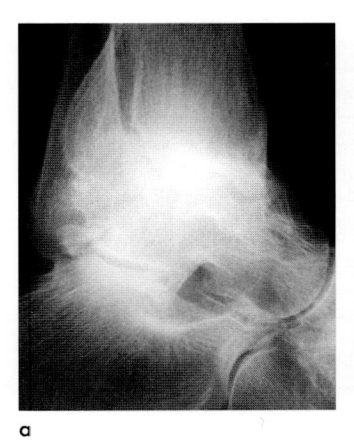

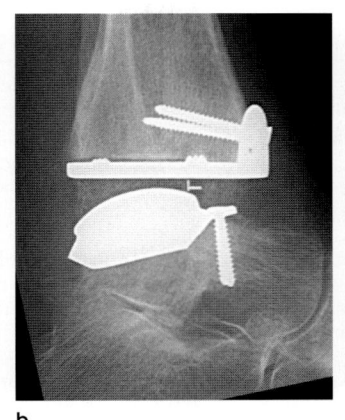

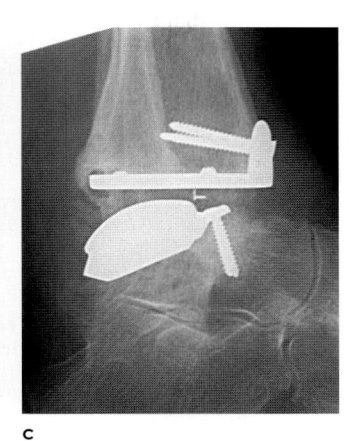

11.4 Implant- and Implantation-Related Complications

Fig. 11.9. Posterior malpositioning of the talar component.
Painful primary osteoarthrosis with remaining range of motion for dorsiflexion/plantar flexion of 20° – 0° – 30° (female, 74 years old) (**a**). The patient was treated with a HINTEGRA® total ankle replacement. Posterior positioning of the talus has exposed the talar component to a posteriorward moment during dorsiflexion of the foot, which provoked a posterior tilt and posterior subsidence of the talar component at 12 months (**b**). Although talar tilt and subsidence were progressing during the second year (**c**), the patient was still extremely satisfied with the result after 24 months, particularly because of the regained range of motion (dorsiflexion/plantar flexion 25° – 0° – 40°). These X-rays were performed under weight-bearing conditions

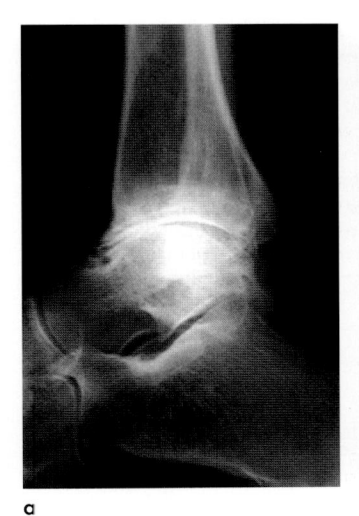

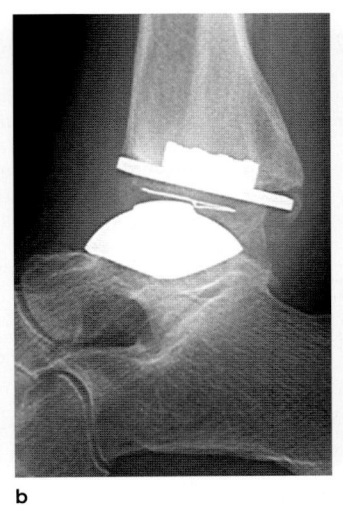

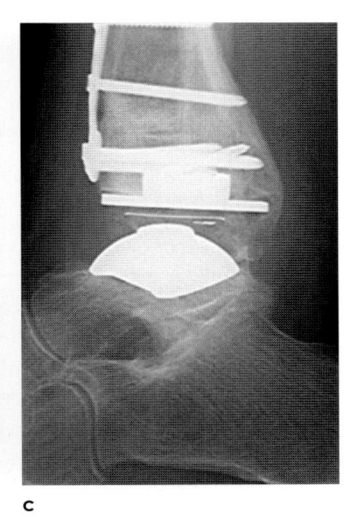

Fig. 11.10. Anterior malpositioning of the talar component.
Post-traumatic end-stage osteoarthrosis 24 years after ankle fracture (female, 58 years old) (**a**). Anterior tilt of the tibial component occurred in the first four months but did not continue afterwards (**b**). The anterior tibial metaphysis was obviously not strong enough to resist the impaction forces, probably due to the relatively anterior position of the talar component and to the weakening of the anterior cortex by the holes for inserting the fixation bars of the tibial component. At the one-year follow-up, the patient complained of continuous medial pain and a feeling of instability. These symptoms disappeared after a supramalleolar open-wedge osteotomy was performed, and at four months after osteotomy, the ankle showed (radiographically) perfect alignment in the sagittal plane (**c**)

Table 11.1. Effects of malpositioning of the ankle prosthesis

Malpositioning	Resulting Problem	Resulting Complications
Proximal displacement	Shortening of the gastrocnemius-soleus complex Proximal migration of the talus Seating the prosthesis on softer metaphysial bone Overtightening of the collateral ankle ligaments	Plantar flexion weakness Medial and lateral gutter impingement Greater risk of subsidence Ligament overstress and range of motion restriction
Distal displacement	Lengthening of the gastrocnemius-soleus complex Excessive bone resection of the talus Seating the prosthesis on softer cancellous bone Slackening of the collateral ankle ligaments	Loss of dorsiflexion motion and altered gait Critical loss of bone stock Greater risk of subsidence Ankle instability
Varus malpositioning	Varus position of the ankle Varus position of the foot Abnormal stress on the polyethylene Overstressing of lateral ankle ligaments	Medial gutter pain from impingement Painful excessive load on the fifth metatarsal Increased polyethylene wear from edge loading Pain and lateral ankle instability
Valgus malpositioning	Valgus position of the ankle Valgus position of the foot Abnormal stress on the polyethylene Overstressing of medial ankle ligaments	Lateral gutter pain from subfibular impingement Pronation deformity and arch discomfort Increased polyethylene wear from edge loading Pain, medial ankle instability, and posterior tibial dysfunction
Medial malpositioning	Thin medial shoulder on distal tibia Overstressing of lateral ankle ligaments	Greater risk of fracture of the malleoli Pain and lateral ankle instability
Lateral malpositioning	Fibular impingement of the implant Overloading of weak anterolateral tibia Overstressing of medial ankle ligaments	Fibular osteolysis Greater risk of subsidence and valgus tilt Pain, medial ankle instability, and posterior tibial dysfunction
Anterior malpositioning	Anterior dislocation of center of rotation Eccentric loading of distal tibia Seating the talar component on weaker anterior bone Anisometric loading of the collateral ankle ligaments	Increased push-off strength, but decreased dorsiflexion Subsidence and anterior tilting of the tibial component Subsidence and tilting of the talar component Instability in plantar flexion, restricted dorsiflexion
Posterior malpositioning	Posterior dislocation of center of rotation Eccentric loading of distal tibia Seating the talar component on harder posterior bone Anisometric loading of the collateral ankle ligaments	Decreased push-off strength, but increased dorsiflexion Subsidence and posterior tilting of the tibial component Decreased risk of subsidence and tilting Instability in dorsiflexion, restricted plantar flexion

cal failure [2, 16]. Pyevich et al [32] found that patients with more than 4° of malalignment had more pain after total ankle arthroplasty. Myerson and Mroczek [30] reported that 48% of patients had a postoperative coronal plane deformity greater than 4°. Saltzman et al [36] reported an average absolute value of deviation from neutral placement in the coronal plane of between 2.4° and 5.3°. Wood [43] reported that 35% of patients had a postoperative coronal plane deformity greater than 5°, and that 18% (seven of 39) of patients with a preoperative coronal plane deformity greater than 15° developed edge loading of the polyethylene bearing (Fig. 11.3).

11.4.2.2 Improper Sizing of Prosthetic Components

In addition to correct positioning, proper sizing of components is mandatory in order to restore the anatomy and biomechanics of a diseased ankle as much as possible (Fig. 11.11). To achieve this goal, implants must allow the ankle to move about a center of rotation, as close to the given center of rotation as possible. This respects the isometric position of the ligaments and exposes them to physiological load only. Proper sizing is also important for preventing impingement, soft-tissue problems, syndesmosis nonunion (if required), and late migration of the components. Improper sizing

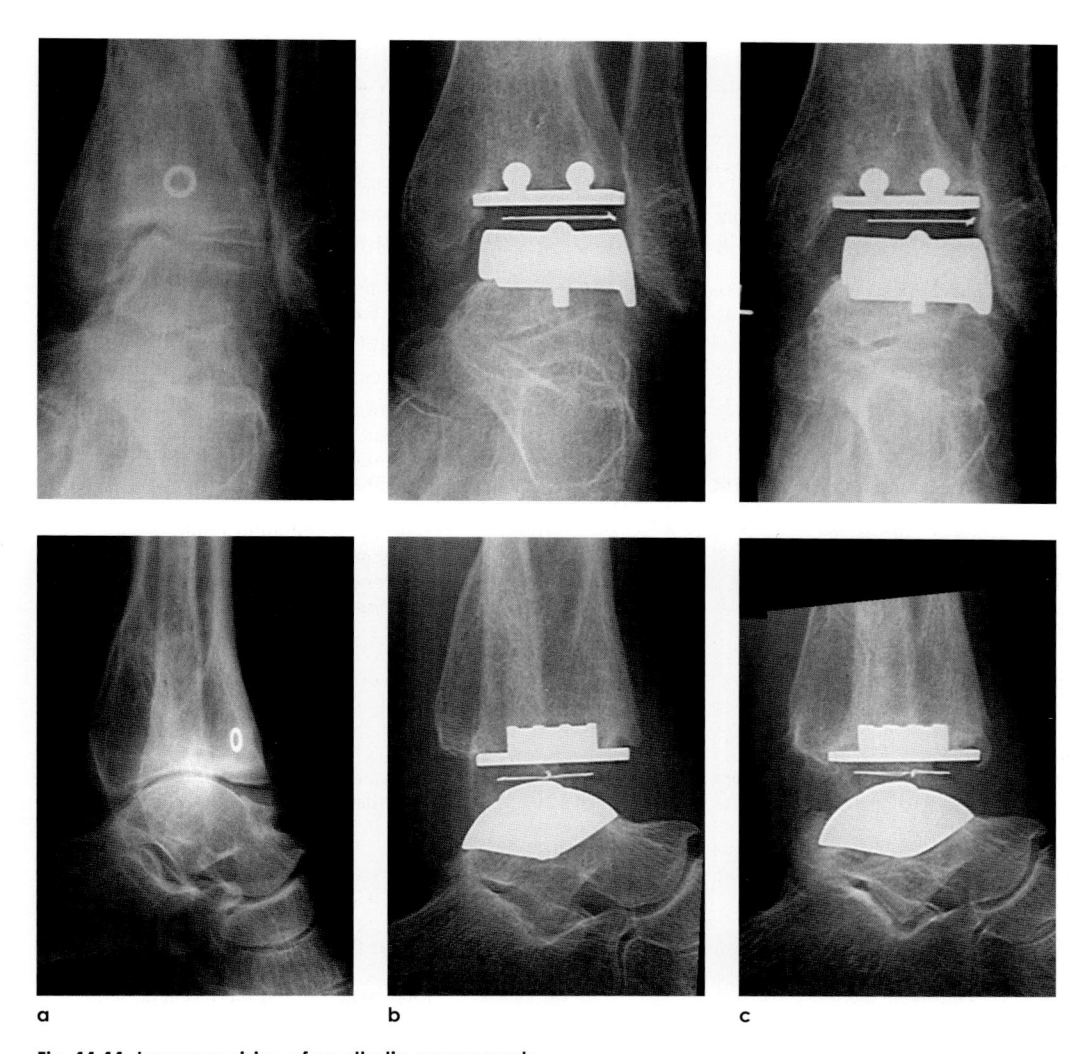

11.4 Implant- and Implantation-Related Complications

Fig. 11.11. Improper sizing of prosthetic components.
End-stage osteoarthrosis with fixed equinus position and enlargement of the distal tibia 12 years after tibial pilon fracture (female, 38 years old) (**a**). The size of the tibial component was chosen with regard to the medial-lateral dimension of the tibiotalar joint, and this decision resulted in undersizing the tibial component in the anteroposterior dimension by more than 20% (**b**). The use of a bigger implant would have required additional bony resection of the medial malleolus (at 12 months). Although the implants are still stable after 58 months, the patient complains of increasing impingement problems and some loss of mobility, which might be explained by the formation of new periarticular bone (**c**)

of components can result in complications similar to those from malpositioning due to displacement.

11.4.2.3 Improper Use of Distraction

The use of distraction for bone resection at the tibial and talar side may also be a source of potential complications. Underdistraction results in excessive bone resection, whereas overdistraction allows for minimal bone resection, but with resultant overstuffing of the joint, which causes pain and loss of motion.

11.4.2.4 Fractures of Malleoli

Malleolar fractures may occur during or shortly after total ankle arthroplasty in up to 22% of cases

(Fig. 11.6) [30, 36]. Intraoperative fractures are related to the limited space between the malleoli for component insertion. Errant placement of cutting jigs, excessive bone resection, overdistraction with the external fixator or spreader, and actual insertion of the components (particularly if the tibial component is oversized and/or positioned too medially) may all contribute to these fractures.

Alternatively, fractures may result from an episode of excessive force placed across the narrowed medial or lateral malleoli, or repeated episodes of lesser force that exceed the strength gained by the remodeling process of the malleoli (Fig. 11.12). Saltzman et al [36] reported eight medial and five lateral malleolus fractures intraoperatively, as well as two medial, four lateral, and one distal tibial fracture postoperatively in 90 total ankle replacements. Two of these patients underwent secondary surgery for repair. Myerson and Mroczek [30] reported five medial, one lateral, and one combined medial and lateral fracture in 50 total ankle replacements. Three of these patients underwent secondary surgery for repair. Wood [43] reported one lateral and eight medial

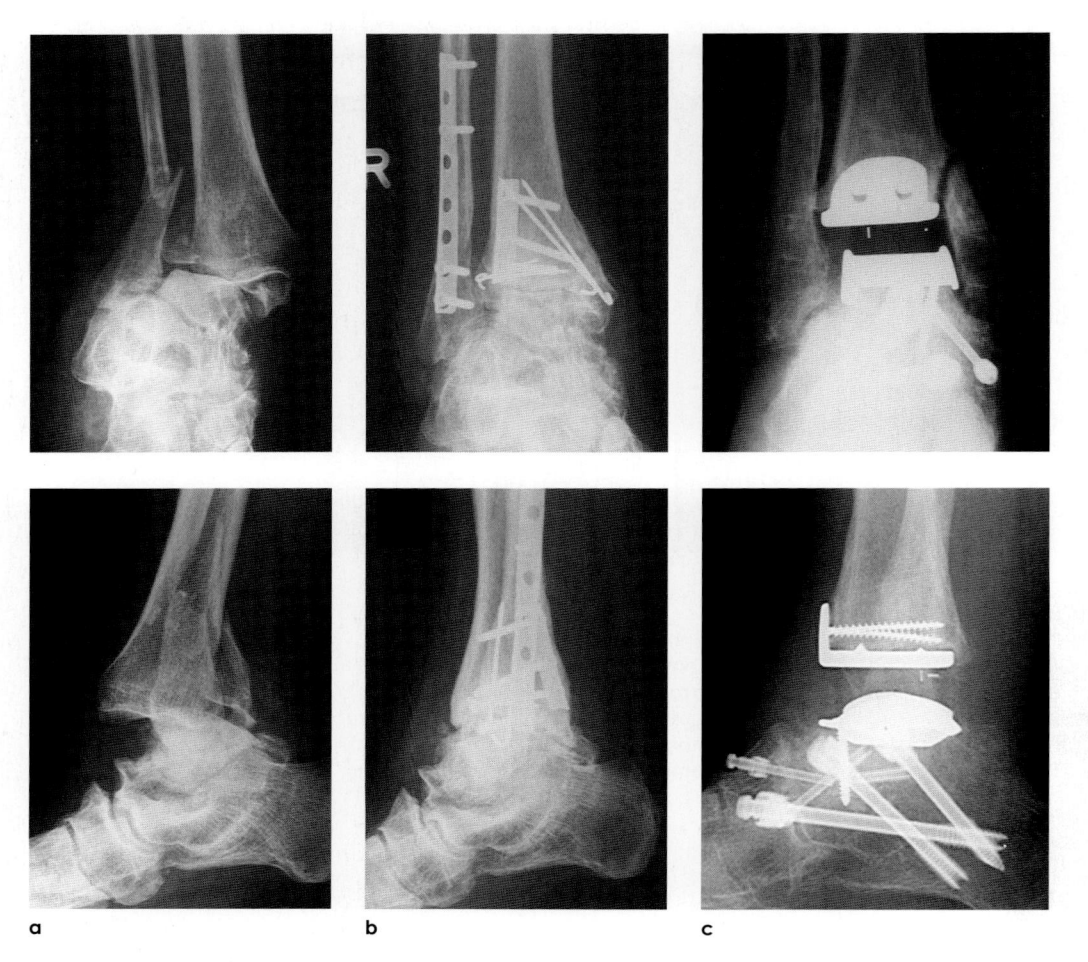

Fig. 11.12. Fracture of the medial malleolus.
Complex dislocation fracture of the ankle with pre-existing osteoarthrosis of the subtalar and talonavicular joints (**a**). Four years later, development of painful end-stage osteoarthrosis with bad bone stock, particularly on tibial side (female, 63 years old) (**b**). As a result, the bony resection was made more proximally, causing a fatigue fracture at the medial shoulder of the distal tibia, which was already weakened by the original fracture (**c**). In spite of the nonunion, the ankle was stable and the patient reported no pain at the three-year follow-up

malleolus fractures during ankle replacement, and one lateral and 10 medial malleolus fractures postoperatively in 200 total ankle replacements. One intraoperative and three postoperative fractures underwent secondary surgery for repair.

11.4.2.5 Tendon Injuries

During surgery, injuries can occur to the posterior tibial, peroneal, flexor digitorum longus, or flexor hallucis longus tendons.

11.5 Early Postoperative Complications

The following complications may be seen in the early postoperative stages after total ankle arthroplasty:
— wound healing problems,
— swelling,
— infection,
— deep venous thrombosis,
— syndesmotic nonunion / instability,
— fractures of malleoli.

These issues are discussed in the sections that follow.

11.5.1 Wound Healing Problems

Wound healing problems were probably the most perplexing complications encountered during first-generation prosthetic surgery. The injured soft-tissue envelope after trauma and/or previous surgery and the thin skin associated with rheumatoid arthritis made wound healing problems in the ankle more likely than in the hip or knee.

Early wound problems range from minor delays in wound healing with superficial infection (Fig. 11.13) to deep infection requiring implant removal. The soft-tissue envelope over the ankle region is unforgiving and care must be taken during surgery to protect the skin and underlying structures. An adequate incision should be made and hooks or self-retaining retractors that attach directly to the skin should be avoided to prevent wound-edge necrosis. Closure of the joint capsule and of the extensor retinaculum, if possible, may prevent a superficial wound problem from becoming a deep infection. Postoperatively, the use of a drain, supplemental oxygen [19], immobilization, and elevation may speed wound healing [24].

Minor delays in wound healing and superficial infections occur in 2% to 24% of cases and are effectively treated with local measures, with or

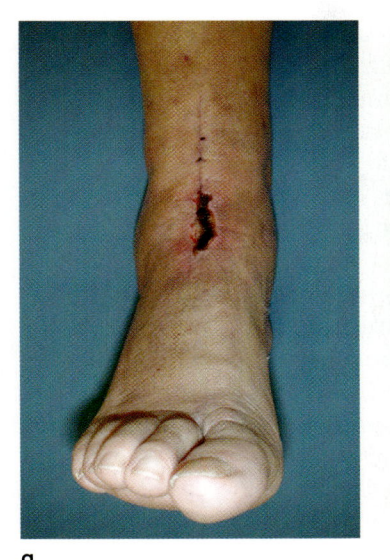

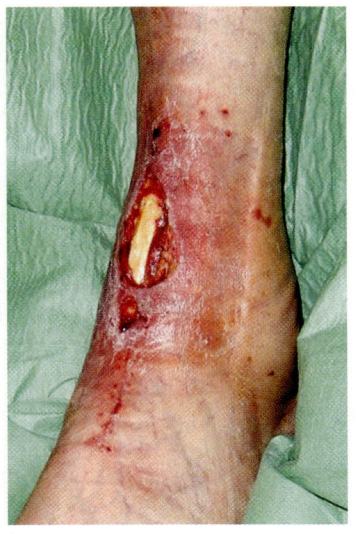

Fig. 11.13. Superficial wound healing problems.
A case with a superficial wound problem with delayed healing within eight weeks (**a**). A case with an extensive superficial wound problem (without deep infection) that required a vascularized flap, but then healed uneventfully (**b**)

without antibiotics [30, 32]. Wood [43] reported a 1% rate of major wound problems with the S.T.A.R. ankle, resulting in skin grafting in one patient and implant removal and ankle fusion in another patient. Saltzman et al [36] reported a 7% rate of major wound problems. Three patients eventually underwent below-the-knee amputation. Two patients underwent implant removal, with one resulting in fusion and the other resulting in a permanent cement spacer.

Delayed wound healing, skin necrosis, and superficial wound infection are still the most common postoperative complications in total ankle arthroplasty.

11.5.2 Swelling

Swelling is a major problem in ankles that have undergone multiple surgeries. Often, significant soft-tissue damage accompanies the initial fracture in patients with post-traumatic osteoarthrosis. Then, multiple subsequent surgeries may obliterate tissue planes and additionally injure the lymphatic system in the area, and chronic edema may develop with long-standing osteoarthritis. Finally, total ankle arthroplasty may additionally damage the soft tissue and increase movement about a preoperatively stiff joint. The result is swelling that may persist for one to 1.5 years after surgery.

11.5.3 Infection

Infection is an uncommon complication after total ankle arthroplasty. Adherence to good surgical technique and appropriate perioperative antibiotic use should limit the incidence of infection.

11.5.4 Deep Venous Thrombosis

The incidence of deep venous thrombosis after total ankle arthroplasty is unknown. A standard prophylaxis, however, seems to be appropriate to lessen the chance of this complication.

11.5.5 Syndesmotic Nonunion / Instability

Syndesmotic nonunion, if required, is another early complication after total ankle arthroplasty. It can be the result of an oversized implant, an inappropriate fusion technique, or insufficient internal fixation. The use of an additional plate for fixation may reduce the incidence of syndesmotic nonunion [38].

11.5.6 Fractures of Malleoli

Fractures may result from an episode of excessive force placed across the narrowed medial (Fig. 11.12) or lateral malleoli, or repeated episodes of lesser force that exceed the strength gained by the remodeling process of the malleoli (see also Chap. 11, Sect. 11.4.2: Problems with Second-generation Total Ankle Prosthesis, Sect. 11.4.2.4: Fractures of Malleoli).

11.6 Late Postoperative Complications

The following complications may be seen in the late postoperative stages after total ankle arthroplasty:
– loss of motion,
– aseptic loosening,
– subsidence,
– polyethylene wear.

These issues are discussed in the sections that follow.

11.6.1 Loss of Motion

Postoperative plantar flexion contracture can occur because of an existing preoperative contracture. Many patients lose range of motion because of soft-tissue injury and casting after their original injury. It is most important, therefore, to completely release the posterior capsule of the ankle joint before implanting the components. In the case of varus deformity, the posterior aspect of the deltoid ligament may also be released to sufficiently address the contracture.

Many surgeons consider heel cord lengthening to be an integral part of total ankle arthroplasty [15, 20, 33, 38]. Leaving a patient with a plantar flexion contracture after total ankle arthroplasty causes abnormal gait and can lead to increased stress in and osteoarthrosis of the midfoot over time. Patients with a positive Silverskjold test [14] may

11.6 Late Postoperative Complications

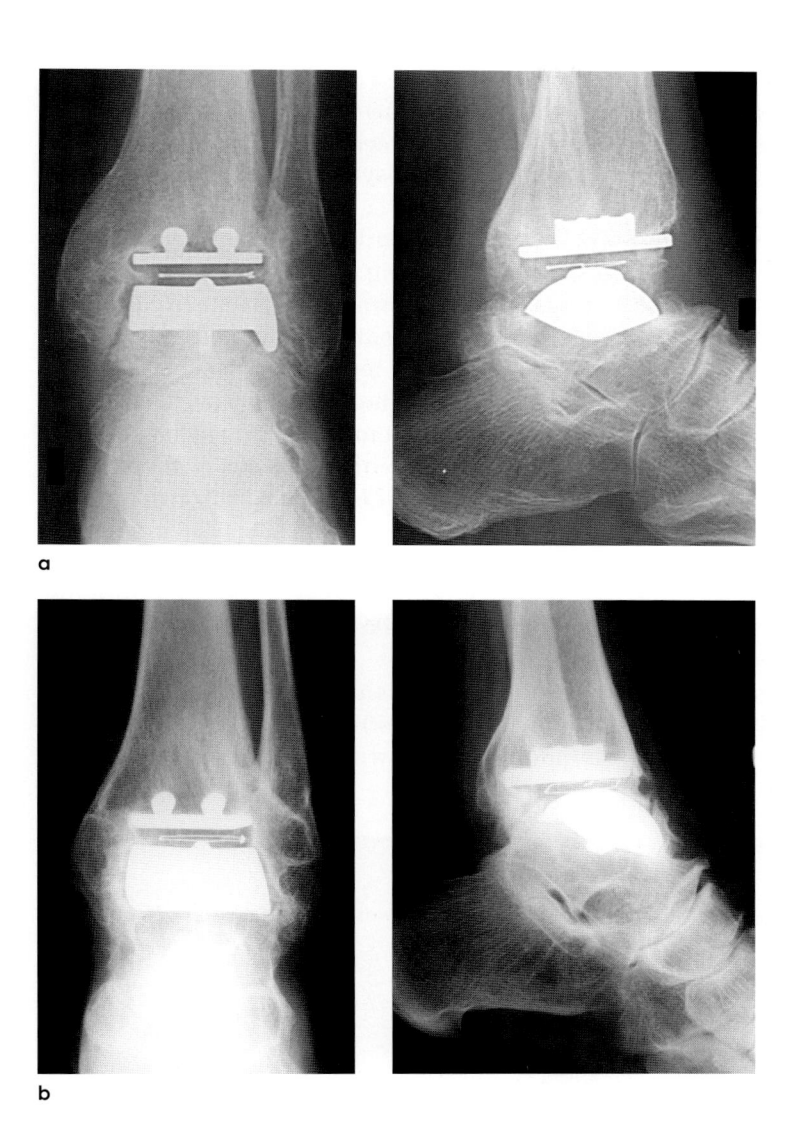

Fig. 11.14. Loss of motion due to progressive periarticular bone formation.
A case with a progressive ossification of the posterior capsule. At the two-year follow-up, the patient (female, 59 years old) was suffering from increased stiffening and pain (**a**). A case with complete ankle stiffness 8.2 years after total ankle replacement (female, 48 years old) (**b**)

undergo either a selective gastrocnemius lengthening (performed at the musculotendinous junction through a posteromedial midline incision), or a percutaneous or open distal Achilles tendon lengthening (using a three-incision technique). Great care must be taken, however, when deciding whether or not to lengthen the Achilles tendon. Distal Achilles tendon lengthening will increase dorsiflexion, but it may also cause push-off weakness during gait. Without proper push-off strength, the terminal plantar flexion that normally occurs during stance phase is lost, resulting in a gait pattern resembling that of a fused ankle. Selective gastrocnemius release causes only a temporary lost of muscular strength [7], and may theoretically cause less plantar flexion strength deficit than distal Achilles tendon lengthening.

Progressive periarticular ossifications can also cause ankle joint contracture (Fig. 11.14). Ossifications of the posterior capsule have been reported in up to 30% of post-traumatic ankles at a mid-term follow-up after total ankle replacement [1, 41, 42]. Pre-existing contracture because of soft-tissue injury and casting after an original injury, and extensive scarring because of repeated surgeries possibly increases the risk of ossifications when regained motion exposes the damaged soft tissue to increased stress. Additional stress to the capsular and ligamentous structures may also result, because proper ligament balancing can often not be achieved in these damaged ankles. Valgus malalignment and the use of a non-anatomically shaped talar component (for example, a cylindrically shaped talus), may cause a chronic medial stress syndrome that has been often associated with progressive ossification of the posteromedial capsule (Figs. 11.5 and 11.14) [41]. The use of a non-anatomically shaped tibial component that does not cover the whole resection surface (that is, the cancellous bone area) may also cause ossifications of the posterior ankle (Figs. 11.11 and 11.14) [8].

11.6.2 Aseptic Loosening

Failure of porous ingrowth and aseptic loosening can be the result of improper implantation of the components, poor bone quality (for example, avascular osteonecrosis, post-traumatic osteosclerosis), inappropriate stress applied to the bone-implant interface (for example, shear forces), and the use of inappropriate prosthetic coating materials. Primary stability of the implant is mandatory for bony ingrowth; therefore attention must be paid (regardless of the prosthetic design) to ensuring that the component is both stably and firmly implanted. Allowing patients to bear weight (with cast protection) starting on the first day after surgery may increase porous ingrowth and proper seating of the components. The use of new coating techniques (such as hydroxyapatite, tricalcium phosphate, porous-coated titanium layer) may improve the speed and quantity of osseointegration of the prosthesis. Applying platelet-rich material from centrifuged patient's blood to the porous-coated portion of the prosthesis may also increase porous ingrowth of the prosthesis [15]. Similarly, the use of stem cells may be effective for improving porous ingrowth (Y. Takakura, personal communication, 2003).

Periprosthetic radiolucent lines are poorly defined around ankle prostheses, and their occurrence is often not associated with loosening [1, 26, 32, 41,

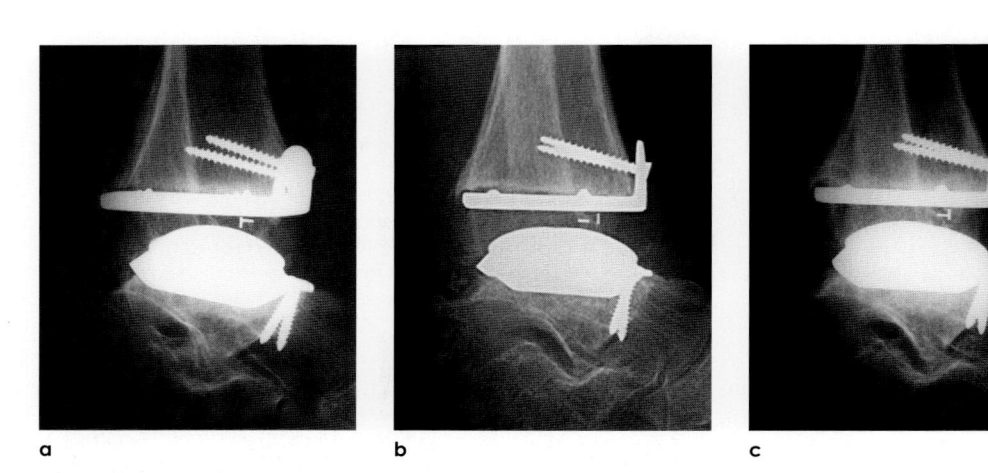

Fig. 11.15. Periprosthetic radiolucency.
This ankle showed periprosthetic lucencies that resolved with time: at six weeks (**a**); at six months (**b**); and at 12 months (**c**)

Fig. 11.16. Revision arthroplasty as salvage procedure for failed total ankle arthroplasty.
X-ray of a painful post-traumatic osteoarthrosis (female, 52 years) (**a**). Regular position of the implants after six weeks (**b**). Some settling of the talar component, but regular position and no pain after 12 months (**c**). Unchanged position of the implants after 48 months (**d**), and no pain. After 60 months, however, marked subsidence of the talar component with painful fibulotalar impingement, and some ballooning loosening at the anterior tibia (**e**). Intraoperative *situs* showing talar osteonecrosis after component removal (**f**). Flat cut of the tibia showing some sclerotic but regular remaining bone (**g**). Final *situs* view of the implanted prosthesis (**h**) with the use of a custom-made talar component (**i**) that uses more bone for support, both anteriorly and posteriorly. Well-aligned and stable position of the implants after eight weeks (**j, k**)

11.6 Late Postoperative Complications

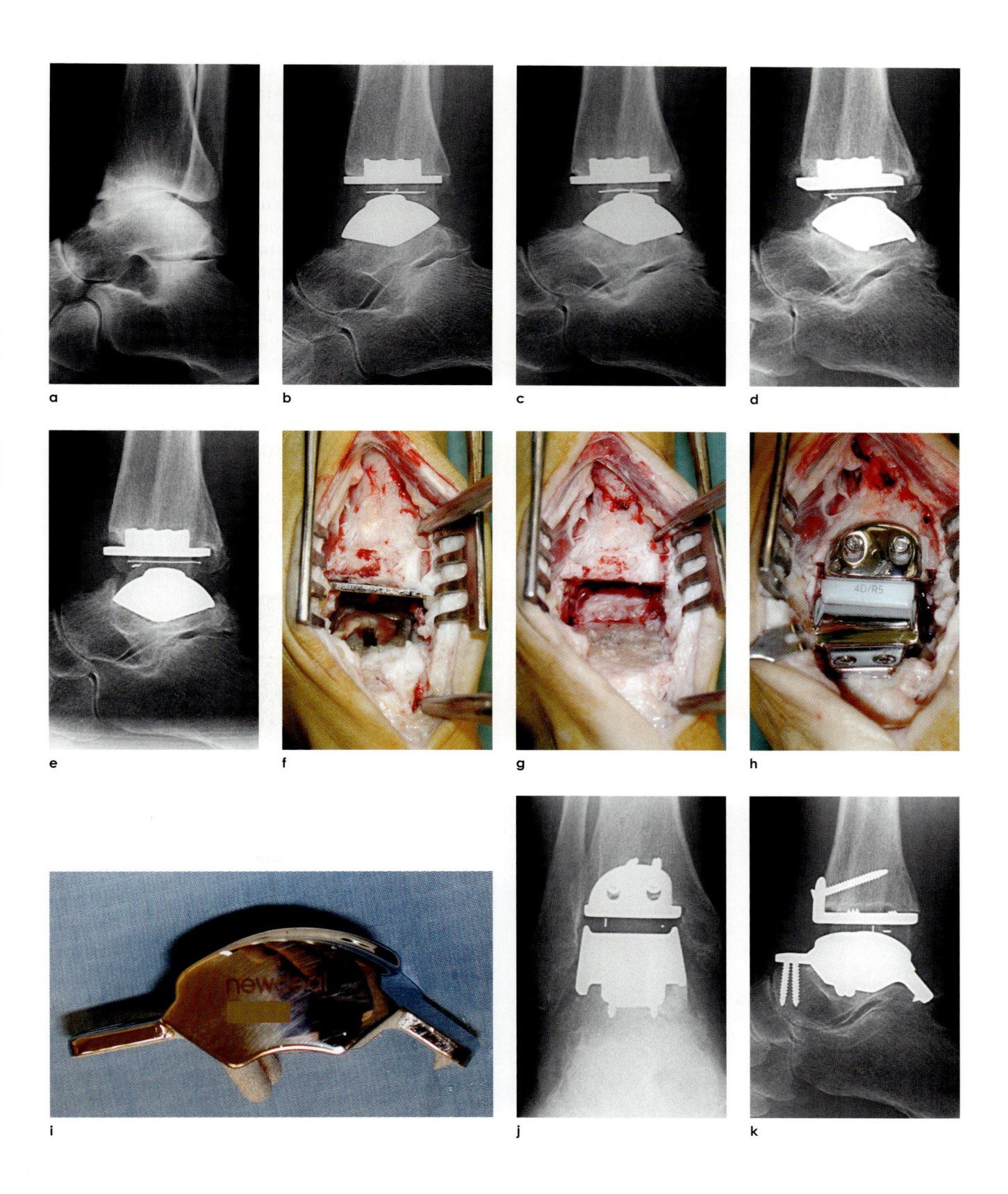

a b c d

e f g h

i j k

42, 44]. Sometimes periprosthetic lucencies even resolve with time (Figs. 4.16 and 11.15).

11.6.3 Subsidence

Subsidence is primarily the result of inappropriate bony support (Fig. 11.16). Weakening of the bone due to extensive resection of the subchondral bone, and failure to use the entire available bone for support of the prosthesis (for example, by using undersized components or non-anatomic prosthetic designs) may result in subsidence of the prosthesis. Early exposure of the prosthesis to excessive load (that is, before stress adaptation of the bone has occurred) may be another reason for subsidence of the prosthesis. Finally, poor bone quality (as with osteoporosis and particularly avascular necrosis) may result in subsidence of the prosthesis with time.

In addition to proper positioning the prosthesis, the use of implants that take advantage of the available surface contact area and require minimal bone

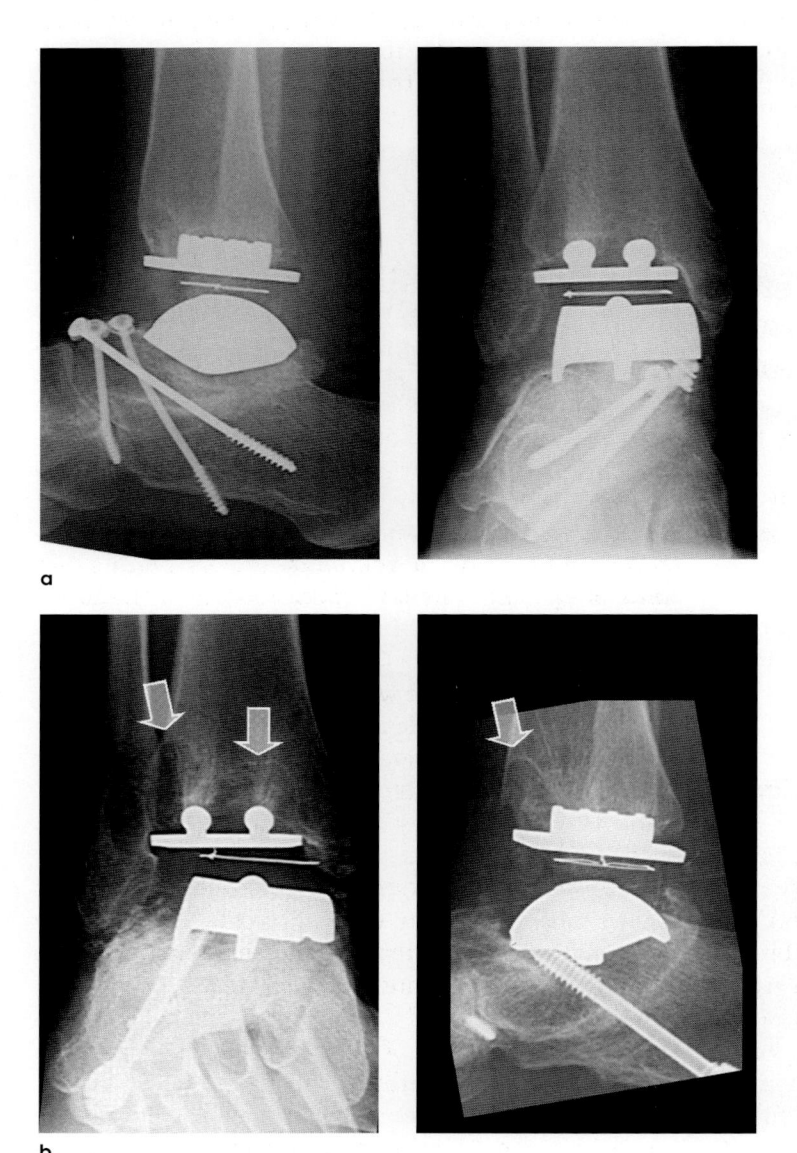

Fig. 11.17. Polyethylene wear and ballooning loosening. Severe valgus deformity four months after simultaneous subtalar fusion and total ankle replacement following breakdown of the talar body in a patient suffering from lupus erythematosus (female, 34 years old) (**a**). The valgus deformity was not fully corrected by re-arthrodesis combined with a medial sliding osteotomy, and this caused edge loading, polyethylene wear, stress shielding (arrows in anteroposterior X-ray), ballooning loosening (arrow in lateral view), and, ultimately, subsidence of the talar component at 58 months (**b**)

resection will theoretically lessen the risk of subsidence.

11.6.4 Polyethylene Wear

The physical properties of polyethylene can vary according to the specific type of polyethylene used and because of a number of other variables. The durability of polyethylene is improved with increasing thickness [3, 4, 5]. Theoretically, thicker polyethylene components in the ankle may help to prevent polyethylene failures, but at the expense of more generous bone cuts. The fundamental importance of bone conservation in the ankle, however, has been widely recognized, since the bone may be weak and the surface areas for support small. Polyethylene requirements for the ankle are, therefore, contradictory to what is necessary for conserving bone strength.

There are also several potential risks for polyethylene wear and weakening related to implant design, including:
- when the polyethylene is not fully congruent with the metal tibial and talar components,
- when the polyethylene component extends past the surface of the tibial components,
- when there is an inappropriate capture mechanism on the tibial or talar component to guide the polyethylene component.

Polyethylene wear may result in ballooning loosening (Fig. 11.17), and fracturing of the inlay (Fig. 11.3) [1, 22, 34, 41, 42].

11.7 Salvage of Failed Total Ankle Arthroplasty

Salvaging a total ankle arthroplasty that has failed and/or become complicated by infection is a tremendous challenge. Failure is likely to be associated with loss of bone stock, malalignment, wound breakdown, or a combination of these problems [14, 15].

First, the prosthesis should be removed and the infection, if present, eradicated. Then, the choice between revision arthroplasty or arthrodesis must be made [11, 25, 39]. Below-the-knee amputation may be another option for disasters where secondary reconstruction seems to be impossible. Arthrodesis may be the first option after implant removal, when bone stock is insufficient to support a new prosthesis (Fig. 11.18). The goals of arthrodesis are to maintain and restore limb length and to correct malalignment, if present. A variety of internal and external fixation techniques may be used, and bone graft may be required to restore limb length [21, 25, 37]. Salvage procedures are associated with a high risk of failure and morbidity [40].

Very little information about revision arthroplasty is currently available in the literature. In the author's experience, however, special revision implants may help to compensate for bone loss and/or to increase the area of bone contact for increased support (Fig. 11.16).

11.8 Conclusions

Complications can and do occur with ankle prostheses, just as they do with arthroplasties of other joints. Even when the complications are understood and the preventive measures or solutions are well thought out, there is occasionally a problem with no clear answer. Every potential solution will have an effect on another part of the biologic system, possibly creating other or additional problems. Therefore, a surgeon contemplating total ankle arthroplasty must have a thorough understanding not only of the anatomy and biomechanics of the lower extremity, but also of the pathologic processes associated with ongoing osteoarthritis of the ankle (and its involvement of the whole ankle joint complex), as well as the total ankle system to be used.

The reported rate of secondary surgery for any cause after total ankle arthroplasty is between 11% and 34% [1, 36, 41, 43]. It should be emphasized, however, that needing secondary surgery does not mean that the procedure has failed: the majority of these patients go on to a successful result after secondary surgery. Current studies reported a 5% to 7% early to intermediate failure rate [33, 36, 41, 43], and a survival rate of 70% at five years [1], of 93.5% at 10 years [10], and of 73% and 76% at 15 years in patients with osteoarthrosis and rheumatoid arthritis [27]. Comparison of complication and failure rates between different studies using different pros-

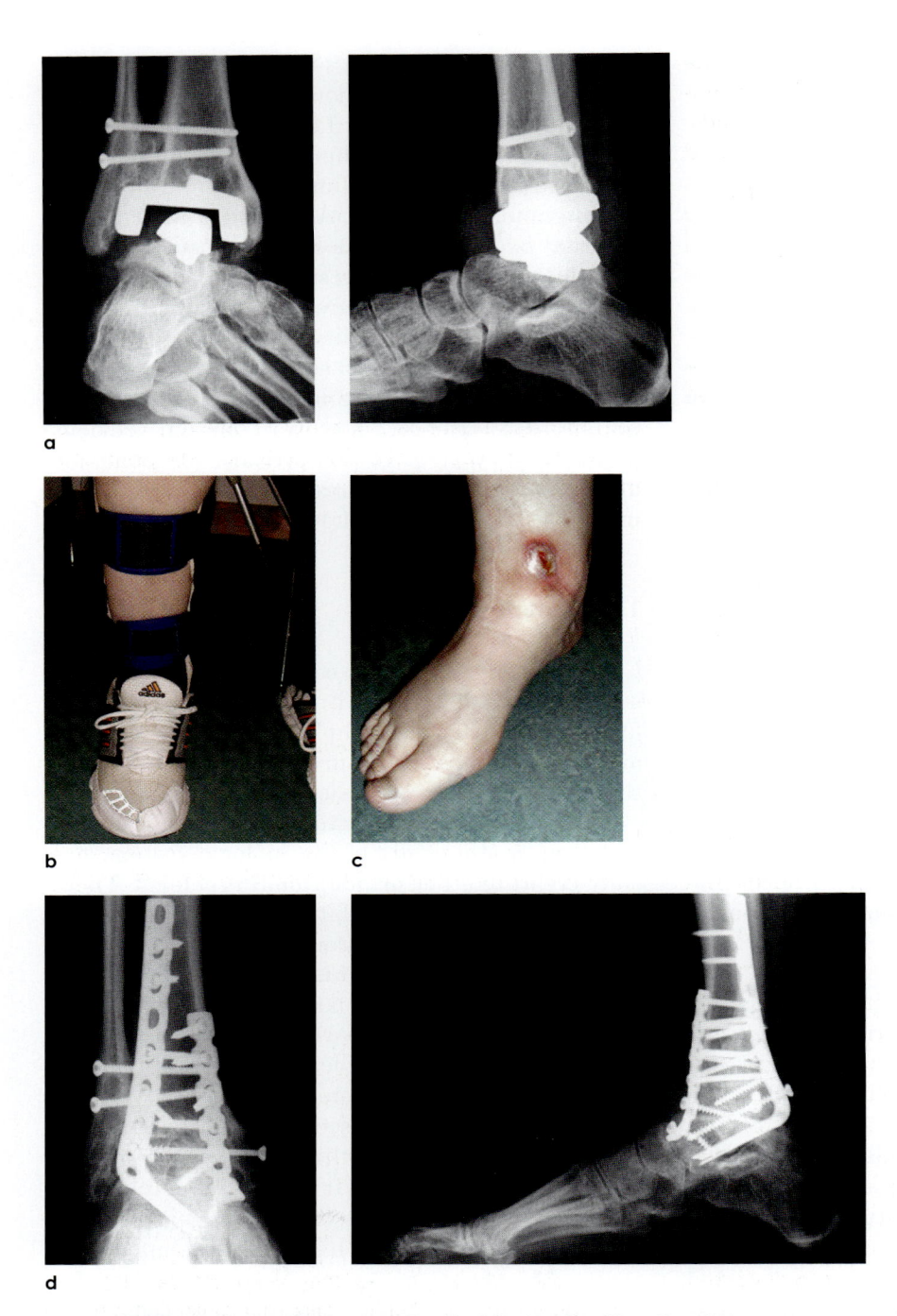

Fig. 11.18. Arthrodesis as salvage procedure for failed total ankle arthroplasty.
Twenty-one months after total ankle replacement using the AGILITY™ ankle (**a**), painful medial instability caused a severe valgus instability of the whole hindfoot that needed bracing for weight-bearing and walking (**b**) (female, 34 years old). The brace caused an ulceration at the anteromedial ankle with local infection and fistula (**c**). Ankle fusion was performed using two tricortical grafts from the iliac crest and two plates in order to save the subtalar joint in this young patient (**d**)

theses should not suggest the superiority of one prosthesis over another. Multiple patient populations and surgeons, varying follow-up periods, variable data collection and reporting practices, and variable thresholds for determining a complication make these sorts of comparisons invalid.

11.8.1 Requirements for Successful Total Ankle Arthroplasty

The following requirements must be met or at the very least considered perioperatively to achieve optimal results in total ankle arthroplasty:
- Meticulous attention must be paid to the soft tissues and careful closure of the extensor retinaculum in order to maintain its function as a protective layer [14].
- Attention must be given to alignment of the lower extremity and foot [12, 17, 20, 22, 35, 38, 40]. A thorough clinical and radiographic analysis of the whole lower extremity is necessary to identify major malalignment. Occasionally, deformities at the hip, femur, knee, or tibia may need to be addressed first.
- Attention must be paid to substantial hindfoot deformities. Weight-bearing radiographs of the foot and ankle, and a hindfoot alignment radiographic view [37] may help to identify varus and valgus deformities of the hindfoot and the longitudinal arch. Such deformities must be corrected with osteotomies or arthrodeses before or at the time of total ankle arthroplasty.
- Attention must be given to ligament imbalance of the ankle due to long-standing deformity or instability. This must be assessed and addressed before or at the time of total ankle arthroplasty.
- Attention must be given to ensuring minimal weakening of the bone stock, as well as to proper sizing and positioning of the selected implants. The use of fluoroscopy during surgery may contribute to the success of total ankle arthroplasty.
- Ankle dorsiflexion must be carefully addressed after the arthroplasty. If 5° of dorsiflexion cannot be achieved while the hindfoot is in a neutral position, then gastrocnemius release may be considered.

11.8.2 Surgeon Experience, Skill, and Training

Recent studies suggest that complication rates decline after a period of surgeon familiarization with the procedure [29, 30, 32]. Other reports have also demonstrated a learning-curve effect for total ankle arthroplasty [1, 23, 42]. While Saltzman et al [36] were able to show a relationship between training method and the rate of perioperative adverse events after total ankle arthroplasty, examining the best way to teach surgeons new to the procedure is critical to its long-term acceptance in the orthopedic community. There is no doubt, however, that surgeons new to the total ankle arthroplasty procedure must understand the hazards they may encounter, and that patients need accurate information about the risks of the procedure.

References

[1] Anderson T, Montgomery F, Carlsson A (2003) Uncemented STAR total ankle prosthesis. Three to eight-year follow-up of fifty-one consecutive ankles. J Bone Joint Surg Am 85: 1321–1329

[2] Bargren JH, Blaha JD, Freeman MA (1983) Alignment in total ankle arthroplasty. Clin Orthop 173: 178–183

[3] Bartel DL, Bicknell VL, Wright TM (1986) The effect of conformity, thickness, and material on stresses in ultrahigh molecular weight components for total joint replacement. J Bone Joint Surg Am 68: 1041–1051

[4] Bartel DL, Burstein AH, Toda MD, Edwards DL (1985) The effect of conformity and plastic thickness on contact stresses in metal-backed plastic implants. J Biomech Eng 107: 193–199

[5] Bartel DL, Rawlinson JJ, Burstein AH, Ranawat CS, Flynn WF, Jr. (1995) Stresses in polyethylene components of contemporary total knee replacements. Clin Orthop 317: 76–82

[6] Bolton-Maggs BG, Sudlow RA, Freeman MA (1985) Total ankle arthroplasty. A long-term review of the London Hospital experience. J Bone Joint Surg Br 67: 785–790

[7] Brunner R, Jaspers RT, Pel JJ, Huijing PA (2000) Acute and long-term effects on muscle force after intramuscular aponeurotic lengthening. Clin Orthop 378: 264–273

[8] Buechel FF, Buechel FF, Pappas MJ (2002) Eighteen-year evaluation of cementless meniscal bearing total ankle replacements. AAOS Instruct. Course Lect., chap 16, pp 143–151

[9] Buechel FF, Pappas MJ, Iorio LJ (1988) New Jersey low contact stress total ankle replacement: biomechanical rationale and review of 23 cementless cases. Foot Ankle 8: 279–290

[10] Buechel FFS, Buechel FFJ, Pappas MJ (2003) Ten-year evaluation of cementless Buechel-Pappas meniscal bearing total ankle replacement. Foot Ankle Int 24: 426–472

[11] Carlsson AS, Montgomery F, Besjakov J (1998) Arthrodesis of the ankle secondary to replacement. Foot Ankle Int 19: 240–245

[12] Clare MP, Sanders RW (2002) Preoperative considerations in ankle replacement surgery. Foot Ankle Clin 7: 709–720

[13] Coester LM, Saltzman CL, Leupold J, Pontarelli W (2001) Long-term results following ankle arthrodesis for post-traumatic arthritis. J Bone Joint Surg Am 83: 219–228

[14] Conti SF, Wong YS (2001) Complications of total ankle replacement. Clin Orthop 391: 105–114

[15] Conti SF, Wong YS (2002) Complications of total ankle replacement. Foot Ankle Clin 7: 791–807

[16] D'Lima DD, Hermida JC, Chen PC, Colwell CWj (2001) Polyethylene wear and variations in knee kinematics. Clin Orthop 392: 124–130

[17] Easley ME, Vertullo CJ, Urban WC, Nunley JA (2002) Total ankle arthroplasty. J Am Acad Orthop Surg 10: 157–167

[18] Fuchs S, Sandmann C, Skwara A, Chylarecki C (2003) Quality of life 20 years after arthrodesis of the ankle. A study of adjacent joints. J Bone Joint Surg Br 85: 994–998

[19] Gottrup F (2002) Oxygen, wound healing and the development of infection. Present status. Eur J Surg 168: 260–263

[20] Greisberg J, Hansen ST, Jr. (2002) Ankle replacement: management of associated deformities. Foot Ankle Clin 7: 721–736

[21] Groth HE, Fitch HF (1987) Salvage procedures for complications of total ankle arthroplasty. Clin Orthop 224: 244–250

[22] Hintermann B, Valderrabano V (2003) Total ankle replacement. Foot Ankle Clin 8: 375–405

[23] Hintermann B, Valderrabano V, Dereymaeker G, Dick W (2004) The HINTEGRA ankle: rationale and short-term results of 122 consecutive ankles. Clin Orthop 424: 57–68

[24] Johnson DP, Eastwood DM, Bader DL (1991) Biomechanical factors in wound healing following knee arthroplasty. I Med Eng Technol 15: 8–14

[25] Kitaoka HB (1991) Salvage of nonunion following ankle arthrodesis for failed total ankle arthroplasty. Clin Orthop 268: 37–43

[26] Kofoed H, Lundberg-Jensen A (1999) Ankle arthroplasty in patients younger and older than 50 years: a prospective series with long-term follow-up. Foot Ankle Int 20: 501–506

[27] Kofoed H, Sorensen TS (1998) Ankle arthroplasty for rheumatoid arthritis and osteoarthritis: prospective long-term study of cemented replacements. J Bone Joint Surg Br 80: 328–332

[28] Liau JJ, Cheng CK, Huang CH, Lo WH (2002) The effect of malalignment on stresses in polyethylene component of total knee prostheses – a finite element analysis. Clin Biomech 17: 140–146

[29] Mann RA, Haskell A. (2004) Perioperative complication rate of total ankle arthroplasty is reduced by surgeon experience. In: Proc. AAOS Congress, San Francisco, USA

[30] Myerson MS, Mroczeck K (2003) Perioperative complications of total ankle arthroplasty. Foot Ankle Int 24: 17–21

[31] Praemer A, Furner S, Rice DP (1992) Arthritis. In: Musculoskeletal conditions in the United States (Park Ridge I, ed), 1st ed. American Academy of Orthopaedic Surgeons

[32] Pyevich MT, Saltzman CL, Callaghan JJ, Alvine FG (1998) Total ankle arthroplasty: a unique design. Two to 12-year follow-up. J Bone Joint Surg Am 80: 1410–1420

[33] Rippstein PF (2003) Clinical experiences with three different designs of ankle prostheses. Foot Ankle Clin 7: 817–831

[34] Rudigier J, Grundei H, Menzinger F (2001) Prosthetic replacement of the ankle in posttraumatic arthrosis. Europ J Trauma 2: 66–74

[35] Saltzman CL (2000) Perspective on total ankle replacement. Foot Ankle Clin 5: 761–775

[36] Saltzman CL, Annunziato A, Coetze JC, Gall RJ, Haddad SL, Herbst S, Lian G, Sanders RW, Scioli M, Younger AS (2003) Surgeon training and complications in total ankle arthroplasty. Foot Ankle Int 24: 514–518

[37] Saltzman CL, El-Koury GY (1995) The hindfoot alignment view. Foot Ankle Int 16: 572–576

[38] Stamatis ED, Myerson MS (2002) How to avoid specific complications of total ankle replacement. Foot Ankle Clin 7: 765–789

[39] Stauffer RN (1982) Salvage of painful total ankle arthroplasty. Clin Orthop 170: 184–188

[40] Thomas RL, Daniels TR (2003) Current concepts review: ankle arthritis. J Bone Joint Surg Am 85: 923–936

[41] Valderrabano V, Hintermann B, Dick W (2004) Scandinavian total ankle replacement: a 3.7-year average follow-up of 65 patients. Clin Orthop 424: 47–56

[42] Wood PL, Deakin S (2003) Total ankle replacement. The results in 200 ankles. J Bone Joint Surg Br 85: 334–341

[43] Wood PLR (2002) Experience with the STAR ankle arthroplasty at Wrightington Hospital, UK. Foot Ankle Clin 7: 755–765

[44] Wood PLR, Clough TM (2004) Mobile bearing ankle replacement: clinical and radiographic comparison of two designs. In: Proc. AAOS Congress, San Francisco, USA

Chapter 12

FUTURE DIRECTIONS

The ideal total ankle prosthesis has yet to be determined, but much has been learned from early experiences in total ankle arthroplasty. Modern implants are typically more respectful of anatomic concerns, and have found new approaches to decrease interface stress. Biologic fixation has improved upon cemented results. Surgical techniques and understanding of associated ligamentous deficiency, malalignment, and deformity have advanced. Current series still have varied results, and longer follow-up is needed. Despite this, some modern ankle replacements represent significant progress, with improved results and survival rates challenging those of arthrodesis. Further, benefits of preserved motion and avoidance of foot osteoarthritis outstrip the "gold standard."

12.1 Current Concerns to be Addressed

Currently, many patients with painful ankle osteoarthrosis and arthritis can be offered a total ankle replacement as a viable alternative to ankle arthrodesis. Although great progress has been made in recent years, total ankle replacement is still plagued by a relatively high rate of perioperative complications and revisions, and some concerns remain with respect to its long-term success.

12.1.1 Prospective Studies

A major concern is the paucity of well-documented prospective studies, in spite of the numerous prosthetic designs introduced on the market. To learn from the successes and failures by meticulous analysis of each case would help to increase current knowledge, and would allow further improvement of total ankle replacement.

Another issue is the selection of patients, which differs markedly among surgeons. Consequently, obtained results can only be compared with caution.

There is, therefore, a need for extensive, well-documented prospective studies that use standardized protocols with comparable parameters.

12.1.2 Prosthetic Design

Each prosthetic design introduced on the market has been an attempt to address the specific demands of the ankle joint. The fact that each new prosthesis has included several new features and/or changes compared to previous designs, however, has made it extremely difficult to evaluate new ideas and changes with respect to their success. Nevertheless, the current concepts have supported the belief that anatomy should be respected as much as possible.

As the mechanical demands on an ankle prosthesis completely change in the hindfoot after extensive fusion, there is probably a need for special designs to address these cases.

Custom-made ankle prostheses based on CT scan data could also have potential advantages for severely traumatized ankles, and particularly for total ankle revisions.

12.1.3 Preoperative Planning and Implantation Technique

The techniques for implantation can still be improved by more accurate instrumentation, and by better pre- and intraoperative planning tools to help in achieving optimal component positioning. Computer-assisted preoperative planning may be particularly sought after to enhance surgical implantation and to improve the clinical outcomes of total ankle replacement. Such planning may be based on minimizing changes in ligament length and the amount of bone stock to be removed. The main output report might be a detailed picture of the replaced ankle, with indications for component locations and quantitative measures for bone cuts. In all likelihood, future design improvements may help to reduce ligament strain, restore normal axes of rotation, and maintain mobile bearing stability.

12.1.4 Polyethylene Wear

As experience with total ankle replacement broadens, ankle component wear and related long-term durability will become the next major concern. In a recent study, polyethylene wear particles retrieved in joint fluid did not show differences in particle number and size between well-functioning total ankle replacements and total knee replacements, however, total ankle replacement generated rounder particles than total knee replacement. The authors concluded that the long-term result of total ankle replacement might be expected equal to total knee replacement in terms of polyethylene wear and the prevalence of osteolysis. Further studies are needed to elucidate polyethylene wear in more detail.

12.1.5 Stability of Bone-Implant Interface

Another issue to be addressed is the long-term stability of the bone-component interface. It is not yet clear whether double-coated surfaces (with or without hydroxyapatite coating) can create stable bony ingrowth and thereby long-term interface stability, as has been the case in total hip and knee replacements. Recently, osteoblast culture coating has been tested in a clinical trial (Dr. Yoshinuri Takakura, Nara, Japan, personal communication 2002), however, longer follow-up is needed to assess this method.

Although early results with semi- and nonconstrained ankle designs are encouraging, it is not yet clear to what extent the current designs can dissipate rotational forces while maintaining the stability of the joint. Careful assessment of long-term follow-up will determine how closely the present designs are mimicking the unique requirements of the arthritic foot and ankle. Further work in biomechanics is necessary to better understand the kinematic changes of the arthritic ankle joint and to estimate the forces acting on the implant-bone interface.

12.2 Further Success will Increase Patient Demand

Successful total ankle replacement may relieve pain and restore some motion, allowing patients to return to certain physical activities that they were not able to perform prior to implantation. Consequently, the physical demands of patients may increase, and successful primary replacements may fail because the replaced ankle is subjected to too much stress.

Analogously, increased success may lead to indications for total ankle replacement being extended to pathologic conditions that are probably not suitable for replacement surgery.

On the other hand, total ankle replacement may be, in some instances, a viable intermediate solution prior to fusion. If, for example, a severe osteoarthritis has developed in a young patient after a trauma, total ankle arthroplasty may allow him or her to regain some motion and to properly bear the affected ankle, which, in turn, may protect the foot from further degenerative joint disease. When the replaced ankle wears out and revision of the prosthesis is no longer possible, ankle arthrodesis remains an option for salvage. The patient, nevertheless, may have benefited greatly from this intermediate solution, which allowed continued participation in some activities (including professional activities) during a significant period of his or her life that would not have been possible with a primary ankle arthrodesis. The intermediate total ankle arthroplasty may additionally have preserved his or her foot from the development of secondary osteoarthritis. Further clinical research is needed, however, to understand the pathologic changes taking place in the neighboring joints of a replaced and fused ankle, respectively, and how they can be influenced.

12.3 Further Research

More accurate research is necessary for a better understanding of the mechanics of the intact and replaced ankle joint complex. First, this should help to further improve the implants, and second, it should help to elaborate guidelines for better planning and more accurate implantation techniques, which would result in more reliable and effective total ankle replacement. Future studies with an emphasis on the objective analysis of long-term clinical results are also necessary to define and delineate the role of total ankle arthroplasty.

12.4 Conclusions

As total ankle arthroplasty continues to evolve as a viable treatment option for end-stage ankle osteoarthritis, the adverse clinical and biomechanical consequences of ankle arthrodesis are far more apparent. Proper patient selection is a critical aspect of promoting successful results. Acceptable results have been reported in older, low-demand patients who have osteoarthritis or rheumatoid arthritis. A significant percentage of patients with end-stage ankle osteoarthritis, however, are younger patients with post-traumatic osteoarthritis. The use of ankle replacement in younger, more physically active patients, and in those with significant deformity in the ankle or hindfoot remains a question to debate. More studies must be completed and further developments must be made to maximize the longevity and functional results of total ankle arthroplasty in future designs and applications.

Along with improved implants that are typically more respectful of anatomic concerns, proper positioning of the implants (particularly of the talar component with respect to the center of rotation of the talus), accurate balancing of the soft tissues, and appropriate correction of malalignment are far more important for the success of total ankle arthroplasty than previously believed. Careful clinical investigation and reliable diagnostic tools should thus be used to identify all of the associated problems so that they can be properly addressed during ankle replacement.

SUBJECT INDEX

A

Adult flatfoot 140
  lateral column lengthening 141
AES ankle
  background 44, 59
  characteristics 52
  complications 60
  concerns 60
  design 44, 59
  loosening rate 46–47, 60
  results 44, 60
  revision rate 46–47, 60
  satisfaction rate 46–47, 60
Age of the patient
  patient selection 165
  specific problems with total ankle arthroplasty 101–102
  the author's approach 102
AGILITY ankle
  background 44, 61
  characteristics 52
  complications 63
  concerns 63–64
  design 44, 51–52, 61–62
  implantation technique 62
  loosening rate 46–47, 63
  kinematics, *in vitro* 38–39
  range of motion, *in vitro* 38–39
  results 44, 51, 62–63
  revision rate 46–47, 63
  satisfaction rate 46–47, 62–63
  syndesmotic arthrodesis, nonunion 64
  talar motion, *in vitro* 38–39
Anatomy, ankle of 25–28
Ankle
  anatomic characteristics, see *Anatomy, ankle of*
  biomechanical characteristics, see *Biomechanics, ankle of*
  instability, see *Instability*
Ankle arthritis
  characteristics of 5–9, 163–164
  epidemiology of 5
  primary, see *Primary osteoarthrosis*
  post-traumatic, see *Post-traumatic osteoarthrosis*
  psoriatic, see *Psoriatic arthritis*
  rheumatoid, see *Rheumatoid arthritis*
  septic, see *Septic arthritis*
  systemic, see *Systemic arthritis*
Ankle arthrodesis
  biomechanical changes after, see *Biomechanics*
  comparison with total ankle arthroplasty 2, 21

  complications after 12, 18–21
  degenerative changes of adjacent joints, see *Osteoarthrosis of adjacent joints*
  failed arthrodesis 158–159
  failures of 15–17
  historical background of 11–12
  functional outcome after 17–18
  fusion rate of 12
  fusion time of 12
  gait analysis 13, 19
  loss of motion 13
  nonunion developed after 17
  outcome of 2
  position of 13
  stress fracture after, see *Stress fracture*
  take down, see *Disarthrodesis*
  techniques of, see *Arthrodesis techniques*
Ankle osteoarthritis, see *Ankle arthritis*
Ankle osteoarthrosis, see *Ankle arthritis*
Ankle prosthesis, see also *Total ankle arthroplasty*
  constrained 44–45
  custom-made implants 152–154, 159, 185
  design 185
  fixed-bearing 45
  list of designs 44
  mobile-bearing 45
  nonconstrained 44–45
  polyethylene-bearing 45
  revision implants 159
  semiconstrained 44–45
  two-component design 44
Arthritis, see also *Osteoarthrosis*
Arthrodesis techniques 11–17, 120–121
  arthroscopic 12–13, 15
  mini-open 12
  open 12
  salvage of failed total ankle arthroplasty 181
  with internal fixation 14–17
  without internal fixation 14
Aseptic loosening 178–181
  radioluscent lines, periprosthetic 178–180
  subsidence 180–181
Avascular necrosis of the talus 152–154, 159
  contraindications 92
  custom-made talar component 152–154
  indications 92
  the author's recommendation
    (for total ankle arthroplasty) 152–153

B

Bath-Wessex
  background 44
  design 44
  failures 49
  loosening rate 46
  results 44
  revision rate 46
  satisfaction rate 46
Biologic fixation 36, 185
Biomechanics, ankle of 29–34
  after ankle arthrodesis 21
  axial load 34
  center of rotation 29–30
  contact area 34
  joint axis 28–29
  motion 29–30
  motion, sagittal plane 30
  motion, restraint 30
  motion, transverse plane 30
  stress forces 34
Blade plate
  for arthrodesis 12
Bone ingrowth 36
Bone stock 186
  loss of 162
Buechel-Pappas ankle
  background 44, 64–65
  characteristics 52
  complications 66
  concerns 66–68
  design 44, 51, 64–65
  loosening rate 46–47
  results 44, 51, 65–66
  revision rate 46–47
  satisfaction rate 46–47

C

Calandruccio device
  for arthrodesis 12
Calcaneal osteotomy
  lateral column lengthening 141
  medial sliding osteotomy 120, 141
  valgisation 120, 135
Calcaneal malunion 145–149
Cement fixation 36, 43
Cerebral palsy
  arthrodesis 11
Charcot-Marie-Tooth disease
  arthrodesis 11
Charnley external fixator
  for arthrodesis 11–12, 14
Clamps
  for arthrodesis 12
Clubfoot deformity 152
  arthrodesis 11
  the author's recommendation
    (for total ankle arthroplasty) 152

Complications of total ankle arthroplasty 2, 163–184, 185
  deep venous thrombosis 176
  early postoperative complications 175–176
  fractures of malleoli 173–176
  heelcord contracture 176
  implant-related complications 168–175
  implantation-related complications 168–175
  improper sizing of prosthetic components 172–173
  improper use of distraction 173
  infection, postoperative 176, 181
  injuries to the neurovascular bundle 108
  late postoperative complications 176–181
  loosening, aseptic 178–180
  malpositioning of prosthetic components 166–172
  motion, loss of 176–178
  ossifications, periarticular 177–178
  polyethylene wear 181
  swelling, postoperative 176
  syndesmotic nonunion / instability 176
  tendon injuries 175
  wound healing problems 108, 175–176
Computer-assisted planning 185
CONAXIAL ankle
  background 44
  design 44
  loosening rate 46
  results 44
  revision rate 46
  satisfaction rate 46
Contact area size 35
Contact stress 35
Contraindications for total ankle arthroplasty
  absolute 92
  preoperative conditions 165–168
  relative 92
Cortico-cancellous peg
  for arthrodesis 14
Custom-made prostheses 152–154, 159, 185

D

Deep venous thrombosis 176
Deformity
  clubfoot 11, 152
  preoperative conditions 167–168
  paralytic 152
  valgus 139–141, 150
  varus 135–138
Design of component 2–3, 37–40
Diabetic neuropathy
  arthrodesis 11
  contraindications 92
  neuroarthropathic degenerative disease 92
Disarthrodesis
  specific problems of 158–159
  the author's recommendation 158–159
Distraction, improper use of 173
Dorsiflexion osteotomy of the first metatarsal 119, 135
Double-coated surfaces 186
Dowel
  for arthrodesis 12

E

ESKA ankle
  background 44, 68
  characteristics 52
  complications 68–70
  concerns 70
  design 44, 51, 68
  loosening rate 46–47
  results 44, 47, 68–70
  revision rate 46–47
  satisfaction rate 46–47

F

Failed total ankle arthroplasty 181
  salvage of 181
Failure rate of total ankle arthroplasty 46–47, 181–183
Fibular malunion 142–144
First-generation prostheses 45–49
  specific problems of 168
  results 48–49
  specific problems 48–49
Follow-up examination
  alignment of the ankle 128
  function 128
  pain 128
  radiographic examination, see Radiographic examination
  range of motion, clinical 128
  range of motion, radiographic 129
Fractures of malleoli
  intraoperative 173–175
  postoperative 176

G

Graft for arthrodesis 12–13

H

Heel cord
  contracture, postoperative 176
  lengthening 121, 176–177
  specific problems for total ankle arthroplasty 101
  the author's approach 101
Hemochromatosis
  indications for total ankle arthroplasty 92
HINTEGRA ankle
  background 44, 70
  characteristics 52
  complications 72
  concerns 72–75
  design 44, 70–72
  kinematics, in vitro 38–39
  loosening rate 46–47
  range of motion, in vitro 38–39
  results 44, 47, 72
  revision rate 46–47
  satisfaction rate 46–47
  talar motion, in vitro 38–39
Hoffmann external fixator
  for arthrodesis 12
Hydroxyapatite coating 36

I

ICLH ankle
  background 44
  design 44
  loosening rate 46
  results 44–47
  revision rate 46
  satisfaction rate 46
Improper sizing of prosthetic components 172–173
Improper use of distraction 173
Indications for total ankle arthroplasty 92
  preoperative conditions 165–168
Infection, postoperative 176, 181
Instability
  lateral ligament reconstruction 117–119
  post-traumatic osteoarthrosis 141
  specific problems for total ankle arthroplasty 98–101
  the author's approach 100–101
  tibiofibular (syndesmostic) instability 144–145
Interface, bone-component 186
Intramedullary nail
  for arthrodesis 12

L

Lateral ankle ligaments
  anatomic configuration 27–28
  function 27
  reconstruction 117–119, 135, 159
Ligament balancing 31, 162
Ligaments, ankle of
  lateral, see Lateral ankle ligaments
  medial, see Medial ankle ligaments
Loosening, aseptic 178–181
  radioluscent lines, periprosthetic 178–180
  subsidence 180–181
Loosening rate 46–47
Lord ankle
  background 44
  design 44
  loosening rate 46
  results 44–47
  revision rate 46
  satisfaction rate 46

M

Malalignment
  preoperative conditions 165–167

reconstruction of the ankle 135–141
sagittal plane malalignment 141
specific problems for total ankle arthroplasty 98
the author's approach 98
valgus malalignment 139–141
varus malalignment 135–138
Malpositioning of prosthetic components 166–172
Malunion
calcaneal malunion 145–149
fibular malunion 142–144
preoperative conditions 165–167
post-traumatic osteoarthrosis 141–142
the author's recommendation 143–145
Mayo ankle
background 44
design 44
loosening rate 46
results 44, 46–47
revision rate 46
satisfaction rate 46
Medial ankle ligaments
anatomic configuration 27–29
function 29
reconstruction 120, 159
recurrent sprains, stretching of 140
Mixed connective tissue disorders
indications for total ankle arthroplasty 92
Medial sliding osteotomy 120, 141
Motion, postoperative loss of 176–178
Muscular balance
restoration 135

N

Neuromuscular disorders
arthrodesis 11
deformity 152
the author's recommendation
(for total ankle arthroplasty) 152
Neurovascular bundle, injuries to 108
New Jersey ankle
background 44
design 44
loosening rate 46
results 44, 46–47
revision rate 46
satisfaction rate 46
Newton ankle
background 44
design 44
loosening rate 46
results 44–45
revision rate 46
satisfaction rate 46

O

Ossifications, periarticular 177–178
Osteoarthrosis of adjacent joints

after ankle arthrodesis 14, 17–19
specific problems for total ankle arthroplasty 97–98
the author's approach 97–98
Osteoblast culture 186
Osteonecrosis
arthrodesis 11
Osteoporosis, osteopenia
contraindications 92
Osteotomies 169
calcaneal osteotomy for valgisation 120, 135
calcaneal osteotomy for varisation 120, 141
first metatarsal for dorsiflexion 119, 135

P

Patient selection 165
age of patient 165
weight of patient 165
Physical activities
specific problems for total ankle arthroplasty 102–103, 186
the author's approach 103
Pins
for arthrodesis 12
Planning, computer-assisted 185
Poliomyelitis
arthrodesis 11
Polyethylene
durability 37
physical properties 37
risks 37
wear 181, 186
Posterior tibial dysfunction
arthrodesis 11
revision of the tendon 121
Postoperative care
follow-up examination, see Follow-up examination
immobilization, brace 128
immobilization, cast 128
rehabilitation program 128
weight-bearing 127–128
Post-traumatic ankle osteoarthrosis
bone loss 141
characteristics 8–9, 163
damage to soft-tissue mantle 142
loosening rate 46–57
instability, collateral ligaments 141
instability, syndesmosis 144–145
malunion 141, 142, 145
revision rate 46–47
reconstruction 141–149
satisfaction rate 46–47
Preoperative conditions 165–168
foot deformity 167–168
malalignment 165–167
malunion 165–167
soft-tissue conditions 165
Primary ankle osteoarthrosis
characteristics 8, 163
indications for total ankle arthroplasty 92
loosening rate 46–57
revision rate 46–47

Subject Index

satisfaction rate   46–47
Prosthesis of the ankle, *see Ankle prosthesis*
Psoriatic arthritis
   characteristics   9
   indications for total ankle arthroplasty   92

R

Radiographic examinations
   techniques   129
   sequential radiographs   129
   loosening of talar implant   129
   loosening of tibial implant   129
   talar subsidence   129
Radioluscent lines, periprosthetic   178–180
Ramses ankle
   background   44, 75
   characteristics   52
   complications   77
   concerns   77
   design   44, 75–77
   loosening rate   46
   results   44, 77
   revision rate   46
   satisfaction rate   46
Requirement for successful total ankle arthroplasty   39–40, 183
Revision arthroplasty   181
   arthrodesis   159, 181
   avascular necrosis   159
   re-arthroplasty   159–181
   revision implants   159
   specific problems of   159–162
   the author's recommendation   162
Revision rate of total ankle arthroplasty   46–47, 181–183
Rheumatoid arthritis
   characteristics   9, 153–154
   indications for total ankle arthroplasty   92
   specific problems for total ankle arthroplasty   93–94, 150
   the author's approach   93
   the author's recommendation   150
   triple arthrodesis   150
   valgus deformity   150

S

Sagittal plane malalignment
   recurvatum malalignment   141
   the author's recommendation   141
SALTO ankle
   background   44, 78
   characteristics   52
   complications   78
   concerns   78–80
   design   44, 78
   loosening rate   47
   results   44, 78
   revision rate   47
   satisfaction rate   47
Salvage arthroplasty   181

Satisfaction rate of total ankle arthroplasty   46–47
Screw fixation
   for arthrodesis   11–14
Second-generation prostheses   49–53
   constraint-conformity/congruency conflict   49
   critical issues   52–53
   specific problems   168–175
   three-component designs   51–52
   two-component designs   50–51
Selection of patients   185
Septic arthritis
   active, recent infection   93
   characteristics   9
   indications for total ankle arthroplasty   92
   specific problems for total ankle arthroplasty   92–95, 155–158
   the author's approach   95
   the author's recommendation (for total ankle arthroplasty)   158
Smith ankle
   background   44
   design   44
   loosening rate   46
   results   44
   revision rate   46
   satisfaction rate   46
Smoking
   specific problems with ankle arthrodesis   17
   specific problems with total ankle arthroplasty   103
Soft-tissue problems
   contraindications   92
   damage to   142
   preoperative conditions   165
   specific problems for total ankle arthroplasty   101
Sports activities
   specific problems for total ankle arthroplasty   102–103, 186
   the author's approach   103
S.T.A.R. ankle
   background   44, 80
   characteristics   52
   complications   81–82
   concerns   82–84
   design   44, 80–81
   kinematics, *in vitro*   38–39
   loosening rate   46–47
   range of motion, *in vitro*   38–39
   results   44, 52, 81–82
   revision rate   46–47
   satisfaction rate   46–47
   talar motion, *in vitro*   38–39
St. Georg ankle
   background   44
   design   44
   loosening rate   46
   results   44–45
   revision rate   46
   satisfaction rate   46
Stress fracture
   after ankle arthrodesis   19
Strut graft
   for arthrodesis   14
Subfibular pain/impingement   139
Subsidence   180

Subtalar arthrodesis
    technique   120–121
Success for total ankle arthroplasty, requirements of   39–40, 183
Surgeon experience / skill / training   183
Surgical techniques for total ankle arthroplasty
    additional surgeries, see Varus deformity, Valgus deformity, and Arthrodesis techniques
    alignment, frontal (coronal) plane   108
    alignment, sagittal plane   108
    approaches of the ankle   53, 106–108
    approach, anterior   106–108
    approach, lateral   108
    complications, see Complications of total ankle arthroplasty
    exposure of the ankle   108
    implants, insertion of   113–116, 186
    implants, fluoroscopic control   116
    planning   186
    positioning of the patient   108
    talar resection   109
    tibial resection, technique   108–109
    tibial resection, angle of   108
    wound closure   116
Surfaces
    double-coated   186
    osteoblast-culture   186
Swelling, postoperative   176
Syndesmotic (tibiofibular) instability   144–145, 176
    the author's recommendation   145
Systemic ankle arthritis
    characteristics   9, 150, 163–164
    loosening rate   46–57
    revision rate   46–47
    satisfaction rate   46–47

T

Talonavicular arthrodesis
    technique   120–121
Talus
    avascular necrosis, see Avascular necrosis of the talus
    anterior extrusion   135, 144
    bony configuration   25–26
    bone support   31
    cortical shell   32
Techniques for implantation, see Surgical techniques
Tendon
    injuries   175
    reconstruction   159
    release   159
    transfer peroneus longus-to-brevis   119, 135
Tibial plafond
    bony configuration   26–27
    bone strength   32
    bone support   31
    cortical shell   33
    force transmission   33
    lateral tibial plafond, wear away of   141, 144
Tibiotalar angle   27
TNK ankle
    background   44, 84

characteristics   52
complications   84
concerns   87
design   44, 51, 84
loosening rate   46
results   44, 51, 84
revision rate   46
satisfaction rate   46
TPR ankle
    background   44
    design   44
    loosening rate   46
    results   44
    revision rate   46
    satisfaction rate   46
Total ankle arthroplasty
    biologic fixation   36, 185
    bone ingrowth   36
    cement fixation   36, 43
    classification of   43
    comparison with ankle arthrodesis   2, 21
    complications of   2, 163–184, 185
    component design   2–3, 37–40
    contact area size   35
    contact stress   35
    contraindications, see Contraindications for total ankle arthroplasty
    difficulties related to   43
    failure rate   46–47, 181–183
    failures of   3, 159, 181
    first-generation, see First generation prostheses
    fixation of prosthesis   34–37
    fractures   35
    hydroxyapatite coating   36
    indications, see Indications for total ankle arthroplasty
    ligament balancing   31
    loosening rate   46–47
    second-generation, see Second generation prostheses
    needs for success   39–40, 183, 186
    planning, computer-assisted   185
    postoperative care, see Postoperative care and follow-up
    revision rate   46–47, 181–183, 185
    satisfaction rate   46–47
    shear forces   34
    uncemented fixation   43
Talonavicular arthrodesis   120–121
Triple arthrodesis
    loss of motion   13
    rheumatoid arthritis   150
    technique   120–121

U

Uncemented fixation   43

V

Valgus deformity   139–141, 150
    anterior extrusion of the talus   144

Subject Index

    calcaneal osteotomy, medial sliding   120, 141
    lateral tibial plafond, wear away of   139, 144
    lateral column lengthening   141
    medial ligament reconstruction   106
    recurrent sprains, stretching of   140
    subfibular pain/impingement   139
    the author's recommendation   141
Valgus malalignment, *see Valgus deformity*
Varus deformity   135–138
    anterior extrusion of the talus   135
    calcaneal osteotomy, valgisation   120, 135
    dorsiflexion osteotomy of the first metatarsal   119, 135
    lateral ligament reconstruction   106, 117–119, 135
    medial ligament release   106, 135
    peroneal longus-to-brevis transfer   119, 135
    the author's recommendation   136–137
Varus malalignment, *see Varus deformity*
Venous thrombosis, deep   176

W

Weight restrictions
    patient selection   165
    specific problems for total ankle arthroplasty   95–97
    the author's approach   97
Wound healing problems   108, 175–176

SpringerMedicine

Peter Brenner, Ghazi M. Rayan

Dupuytren´s Disease

A Concept of Surgical Treatment
Foreword by Hanno Millesi

Translated from German by Birte Twisselmann.
With illustrations by Jakob Gratzer and Hanna Schimek.

2003. XIV, 233 pages. 57 figures, partly in colour.
Hardcover **EUR 229,–**
(Recommended retail price)
Net-price subject to local VAT.
ISBN 3-211-83656-X

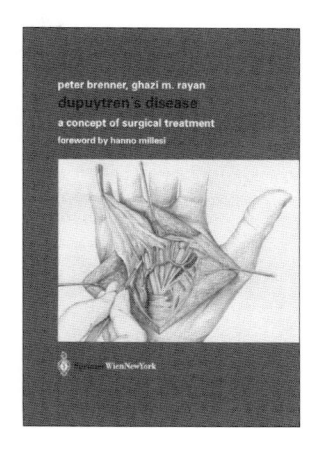

Dupuytren's Disease is particularly widespread among northern Europeans, but the therapeutic success-rate often leaves much to be desired. A 50% recurrence-rate after surgery indicates that the disease cannot be treated by surgery alone. This book therefore adopts two parallel approaches: first of all emphasis is placed on the systemic character of Dupuytren's Disease in context with other connective tissue diseases by a description of the biochemical and molecular-biological changes in the diseased connective tissues; and secondly, a diversified picture of the given anatomical facts serves to explain the employment of the various therapeutic approaches. In addition to the aspects of conservative therapy, a description is given of the current surgical procedures including the complications typical of the same, and accompanied by basic drawings.

The book is intended for all those interested in a comprehensive up-to-date survey of Dupuytren's Disease, and in instructive information on the established therapeutical concepts.

SpringerWienNewYork

P.O. Box 89, Sachsenplatz 4–6, 1201 Vienna, Austria, Fax +43.1.330 24 26, books@springer.at, **springer.at**
Haberstraße 7, 69126 Heidelberg, Germany, Fax +49.6221.345-4229, orders@springer.de, springeronline.com
P.O. Box 2485, Secaucus, NJ 07096-2485, USA, Fax +1.201.348-4505, orders@springer-ny.com, springeronline.com
Eastern Book Service, 3–13, Hongo 3-chome, Bunkyo-ku, Tokyo 113, Japan, Fax +81.3.38 18 08 64, orders@svt-ebs.co.jp
Prices are subject to change without notice. All errors and omissions excepted.

SpringerMedicine

Walter Hruby (ed.)

Digital (R)Evolution in Radiology

Bridging the Future of Health Care

Second, revised and enlarged edition.
2005. Approx. 280 pages. Approx. 100 figures.
Hardcover approx. **EUR 160,–**
Subscription price, valid until 3 Months after publication:
Approx. EUR 140,–
(Recommended retail prices)
Net-prices subject to local VAT.
ISBN 3-211-20815-1
Due April 2005

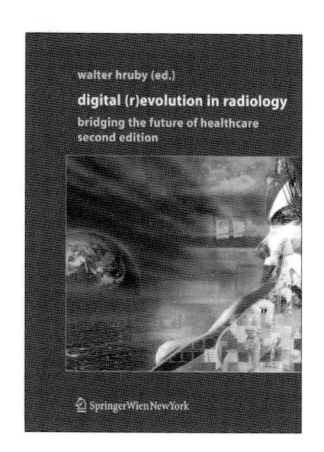

According to a statement of Gordon Moore computer performance doubles every 18 months. So it is not surprising that the "half-time" of modern computers is rapidly decreasing. Increasing demands of public health for radiology together with a rapid development of information technology and innovations result in a digital environment, where thorough guidance is necessary. This book is such a solid guidance for radiologists and other medical staff working in this field.

The second edition has been brought up-to-date, revised and new aspects have been incorporated that focus on the synergy that results from the integration of digital systems used in radiology such as image fusion, "functional" imaging, electronic patient records and health networks, etc. It is intended for radiologists and all other physicians, as well as technicians, scientists, IT-experts, health care providers and health maintenance organisations. The IT-market now has changed so much that Integrated Health Care Enterprise becomes reality.

SpringerWien NewYork

P.O. Box 89, Sachsenplatz 4–6, 1201 Vienna, Austria, Fax +43.1.330 24 26, books@springer.at, **springer.at**
Haberstraße 7, 69126 Heidelberg, Germany, Fax +49.6221.345-4229, orders@springer.de, springeronline.com
P.O. Box 2485, Secaucus, NJ 07096-2485, USA, Fax +1.201.348-4505, orders@springer-ny.com, springeronline.com
Eastern Book Service, 3–13, Hongo 3-chome, Bunkyo-ku, Tokyo 113, Japan, Fax +81.3.38 18 08 64, orders@svt-ebs.co.jp
Prices are subject to change without notice. All errors and omissions excepted.

SpringerMedicine

Thomas P. Sculco,
Ermanno A. Martucci (eds.)

Knee Arthroplasty

2001. VI, 250 pages. Numerous figures.
Hardcover **EUR 127,–**
(Recommended retail price)
Net-price subject to local VAT.
ISBN 3-211-83531-8

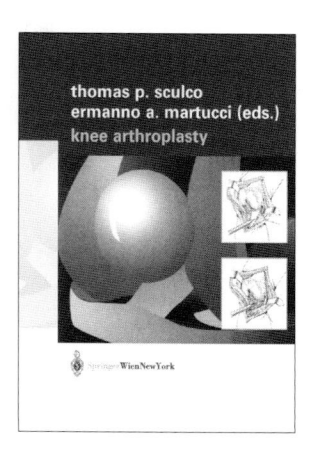

The number of patients submitted each year to knee replacement surgery has constantly risen, until it has even exceeded that of patients submitted to hip replacement. The development of studies on biomechanics, on prosthetic design, and on materials used, has led to further improvement of implants.

The volume has been divided into five parts, each including several chapters assigned to renowned specialists who deal in an organic and modern manner with the most significant problems of knee replacement surgery. The authors have taken into consideration the biomechanical features, the indications, and the surgical methods used. Furthermore, particular attention is paid to the selection of prostheses and to the attempts to reduce polyethylene wear and stress at the prosthesis/bone or prosthesis/cement/bone interface. A rise in indications for the treatment of degenerative pathology of the knee through the prosthesis has inevitably led to a rise in surgical and mechanical complications, and thus to a rise in the number of revisions.

Therefore, a wide review of the most common complications and surgical techniques that may be adopted in these cases is presented. The editors have gathered the experience of internationally renowned authors who present the current state of the art on knee arthroplasty.

SpringerWienNewYork

P.O. Box 89, Sachsenplatz 4–6, 1201 Vienna, Austria, Fax +43.1.330 24 26, books@springer.at, **springer.at**
Haberstraße 7, 69126 Heidelberg, Germany, Fax +49.6221.345-4229, orders@springer.de, springeronline.com
P.O. Box 2485, Secaucus, NJ 07096-2485, USA, Fax +1.201.348-4505, orders@springer-ny.com, springeronline.com
Eastern Book Service, 3–13, Hongo 3-chome, Bunkyo-ku, Tokyo 113, Japan, Fax +81.3.38 18 08 64, orders@svt-ebs.co.jp
Prices are subject to change without notice. All errors and omissions excepted.

SpringerMedicine

Mario Campanacci

Bone and Soft Tissue Tumors

Clinical Features, Imaging, Pathology and Treatment

Foreword by William F. Enneking.
Second, completely revised edition.
1999. XX, 1319 pages. 1120 figures.
Hardcover **EUR 369,–**
(Recommended retail price)
Net-price subject to local VAT.
Jointly published with Piccin Nuova Libraria, Padova
ISBN Co-Publisher: 88-299-1141-0
ISBN 3-211-83235-1

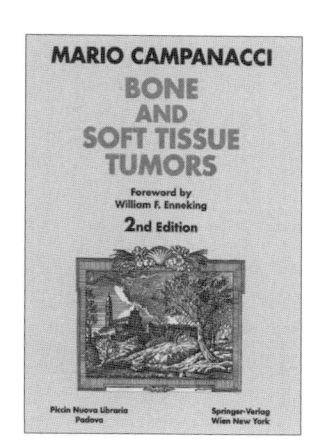

This is an extraordinary book by an extraordinary author. Dr. Campanacci brings to the readers the vast experience in musculoskeletal oncology of the Rizzoli Orthopaedic Institute in Bologna. As such, he has had at his disposal the patient records, radiographs and pathologic material dating back to 1905. The wealth of clinical material that has been accumulated at the Rizzoli Institute, with exquisite documentation and maintenance is a unique resource and testimonial to not only the author but his predecessors. This book brings to the reader an almost unparalleled experience from one of the leading centers of musculoskeletal oncology in the world.

From the Foreword of William F. Enneking:
This second english edition is an entirely new book. It has been thoroughly rewritten, from the first to the last word. About 30% of the pictures are new. The new book incorporates the accumulated personal experience of the author, covering over 20.000 inpatients and many more outpatients, the perusal of the literature of the last 10 years, the recent developments in imaging (particularly MRI), microscopic diagnosis (especially immunohistochemistry and electron microscopy) and the ultimate progress in surgical and non-surgical treatment modalities.

Mario Campanacci (1932–1999) was an orthopaedic surgeon and a pathologist with 40 years of experience (started in 1958 in the Laboratory of Pathology and Tumor Center of the Rizzoli Orthopaedic Institute) focused on musculoskeletal oncology. He was Professor of Orthopaedic Surgery and Pathology, University of Bologna, Director of the 1st Orthopaedic Clinic and of the Tumor Centre, Rizzoli Orthopaedic Institute, Bologna and Director of the Graduate School of Orthopaedics, University of Bologna.

SpringerWienNewYork

P.O. Box 89, Sachsenplatz 4–6, 1201 Vienna, Austria, Fax +43.1.330 24 26, books@springer.at, **springer.at**
Haberstraße 7, 69126 Heidelberg, Germany, Fax +49.6221.345-4229, orders@springer.de, springeronline.com
P.O. Box 2485, Secaucus, NJ 07096-2485, USA, Fax +1.201.348-4505, orders@springer-ny.com, springeronline.com
Eastern Book Service, 3–13, Hongo 3-chome, Bunkyo-ku, Tokyo 113, Japan, Fax +81.3.38 18 08 64, orders@svt-ebs.co.jp
Prices are subject to change without notice. All errors and omissions excepted.

Springer and the Environment

WE AT SPRINGER FIRMLY BELIEVE THAT AN INTERnational science publisher has a special obligation to the environment, and our corporate policies consistently reflect this conviction.

WE ALSO EXPECT OUR BUSINESS PARTNERS – PRINTERS, paper mills, packaging manufacturers, etc. – to commit themselves to using environmentally friendly materials and production processes.

THE PAPER IN THIS BOOK IS MADE FROM NO-CHLORINE pulp and is acid free, in conformance with international standards for paper permanency.